Am. Red C____
1140 Vetere___
10/1 - 11/12
Wed.

Lamaze
Ida Byrd 825-5812
                5005
        10/14 Tues.
Nancy Padberg 822-6739
                479-7938
    11/11 Wed.

across from   Chapman Rm.
24139

Pregnancy, Birth, and Family Planning

Pregnancy, Birth, and Family Planning

A GUIDE FOR

EXPECTANT PARENTS IN THE 1970s

ALAN F. GUTTMACHER, M.D.

WITH DRAWINGS BY ANTHONY RAVIELLI

The Viking Press | *New York*

*To the memories of my mother,
Laura, 1873–1955,
and my twin brother, Manfred,
1898–1966.*

Copyright 1937, 1947, 1950, © 1956, 1962, 1965, 1973
by Alan F. Guttmacher
All rights reserved
Published in 1973 by The Viking Press, Inc.
625 Madison Avenue, New York, N.Y. 10022
Published simultaneously in Canada by
The Macmillan Company of Canada Limited
SBN 670-57311-6
Library of Congress catalog card number: 72-79006
Printed in U.S.A.

This volume contains some completely revised and rewritten material from
the following previously published books by Alan F. Guttmacher: *Into
This Universe, Having a Baby,* and *Pregnancy and Birth.*

Foreword

Birth is the most dramatic event in human experience. If a Broadway play could pack into two hours half the drama of this crucial moment, it would be a "sell-out" for years on end. Despite more than forty five years in obstetrics and participation in thousands of deliveries, each birth excites me today as it first did more than four decades ago. As the baby issues forth, questions crowd the mind, some immediate—the sex, condition, and appearance; others remote—longevity, career, progeny, the ultimate proportion of happiness to tragedy.

The sense of responsibility, the emotional involvement doctors feel in the conduct and outcome of each delivery is greater than the uninitiated suspects. A facet which makes the obstetrician's burden unique in the whole field of medicine is his double obligation: he simultaneously cares for two patients, mother and infant. Each has an individual right to life. Fiction suggests that a doctor is frequently faced at the time of birth with the dilemma, which life to save. The fact is that, through the developments of modern medicine, in almost every instance both lives can be and are saved. If the situation were ever to develop that at delivery only one of the two lives could be saved, a situation I have never encountered, I am almost certain the life of a mother would be given primacy.

The author does not intend to deprecate the even greater importance of birth to parents, for he has been a participating father on three happy occasions and a grandfather twice. It is the rare couple which does not face "B" day with a mixture of hope and fear. There is the hope of an easy, safe deliverance of a healthy, normal baby, and the hope of their own superior performance as parents. There is the fear of some obstetric mishap to mother or child, or of an abnormality in the infant. Fortunately, today, with the vast improvements in obstetric care, birth misadventures are uncommon. If congenital abnormalities occur—and they do once or twice in a hundred newborn—they can frequently be corrected by surgical or other medical means.

This book is written to tell the lay reader the facts of conception, pregnancy, birth, and family planning. With the general increase in educational opportunities, widespread interest has arisen concerning science—in particular, medicine. Curiosity about the beginnings of the child is certainly natural to the woman who cradles it within and the man whose seed begot it. Then, too, a first pregnancy is a new and different experience, replete with unusual sensations and vicissitudes which require explanation. The process of birth is like a journey into the unknown; I hope that *Pregnancy, Birth, and Family Planning* will serve as a trusted map of what lies ahead and rob the trip of fear stemming from ignorance and uncertainty. Then too, I hope it will help endow every child with the priceless birthright of being earnestly wanted by responsible parents.

The progenitor of this book, *Into This Universe*, was published in 1937 by The Viking Press. Revised paperback editions were issued in 1947 and 1950 with the title *Having a Baby. Pregnancy and Birth*, a total rewrite of the previous books, was published by The Viking Press in 1956 and completely revised in 1962. *Pregnancy, Birth, and Family Planning* is the latest child of this rather extended book-bearing succession. To be sure, it resembles its siblings, but there are striking differences, largely modernizations. The decade since 1962 has witnessed some remarkable advances—some scientific, others sociomedical—in obstetrics.

Acknowledgments

I want to thank Mrs. Margherita Hawkins, Director of Prenatal Patient Education at the Mount Sinai Hospital, for advising me in regard to the baby's layette and the preparation of the formula. I am grateful to the authors of three books: Mrs. Alice Gerard for *Please Breast-Feed Your Baby*; my former colleague Mrs. Elizabeth Bing for *Six Practical Lessons for an Easier Childbirth*; and most particularly, my two colleagues and friends Dr. Louis Hellman and Dr. Jack Pritchard, who kindly sent me an advance copy of the excellent new edition of their distinguished medical textbook *Obstetrics*.

Contents

Illustrations

Pregnancy, Birth, and Family Planning

1

You Were a Long Shot

When a baby grows up to be a millionaire or a bishop or a president, he is considered to have done so as the result of chance. Yet in none of these happenings does chance play so large a part as in the miracle of birth. The selection of parents is most fortuitous; if your father and mother had not been who they were, you would not be you. Then, too, at the moment of conception any one of 400 million male cells—spermatozoa—had an equal chance of becoming your particular biological father; only one did. And no two of these 400 million spermatozoa were exactly alike. Each had a slightly different chromosomal make-up. The chromosomes containing helixes of deoxyribonucleic acid, DNA, are those constituents of the body cells which carry the blueprint of the offspring. When the two sets of blueprints—one from the father and one from the mother—are followed, a unique product results. In your case, by one chance in 400 million, that unique product was you. If any other of those 400 million spermatozoa had fertilized the ovum from which you were created, you certainly would have been a strikingly different person, perhaps of the opposite sex.

The complex, seemingly magical process of fashioning a baby is by now quite well understood—a process that is a far cry from the primordial beginnings of life on this planet. The earliest life was probably a single-celled organism that reproduced by division into two similar organisms. And when those two organisms had grown to adult size, each of them divided into two. There were no special sex cells and no separate sexes. Some simple animals still adhere to this primitive reproductive pattern.

The Biological Advantage of Two Sexes

Later in the process of evolution sexual differentiation arose, and the fusion and mixing of elements from two separate adult cells were required for the fabrication of a new young cell. The existence of separate sexes is of great advantage to both the survival and development of a species. That advantage lies in variability. If a single parent cell simply divides into two new cells, and they split into two and all the new individuals also reproduce by division, each of the progeny in this species is an exact or almost exact duplicate of the original parent. Then if some adverse environmental influence comes along, such as drought or extreme cold, and the organism is especially susceptible to it, the whole species will be wiped out. This is far less likely if elements from two separate parent cells fuse and this combination of genetic materials then divides; for the progeny is never an exact duplicate of either parent, but has some characteristics of both. When this progeny mates with a similar organism from a set of different parents, still greater variation results.

The process of the union of the sex cells, as it occurs in man and the other mammals, did not just happen; it evolved through many steps, some of which we can trace. More primitive forms of life, simple marine animals like the starfish, have a very wasteful form of sexual reproduction. There are two sexes, but the sperm and eggs are discharged haphazardly without any physical awareness or even propinquity between the two parents. A more advanced stage in the evolution of the union of the sex cells is illustrated by fish. In them there is strong physical awareness between male and female during mating, but absence of physical contact. The male swims above the female, and as she discharges her eggs he discharges his sperm. In the frog, which has a still more advanced pattern of mating behavior, there is not only sex awareness but actual physical contact. The male clasps the back of the female with a specialized clasp organ, and as she discharges her eggs he discharges his sperm upon them. All varieties of external insemination, however, are relatively wasteful and inefficient.

Internal insemination as practiced by man, by the other mammals, and by many submammalian forms, is far more efficient. In this pattern of reproduction a special organ of the male, the penis, is inserted into a special organ of the female, the vagina. In addition to depositing the semen well on the way to the precise area where it is to function, this method of introducing the male ejaculatory organ deep within the body of the female protects the spermatozoa by releasing them in a highly favorable environment. Such conditions as temperature and moisture within the cervical canal, the uterus, and the Fallopian tubes of the female reproductive tract are optimum for the conservation of spermatozoa.

Libido

The ageless, unhurried process of evolution has granted animals immense protection by making vital functions pleasurable. It is pleasant to eat, drink, void, defecate, sleep—and impregnate or be impregnated. This pleasure in sex is termed libido, and the libido is created by body chemicals, the sex hormones. So closely interwoven are reproduction and sexual pleasure that the sex cells which unite to form the embryo and the sex hormones which create the appetite for mating in each of the sexual partners are produced in one and the same organ—in the ovary of the female and in the testis of the male.

Mating among mammals may be restricted to a single annual season, as in deer, bears, and seals; or it may take place in isolated recurrent estrus periods (mating periods), as in cats, dogs, and the domesticated rodent, rats, mice, and rabbits. Still a third type of sexual rhythm is demonstrated by the primates—men, apes, and monkeys—a willingness to mate at all times without restriction of season or estrus period, though, to be sure, with fluctuations of desire, particularly on the part of the female. In many women libido seems to bear a close time relationship to the stage of the menstrual cycle, being most intense just before the menses, during its waning days, and immediately following it. This is difficult to understand from the viewpoint of survival of the species, since these three periods occur during the least fertile days of the month. Another oddity in the sexual behavior of primates is the female's acceptance of the male during pregnancy. Since mating at this time serves no apparent physiologic function one must postulate that primates have discovered its emotional value to both participants. Nonprimate animals do not copulate after pregnancy has begun. However, some species mate almost immediately after birth has occurred.

No doubt through the timeless process of evolution primates have gradually emancipated mating from many of the modifying influences which still affect subprimate species, and in making love man is the most emancipated of the primates. In some baboons the skin of the vaginal area goes through a cycle of color changes dependent upon the ovarian hormones, estrogen and progesterone, and when the color is a scarlet red the female is most receptive to the male. Estrogen and progesterone are hormones produced by the ovary in all mammals, but each at different times and in differing amounts depending upon the stage in the reproductive cycle. In monkeys it has been shown that the male develops sexual interest in a spayed female (one in which the ovaries have been removed) only if she is given estrogen, but remains uninterested if progesterone is injected.

Some subprimate mammals breed only in the spring, the time of breeding regulated by the proportion of light to darkness. If such an animal is captured and artificially subjected to ten hours of light and fourteen of darkness the female's heat period does not occur, but when the proportion of light is increased to fourteen hours, mating occurs. Other animals breed in the fall, the act of breeding triggered by a daily excess of darkness over light. It has been found that the brain measures the light-darkness ratio, and when a proper seasonal mix is reached a message from the brain activates the ovary.

In some animals there are social factors which affect mating. Among several strains of mice if a large group of sexually active females are put into a cage without males, a gradual disappearance of mating cycles occurs. The inhibiting factor was found to be the odor of the other females' urine. Disappearance of mating cycles does not occur if a female is caged alone unless urine from another female is frequently smeared on her nose. The presence of males, due to the sexually stimulating influence of the odor of male urine, will neutralize such inhibiting influences from the smell of female urine. Realization that the mating instinct is so sensitively influenced in many other animals makes it easier to comprehend human sexual difficulties. Dr. William Masters and Dr. Virginia Johnson in their excellent study of human sexual inadequacy underscore the fact that sexual difficulties in man are almost never caused by an organic lesion, but are usually psychogenic in origin. That is why it is so important that adolescents be introduced to the miracle of sexual reproduction in a sensitive, intelligent fashion by the home and the school. The Masters-Johnson study proves that it is dangerous to create an aura of sin, dirt, and taboo about human sexual activity. Sexuality should be viewed as a beautiful gift which when used intelligently with freedom, joy, and consideration greatly enriches all facets of life.

The Sex Cells—Eggs and Spermatozoa

The eggs of all the higher mammals are similar in both size and appearance—round, with a clear, thin, shell-like capsule, as rigid as stiff jelly. The capsule encloses liquid in which are suspended hundreds of fat droplets, protein substances, and other materials, including the nucleus. The egg, the largest cell of the whole body, is approximately 1/200 of an inch in diameter—about one-fourth as large as the period punctuating the end of this sentence. The eggs of mice, rabbits, gorillas, dogs, pigs, whales, and humans are all about the same size. It is incredible but true that the whale's tons and the mouse's ounces spring from a round speck of matter with relatively the same diameter and weight.

The spermatozoa of different species show greater differences in form than do ova. The human spermatozoon consists of an oval head 1/6000 of an inch in diameter, mostly occupied by the nucleus. With the aid of additional magnification bestowed by the electron microscope, it has become evident that the head is loosely enveloped by a veil-like structure called the acrosomal membrane, and is attached by a short neck to a cylindrical middle piece that terminates in a thin tail about ten times as long as the head. The tail, which consists of several hairlike fibrils resembling a horse's tail, is capable of rapid side-to-side lashing movements, by means of which the spermatozoon is propelled. The motor which moves the tail is located in the middle piece. A spermatozoon is 1/600 of an inch long from the top of its head to the end of its flagellum, a short, hairlike structure protruding from the end of the tail. A spermatozoon can swim an inch in four to sixteen minutes depending on whether it is traversing watery uterine or tubal fluid or relatively viscid cervical mucus. Easily blocked by the slightest obstruction because of its small size, its path is seldom in a straight line, and frequently it takes more than the minimum time to progress an inch.

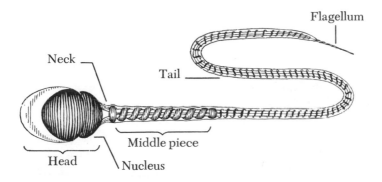

Structure of spermatozoon as seen through electron microscope

When ejaculated, spermatozoa are suspended in seminal plasma, a thick mucoid fluid produced by the male during sexual orgasm. Semen, which arises from the prostate, the seminal vesicles, and the accessory reproductive glands, is not a homogenous fluid immediately upon ejaculation. It is full of tapioca-like mucus lumps that dissolve within five minutes, rendering it a sticky, whitish, uniform secretion with a specific acrid odor. The amount of semen ejaculated depends in part upon the interval between successive ejaculations; in humans the normal quantity varies from one-half to one and one-half teaspoons. In the stallion the quantity is ordinarily two ounces, ten to thirty times as much as in the human. A fresh drop of semen seen under a microscope suggests the rush of traffic in a crowded city street. Myriads of spermatozoa dash here and there, now steering straight ahead, now halted by a speck of dust, now free again to scurry out of the microscopic field. It is a spectacle surcharged with dramatic interest. The average human ejaculation contains almost a half billion spermatozoa—a seemingly extravagant superfluidity of numbers, since only one spermatozoon fertilizes the egg.

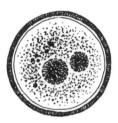

Egg in the process of reducing the number of chromosomes by extrusion of polar body

Fertilization

The essential step in the initiation of a new life is fertilization, the penetration of the ovum by a spermatozoon and the fusion of a portion of the two cells into a new single cell. From this united parent cell originate all the billions of cells which form the infant. The part of each cell which fuses is the nucleus, that glob of material in a cell which stains dark with aniline dyes in properly prepared microscopic slides. The nucleus is not a solid mass of tissue, as it may appear under low magnification, but is made up of a network of little dark-staining rods called chromosomes, which were referred to at the beginning of this chapter. There is a specific number of chromosomes characteristic for each species, and every cell of the body of each animal belonging to the particular animal family contains this number of chromosomes. Chromosomes are paired. One species of primate has its genetic material divided in forty pairs of chromosomes, while in one species of rodent it is divided into seventeen pairs. The famous fruit fly, which has contributed so selflessly to man's knowledge of genetics, possesses only four pairs of chromosomes. In man there are forty-six single chromosomes, but each has a counterpart; thus there are twenty-three different pairs. Before fertilization is accomplished the chromosome number of each parent cell, sperm and ovum, has been halved, in the human from forty-six to twenty-three, one member of each of the twenty-three pairs remaining in the fully mature sex cell. Thus, when the two mature human sex cells fuse, each brings twenty-three chromosomes to the process of fertilization, and their union restores the human species number of forty-six. Research has shown that these minute microscopic rods are the all-powerful agents in the transmission of hereditary characteristics. To them each of us owes not only his sex but his body build, coloring, and, in large measure, his mentality, emotional make-up, and longevity.

Chromosomes in reality are chains of smaller genetic units termed genes. The total number of genes in our twenty-three pairs of chromosomes is estimated between ten and fifty thousand. Since the individual genes are the ultimate determinants of genetic inheritance, the almost infinite variety of combinations explains why all humans differ so markedly, unless they are identical, one-egg twins. One-egg twins have exactly the same chromosome-gene make-up, since the egg after fertilization divides and from each half an independent embryo develops. Thus since a pair of one-egg twin children contain the same chromosomes and genes they are genetic duplicates of each other.

2

Impregnation

For conception to occur it is necessary that a sperm cell makes contact with and penetrates an egg cell. Where are the two sex cells produced, and how is contact between them established?

The Testes and Sperm Production

Throughout a man's reproductive life, which in rare cases continues after the age of eighty or ninety, spermatozoa are constantly being formed by the two testicles suspended in the scrotum, a thin-walled sac of skin. The scrotum is a highly specialized structure which, because of its external location and its large area of skin surface, constantly maintains the testicles at a temperature about six degrees Fahrenheit below that of the interior of the body. In warm weather the scrotum is large and flaccid, exposing a large skin area for heat loss through evaporation, while in a cold temperature the scrotum is small and contracted to conserve heat. In truth, the scrotal pouch is a highly effective air conditioner. The sperm-making cells of the testicle are extremely sensitive to heat, and within twenty-four hours after being exposed to a temperature as high as that of the body's interior, cease producing spermatozoa.

In early fetal life the testicles are situated high up within the abdomen, and they gradually migrate downward, reaching the scrotum about eight weeks before birth. Occasionally boys delivered at full term are born with undescended testicles; in some, the condition corrects itself within the first few months or years of life. If lack of descent persists, at five or six years of age the child is given injections of the gonadotrophic hormone recovered from the urine of pregnant women, or tablets by mouth of the male hormone, testosterone, first isolated from the urine of bulls. Either stimulates the testicles to grow, and because of the resulting increase in weight they may then gravitate spontaneously into the scrotum. Cases in which this does not occur require a surgical operation to guide the testicle into the scrotum and sew it in place. The operation is successful in preserving potential fertility in most but not all cases. The ideal time to perform such an operation is between the ages of nine and eleven years. Otherwise, by the time of full adolescence, the sperm-producing tissue of the testicle is already so irreparably damaged by chronic exposure to the relatively high intra-abdominal temperature that reposition has uncertain value. A few mammals possess no scrotum, notably the bull elephant, whose testicles remain intra-abdominal. As far as I know, the relationship of sperm production to temperature has not been studied in these species.

Another evidence of the sensitivity of human sperm-producing cells to increased temperature is the temporary infertility that often follows bouts of high fever or immersion of the scrotum in water of 130 degrees Fahrenheit for a half hour.

In the human adult the two testicles have the shape and size of plums. Their functions, the production of sperm cells, and the manufacture of the masculinizing hormone, testosterone, are accomplished by separate types of cells.

Spermatogenesis, the creation of sperm cells, is a continuous process commencing in early adolescence and usually not ceasing until death. Each testicle contains hundreds of thousands of little round chambers, lined with cells called spermatogonia from which spermatids, the forerunners of spermatozoa, are derived. When the formation of a spermatozoon has been completed, it is delivered into a collecting duct that interconnects with larger ducts, through which it finally passes into the epididymis, a long, narrow, much-coiled tube lying above each testicle. The canal of the epididymis is continuous with the canal of the *vas deferens*, a tube which runs from the upper scrotum through the body to the urethra of the penis, from which the sperm cells are ejaculated. At the upper end of each *vas*, near the point where it empties into the urethra, is a collecting sac called the seminal vesicle which contains a small amount of viscid fluid. Millions of sperm cells enter this repository daily to be stored there until ejaculation. At ejaculation the muscle cells in the wall of the seminal vesicle go through a series of contractions expelling its fluid swarming with spermatozoa into the urethra. Other glands, most notably the prostate, also contract during orgasm, expelling their fluids as well. All these secretions form the semen. Because of their tiny size, the hundreds of million sperm cells make up a negligible amount of the semen. Therefore, male sterilization, tying and severing each *vas* near the testicle to obstruct the upward journey of the sperm cells from the testicle, does not appreciably diminish the volume of ejaculated semen. The seminal vesicles, prostate, and other glands still discharge their fluids during orgasm, precisely as they did before the operation. The volume and quality of the semen is the same if ejaculated during coitus or masturbation.

The second type of testicular cell, the interstitial, or Leydig, cell, produces testosterone, which is absorbed directly into the blood stream from its place of origin in the testicle. Carried in the blood, it affects such masculine characteristics as body form, libido, sexual potency, voice register, and body and facial hair. Leydig cells are not sensitive to heat and, unlike spermatogonia, continue to function normally in an intra-abdominal testicle. Therefore, males with undescended testicles are wholly masculine except for the absence of spermatozoa in ejaculated semen. In the castrated or eunuchoid male, however, the removal of the testicles causes profound modification of masculine characteristics because of the lack of testosterone in the blood stream.

The Journey of Spermatozoa Up the Male Ducts

From each testicle the spermatozoa slowly pass upward through the epididymis. The trip through the ducts requires two to four weeks, the spermatozoa maturing as the journey progresses. If the male is continent for some time, the spermatozoa that complete the journey are stored in the ducts and epididymis and may suffer effects of senility. Therefore, the first ejaculation after a long interval may produce cells of impaired motility. For this reason, doctors prescribe moderately frequent intercourse for most couples desirous of pregnancy who are having difficulty in conceiving.

Spermatozoa do not make their own way up the male ducts, since they are motionless at this stage, but are propelled upward by imperceptible contractions of the muscular tissue forming the walls of the epididymis and *vas*. It is only after the mass of sperm cells is diluted during orgasm by addition of fluid from the prostate and other glands of the male that they are thrown into vigorous movement. Spermatozoa remain actively motile in the seminal fluid at room temperature for twenty-four hours or longer after ejaculation and as long as seventy-two hours in the upper reaches of the female reproductive tract.

Function and Structure of the Penis

The penis, the male depository organ, has a conical end, the glans, which in the uncircumcised male is partially protected by a thin, elastic, retractile skin cover, the foreskin. The urethra, the tube from which the urine ordinarily flows and from which semen is ejaculated during orgasm, runs through the center of the shaft of the penis and terminates in a small elliptical opening at the tip of the glans. When relaxed and flaccid, the penis of the average man measures about four inches in total length and has a diameter of about an inch. When completely erect under the stimulus of sexual excitement, it measures slightly more than six inches and is an inch and one-half in diameter. Erection is accomplished by the rapid and greatly increased inflow of blood into the special spongy tissue which forms the organ, and by the temporary imprisonment within it of this increased blood under pressure—which comes about through the closure of exit valves in the veins that return the blood from the penis back into the general circulation. Orgasm consists of a series of muscular contractions involving the whole male tract, which drives out the semen in spurts, after which the valves of the veins open, releasing the imprisoned blood and allowing the penis to soften and wilt, a process termed detumescence.

During the process of erection, a temporary valvelike structure forms at the junction of the bladder with the urethra, which prevents urine from being discharged with the semen during ejaculation.

Function and Structure of Female Sex Organs

The reproductive organs of the female serve a fivefold purpose. First, they provide a receptacle for the male semen; second, they produce the ovum; third, they serve as a trysting site for sperm and egg; fourth, they furnish a place where the fertilized ovum can develop into a fetus; and fifth, they manufacture two chemicals, estrogen and progesterone, essential for carrying out the female's role.

The vagina is the body cavity adapted to the reception of the semen. In actuality, the vagina is a potential cavity. Unless distended by the penis or by passage of an infant during birth, the front and rear walls are virtually in apposition to each other. In the virgin, its entrance is, in most cases, partly closed by the hymen, a skinlike membrane that stretches across the vaginal entrance, containing one or more small openings. Normally the membrane is destroyed at the initial sexual intercourse. However, the hymen is a highly variable structure, being absent at birth in some cases and complete without any opening in others; therefore, caution is necessary in attaching medico-legal importance to its condition as evidence of virginity.

The entrance to the vagina is guarded on either side by a small and a large fold of skin, called the labia, or lips, of the vagina. Since one pair is relatively small and the other large, they are termed labia minora and majora. At the outer end of the vagina, just above the urethra from which the urine exits, is the clitoris, the homologue of (i.e., roughly, but not exactly, corresponding to) the male's penis. When unerected, it is usually about a half-inch in length, and when erected, almost twice as long. In its unerected state the clitoris is virtually completely covered by a hood of skin, equivalent to the male foreskin, or prepuce. The sole function of the clitoris is to react to sexual stimulation, enhancing the female's pleasure and response.

The two ovaries, almond-sized and -shaped organs which lie in the lower part of the abdominal cavity, produce the ova. Ordinarily, one ovum matures each month, beginning with the onset of the menses and continuing until the menopause, except during the nine months of pregnancy and a few months thereafter. Since usually there is but one ovum a month, only one of the ovaries matures an egg every four weeks, the two ovaries dividing the task with no discernible plan. Sometimes they alternate; at other times the same ovary produces the ovum several months in succession. If one ovary is surgically removed, the remaining one takes over the complete burden of egg production, maturing an ovum each month, usually with no reduction in fertility.

Perhaps in 5 to 10 per cent of cycles, two eggs are ovulated, one from each ovary or both from the same one. If both eggs are fertilized and then implant and develop, which occurs in less than one per cent of cycles, two-egg, or nonidentical, fraternal twins result. Since two eggs and two sperms are involved, the twins are no more alike than single-born siblings would be at the same age. One could say that fraternal twinning is not true twinning, since the term comes from "getwin," dividing into two. Quite properly fraternal twinning could be termed "littering," a litter of two babies at once.

The two Fallopian tubes, or oviducts, one on either side of the uterus, lead from the abdominal cavity near each ovary to the interior of the uterus. Their length is approximately five inches each. They form the pathway for the upward trek of the spermatozoa and the downward journey of the ovum. The tubal canal, or channel, is constantly moist with secreted fluid, the amount of which increases significantly at the time of ovulation. Finally, there is the pear-sized, pear-shaped, two-to-three ounce, muscular uterus, enclosing a slitlike, highly distensible cavity. It is here that the fertilized ovum embeds and the fetus develops. The ovary, like the testicle, is also an endocrine gland and manufactures the two female hormones, estrogen and progesterone, in varying quantities depending on the phase of the monthly cycle.

After this introduction we are now prepared to discuss the time, the place, and the manner in which sperm and egg meet.

Ovulation

The ripe egg is attached to the interior of the Graafian follicle, which bulges from the surface of one ovary once a month. Through the influence of a hormone from the pituitary gland, LH (Luteinizing hormone), after becoming a ½-to-¾-inch, blisterlike structure, the follicle ruptures. In my first scientific paper, published over fifty years ago, I advanced evidence that contractions of muscle fibers in the follicle wall played a role in causing rupture. Current research has demonstrated that a chemical also appears in the follicular fluid at the appropriate time which digests tissue in the follicle wall, reducing its strength. The exquisite interplay and miraculous coordination of multiple mechanisms to make reproduction work successfully never ceases to amaze me. Another good example is the coordination of activities of the Fallopian tubes with follicular rupture. The Fallopian tube resembles a cornucopia. The wide bowl-like ovarian end is fringed with many fingerlike processes, termed fimbria. During most of the monthly cycle, the fimbria are flaccid and inert. Just preceding ovulation they become erect and constantly lick the surface of the adjacent ovary like hungry tongues seeking to sweep the surface of the freshly ruptured follicle and lick the egg into the open end of the tube. If by mischance the tiny egg is spilled into the abdominal cavity near the vicinity of the tube, the tube acts like a siphon and attempts to suck the spilled egg into it.

In humans ovulation is totally independent of sexual intercourse, occurring with equal frequency in the sexually developed virgin and the sexually active woman. If fertilization does not occur—obviously its occurrence is relatively infrequent—the tiny unfertilized egg quickly dies and fragments into many pieces, which white-blood cells scavenge.

To be fruitful, sexual intercourse must take place within seventy-two hours before ovulation or within twenty-four hours after its occurrence, since a sperm cell is capable of causing fertilization for no more than seventy-two hours after being deposited in the female and an egg if unfertilized survives less than twenty-four hours after ovulation. If we can place ovulation in a definite relationship to some easily observed recurrent phenomenon of the reproductive cycle, such as menstruation, we are well on the track of knowing when sexual intercourse is most likely to result in pregnancy. Significant data on ovulation have been collected by several methods—by the examination of ovaries at the operating table and in surgically removed specimens; by the actual washing of an egg from the Fallopian tube; by observation of pregnancies following a single, accurately dated copulation; and by observation of results from artificial insemination, when the wife is impregnated by mechanical injection into the vagina (or occasionally the uterus) of a single specimen of fertile semen, obtained from the husband or, if he is sterile, from another man, termed a donor. From such observations it appears that ovulation most often occurs between eight and nineteen days after the onset of the menses, the exact day being influenced by the length of the menstrual interval. Women with short menstrual intervals

—for example, twenty-five days—are likely to ovulate early, and those with long intervals—such as thirty-one to thirty-five days—late. Actually, a woman ovulates about fourteen days before the onset of her next menses. However, when an egg is fertilized there is no next menstrual period, ovulation occurring about fourteen days before she would have menstruated had she not become pregnant.

Since most women menstruate approximately every twenty-eight days, if one counts the first menstrual day as day one, the usual time of ovulation is day thirteen or day fourteen, which explains the fact that impregnation is most likely to occur in mid-cycle, midway between the menses. In very rare instances, however, impregnation may result from intercourse at virtually any time during the menstrual month—which implies that ovulation in exceptional cycles occurs at exceptional times. There is evidence that female orgasm infrequently may trigger an aberrant ovulation in some women. Three mammals, the cat, ferret, and rabbit, regularly ovulate only after copulation. They lack the spontaneous ovulation of the human and other mammals which ovulate cyclically, irrespective of copulation. All clinicians of experience can cite examples of patients becoming pregnant at odd periods in the cycle. I recall a young female physician who visited her husband for a week while he was on a temporary research assignment in Puerto Rico. They had intercourse on the sixth day, during the end of her menses, and then parted. Eight weeks later she came to my office with a two-month pregnancy, her husband still being in Puerto Rico.

The two periods in the month when impregnation is least likely, the relatively "safe periods" for sex relations without causing conception, are the first week of the cycle including the menses, and the last week, that is, the week prior to menstruation. The smallest number of conceptions takes place at these times.

The Egg's Journey Down the Tube

After ovulation, the egg, having passed from an ovary into the Fallopian tube, travels down the five-inch tube. The passage takes from three to five days. The muscular walls of the tube encircle a canal which is wide at the ovarian end and at the uterine end narrows to a bore as small as a broomstraw. The mechanism that propels the egg downward through the tube toward the uterus seems to be a combination of fluid currents and rhythmic muscular contractions like those which carry food and excreta through the intestinal tract. Many of the cells lining each Fallopian tube are ciliated: they possess hairlike projections from the surface that beat vigorously. Under the microscope they remind me of a field of wheat being blown by the wind. The beating of the cilia causes a fluid current which mostly flows down the tube from the ovarian toward the uterine end. When the ovum is ovulated from a ripe ovarian follicle, it is surrounded by a thick, loosely adherent covering of some 3000 small cells, the cumulus cells which envelop it completely during its residence in the follicle. Some of the cells are brushed loose by the egg's contact with the sides of the tube, especially with the ciliated cells of the tubal wall.

The Upward Journey of the Spermatozoa

The mid-portion of the tube is the rendezvous for egg and sperm. Explanations of how spermatozoa ascend from the vagina into the uterus, and from the uterus to the meeting place in the tube, have shifted as knowledge of the subject has increased and clarified. A hundred years ago a spermatozoon was believed to be endowed with instinctive, bloodhoundlike qualities which directed it along the proper path to insure fertilization.

Today it is known that the fate of the several hundred million spermatozoa depends in part on the phase of the recipient's menstrual cycle.

During the three or four days before ovulation and the day of ovulation itself, the canal of the cervix, the entrance passage into the uterus from the vagina, is filled with a profuse, transparent, watery mucus which furnishes a highly favorable environment for sperm cells and through which they swim with ease. The appearance of this profuse mucus explains why some women notice a colorless vaginal discharge each month during three to five days in mid-cycle. Some women occasionally stain or even bleed lightly for forty-eight hours in mid-month, this being synchronous with the time of ovulation. Many report pain in occasional cycles for four or five hours on one side or the other of the lower abdomen, depending on whether the egg that particular month was ovulated from the right or left ovary. At all other times of the month except for these several days in mid-cycle, the cervical canal contains a scant, sticky, opaque mucus, much less easily penetrated by spermatozoa, and many are entrapped and halted in it like flies on flypaper.

During intercourse the spermatozoa are catapulted into the upper vagina, into the region of the cervix. When ejaculated, the semen (as we stated before) contains discrete gelatinous material, but rapidly becomes uniformly liquefied. The sperm cells swim haphazardly in all directions, some into the upper recesses of the vagina, some toward the outside, others away from the middle of the vagina far to one side or the other. The bulk of the spermatozoa never reach the protective confines of the cervical canal, but remain in the vagina, exposed to the hostile environment of vaginal secretions, which are quite acid in reaction. Sperm cells are sensitive to an acid medium, and those remaining in the vagina become motionless and dead within a few hours. A relatively few by sheer spatial accident immediately gain the sanctuary of the cervical mucus. This was demonstrated by studies in which cooperating couples notified the physician as soon as male orgasm had been accomplished. The physician then took samples of mucus from high up in the cervical canal. Much to the surprise of the scientific community, the cervical mucus tested was already swarming with sperm cells. The cervical mucus is weakly alkaline and sperm cells thrive in it. Some swim straight up the one-inch, mucus-filled canal with almost purposeful success, while others bog down on the way, getting hopelessly stranded in tissue bays and coves. A small proportion of the total number ejaculated eventually reach the cavity of the uterus and begin their upward two-inch excursion through its length. Whether this progress results solely from the swimming efforts of the spermatozoa or whether they are aided by fluid currents and muscular contractions of the uterus is still unknown. The undaunted ones, those not stranded in this veritable everglade, reach the openings of the two Fallopian tubes—one on each side of the triangular-shaped, slitlike uterine cavity, the base of the triangle being up—and continue their journey upward from the uterus into one of the tubes.

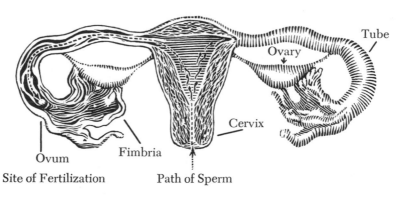

Internal female genital tract, showing site of fertilization

If the egg is discharged from the right ovary and has reached the mid-portion of the right tube, two or three inches above the utero-tubal junction, a spermatozoon swimming up the left tube has, of course, no chance of impregnating it. It is calculated that only a few thousand of the 400 million cells ejaculated ever reach the trysting site, the mid-segment of the Fallopian tube containing the egg. The one sperm that achieves its destiny has won against gigantic odds, several hundred million to one. The baby it engenders has a far greater mathematical chance of becoming president than the sperm had of fathering a baby. No one knows just what selective forces are responsible for the victory. Perhaps the winner had the strongest constitution; perhaps it was the swiftest swimmer of all the contestants entered in the race. Perhaps it was merely the luckiest in finding a fluid current leading straight to the ovum. According to experimental evidence, this total five-inch journey requires approximately thirty or forty minutes. If ovulation occurred within several minutes to twenty-four hours before the sperm's journey ends, the ovum will be in the tube, awaiting fertilization; if ovulation took place more than twenty-four hours before insemination, the egg cell will have already begun to deteriorate and fragment, rendering it incapable of being fertilized by the time the spermatozoon reaches it. On the other hand, if ovulation has not yet occurred, but takes place within two or three days after intercourse, living spermatozoa will be cruising at the tubal site waiting for the egg.

We have followed the sperm and egg to their meeting place, and we can now observe what happens when they meet—that is, the actual process of fertilization.

The Process of Fertilization

The method by which the tiny sperm cells locate the egg is not clearly understood. Because of the few spermatozoa, just a few thousand, in the relatively long tube at the time of fertilization, many investigators feel some process other than random encounter is involved. It has been suggested that the egg exerts a chemical trapping effect increasing sperm concentration by making them swim more rapidly when they are headed toward it and less rapidly when going away from it. When sperm-egg collision occurs the sperm becomes immediately bound to the egg's surface.

There is species specificity in the process of fertilization. All animal groups within the same species interbreed and are normally fertile with each other, as is illustrated by the bizarre results in the crossing, most usually by accident, of diverse canine strains. Related species are occasionally fertile with each other: horse and jackass (mule); zebra and donkey (dobra); cattle and buffalo (cattalo); and lion and tiger (liger). However, offspring from related species are almost invariably infertile.

Before fertilization can be accomplished the sperm must undergo the process of capacitation, that is, gaining the capacity to fertilize. Freshly ejaculated spermatozoa are in fact incapable of causing fertilization, which has nothing to do with their motility, as uncapacitated spermatozoa swim quite handsomely. Capacitation is accomplished by exposure of the sperm to secretions of the uterus, the Fallopian tube, or the ovary's

Graafian follicle. Capacitation requires as little as two hours in the hamster and as long as eleven hours in the rabbit. There is suggestive evidence that it requires eight hours in man. Through electron microscopy, which permits magnification from ten thousand to more than one hundred thousand times, it has been determined that each sperm head is surrounded by two membranes, a plasma membrane closely applied to it and the loose, veil-like acrosomal membrane mentioned earlier. Capacitation permits two very essential activities by the sperm cell, first penetration of the multi-layered halo of cumulus cells, which surround and adhere to the surface of the egg when ovulated, and second, penetration of the jellylike capsule of the egg, the zona pellucida. As far as can be observed, a capacitated sperm appears the same as a sperm before capacitation. However, several hours' exposure to fluids of the female reproductive tract enables it to undergo the acrosomal reaction, which ruptures the outer membrane surrounding the sperm head and releases an enzyme beneath the membrane that can dissolve cumulus cells, cutting a path through the surrounding halo to the egg's surface, where it softens the capsule so that a sperm can penetrate it. In the process of fertilization it is believed that hundreds of sperm cells jointly contribute this essential enzyme material.

The egg capsule, the zona pellucida, is relatively firm and rigid; its thickness is approximately one-tenth the diameter of the egg. Precisely how a spermatozoon penetrates the capsule is not completely known. The sperm does not swim its way through the capsule with the point of its head foremost, but appears to attack the egg with the side of its head. The path it makes through the zona is not straight but oblique. It is possible that the egg cooperates in the process by thrusting out, a streamerlike process that engulfs the sperm head and draws it inward.

In the rat, the whole spermatozoon enters, the lashing tail as well as the head. Following penetration, the sperm progresses to the pole of the egg opposite its point of entry and there comes to rest, the tail ceasing its thrashing movements. Additional spermatozoa have been observed to enter the rat egg after the fertilizing spermatozoon had already assumed its final position and become quiescent. These additional spermatozoa remain in the narrow fluid space between the inside of the egg capsule and the jellylike interior substance, taking no part in fertilization. It is not known whether the penetration of the rat ovum by several spermatozoa occurs only in eggs fertilized under the microscope, or whether it also happens in nature. In the human it is not known whether the head alone or the whole spermatozoon, including the tail, enters the egg. However, supernumerary sperm are often lodged or trapped in the gelatinous zona pellucida. As in the rat, some enter the perivitelline space, the narrow zone between the covering of the egg and its true contents, the cytoplasm with its nucleus. However, only a single sperm penetrates the perivitelline membrane to pair the twenty-three chromosomes of its nucleus with the twenty-three chromosomes of the nucleus of the egg.

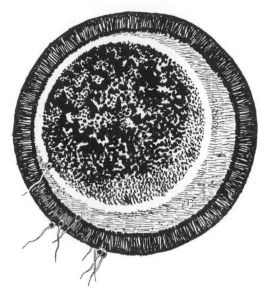

Penetration of egg by fertilizing spermatozoon

Fusion of the Two Nuclei

In the rat during the first nineteen hours after fertilization both the male and female nuclei enlarge and migrate toward the center of the cell. The next step is the fusion of the two nuclei into one parent nucleus. When this has been accomplished, fertilization is completed, and the fertilized ovum then begins to divide into two cells; the two cells divide into four, the four into eight, and so on, creating after

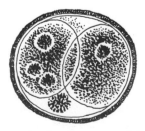

Two-cell stage in development of the egg

twenty-one days a newborn rat weighing less than an ounce. In the human the same process, after an average of 266 days from the moment of fertilization or 280 days from the beginning of the last menstrual period, creates a seven-and-a-half-pound baby. Whether rat or human, the infant animal is formed by a marvelously intricate and orderly arrangement of billions of cells.

The Enigma of When the Fetus First Becomes a Living Being

This problem has confounded philosophers and scientists for millennia and is likely to do so for millennia to come. Some say human life no longer begins; it began a few million years ago and has been a continuum ever since, simply being poured into new individual containers. Others claim life begins with ensoulment, a process defying both definition and assignment of time of occurrence. Some, more biologically oriented, state that human life begins with the union of sperm and ovum, others with the egg's implantation. Thought being the hallmark of the human being, some believe that the fetus first becomes a living human when it becomes capable of thinking, whenever that is. The onset of movement endows the fetus with life for some. A large segment of the population believes that life commences as soon as the fetus is viable, that is, capable of survival outside of the mother (twenty-six to twenty-eight weeks), while another portion feels that life begins only at birth.

Sir Alan Parkes, the British zoologist, differentiates between biological and human life, the former beginning with fertilization, the latter with implantation, when the developing egg assumes dependence upon its mother for its nutrition.

To me this whole discussion is more philosophy than science. Scientifically all we know is that a living human sperm unites with a living human egg; if they were not living there could be no union. The result is continued life of these living cells and fabrication of another human created in the image of, but with differences from, any of its ancestors. Does human life begin before or with the union of the gametes, or with birth, or at a time intermediate? I, for one, confess I do not know.

The Early Hours of the Fertilized Egg

In the mouse the two-cell egg appears twenty-four hours after fertilization, and the four-cell stage after thirty-eight to fifty hours. In the human a two-cell stage has been observed within twelve hours after fertilization and sixty-four-cell development in seventy-two hours. By the fifth day the human ovum is made up of about 500 cells, the cells having doubled their number about every twelve hours since the time of fertilization.

In all mammals the developing egg in its earliest phase, while still a traveler down the Fallopian tube, is a solid mass of cells, aptly termed a morula (from *morum*, Latin for "mulberry," which it resembles). It is still round and has increased little if at all in diameter, its contents merely having divided into smaller units. In this respect it is like a real-estate development. At first a road bisects the whole area; then a cross-road divides it into quarters, and later other roads into eighths and twelfths. This happens without the addition of any land, simply by subdivision of the original tract.

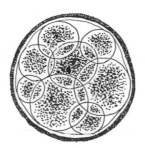

Eight-cell stage in development of the egg, after approximately 60 hours

The egg passes from the tube into the uterus on day four or five, when it is no longer a solid mass of cells, the cells having arranged themselves about the outer surface of the sphere, the center now being occupied by fluid. It is then termed a blastocyst (Greek, "sprouting bladder"). By the fifth day the multicellular conceptus begins to increase in size. It floats about the slitlike uterine cavity for three or four more days and then adheres to its inner cell lining, which has been exquisitely prepared by the special hormone progesterone, fed by the ovary into the bloodstream from whence it reaches the uterus. Progesterone has made the lining succulent and swollen with a network of new and enlarged blood channels coursing through it. The developing egg, possessing an enzyme that digests away the surface cells to which it has adhered, then sinks down into the depths of the uterine lining. The process is something like hoeing the firm, dry earth above to plant the corn in the soft, moist, rich earth beneath. Implantation occurs on the eighth day in man and on the fifth day in the mouse, despite the fact that pregnancy in the mouse is only $\frac{1}{13}$ as long as in man. By the twelfth day the human egg is already firmly implanted, but the damaged, superficial uterine lining cells through which it passed have only partially healed to roof over the tissue nest in which the egg now rests. About two out of three pregnancies implant on the posterior, or rear, wall of the uterine cavity, and one in three on the anterior, or front, wall.

On microscopic study the twelve-day egg already shows a specialized accumulation of cells which later will form the embryo. The remaining cells become the afterbirth and membranes.

Impregnation is now completed, as yet unbeknown to the woman. She has not even had time to miss her first menstrual period, and other symptoms suggestive of pregnancy are still several days distant.

It is important to point out that many more eggs are fertilized than babies born. Fertilization, implantation, and early development of the ovum are each so complex that something frequently goes wrong and then further growth ceases. If this occurs within the first ten to twelve days, the menstrual period is not even late. If development of the ovum is arrested, say around the fifteenth day, the menses are delayed a week or so but no recognizable tissue is passed. However, if pregnancy progresses several weeks before it comes to a halt a discernible miscarriage occurs. It is estimated that at least 30 to 50 per cent of fertilizations never end up as a baby.

3

Are You Pregnant?

Ordinarily diagnosis of pregnancy presents no problem to patient or physician. In contrast to most conditions for which people seek a doctor, pregnancy is usually prediagnosed by the patient. Yet on rare occasions its diagnosis may be puzzling. The correct answer to such a puzzle is then determined from three types of data: the patient's symptoms, certain bodily changes determined by the physician, and specific laboratory tests.

Symptoms

Absence of Menses

Failure to menstruate (amenorrhea) is usually the earliest evidence of pregnancy. A missed menstrual period in a woman between fifteen and forty-five with previously regular cycles who has been having sexual intercourse suggests pregnancy as the most likely possibility, though not the only one, since there are many other causes for a delayed or even a skipped period.

Age must be taken into account, since the periods may be quite irregular toward the onset and the termination of a woman's menstrual career. Recent childbirth, especially when a woman is nursing, may eliminate the menses temporarily or lengthen the interval between them. Illnesses, including severe anemia, tuberculosis, untreated diabetes, disturbances of the thyroid gland, high fever from infection, and a host of other diseased states may create menstrual disturbances. Malnutrition may lead to an absence of menstruation; the failure of many female war prisoners in World War II to menstruate during incarceration was probably mainly for this reason. Amenorrhea may occur in women who have lost weight rapidly on a very strict anti-obesity regimen. Psychological factors may be responsible for absence of menses. Among these one may list adjustment to a new country of residence; a change of jobs; a sudden emotional upset, as death of a loved one; war bombing; and either fear that unwanted conception has occurred or an overpowering mania to become pregnant, tragically met in women with a long history of sterility. I can recall many situations in which fear of pregnancy postponed an expected period. Several decades ago when I was in residency training in New York City my wife was called by a college classmate in a high state of alarm because her period was two days late. It appears that she had given up her virginal status on one occasion several days before. Naturally I was consulted in the crisis. Tongue in cheek I prescribed three doses of a nauseating mixture of quinine, castor oil, and ergot. I knew that if she were pregnant nothing would happen, but if she weren't, unmerited faith in the brew's effectiveness might jolt the psyche, permitting menstruation. The next day at 9:30, our telephone rang to report the therapeutic triumph and to extol my medical acuity. She had just taken the first of the three doses.

Scanty Menses in Early Pregnancy

Women may be pregnant and still appear to menstruate during the early months. On close observation, such menstrual periods are different. Ordinarily they are shorter and scantier. In the typical instance the woman menstruates three days instead of five at the normal time her period is due. A month later she menstruates half a day, the following month for an hour, and then the menses cease entirely during the remainder of pregnancy. Not infrequently women may develop menstrual cramps at the first missed period without any bleeding or staining. They fully expect to menstruate each hour, but do not. The discomfort lasts for three or four days, then ceases.

Breast Changes

Many women suffer a pronounced fullness of the breasts premenstrually, which subsides rapidly just before or with the onset of menstruation. When pregnancy occurs, this fullness continues instead of disappearing, and becomes even more marked. At the same time the pregnant woman may feel a tingling in the breasts, and they may become tender, the nipples being hypersensitive. These sensations usually are of short duration; the breasts remain large, but the feelings of tenseness and tenderness disappear. In preparation for lactation the mammary glands actually continue to increase in size during the remainder of pregnancy, the enlargement in part being due to growth of the milk-secreting glandular tissue and in part to a greatly enriched blood supply. This latter is often manifested in the second half of pregnancy by the appearance of a delicate tracery of blue veins beneath the skin on the chest, especially noticeable in women with very fair skin. The nipple and the colored circle of skin surrounding it—the areola—enlarge, and their pigmentation darkens. Arranged in a circular fashion around the periphery of the areola, near the skin edge, are a number of small, round-ish elevations, oil glands—in the inimitable words of Montgomery, their discoverer, "a constellation of miniature nipples scattered over a milky way." In some women breast enlargement is accompanied by the forma-tion of stretch marks in the skin—striae; since they appear more exten-sively over the abdomen they will be discussed later in this chapter under "abdominal changes."

Nipple Secretion

After the first few months a sticky, yellowish, watery fluid—colostrum—may be expressed from the nipples by gently stripping the breast. This finding is not absolute evidence of pregnancy, for women who have borne and suckled children may retain colostrum in the breasts for years. In the later months of pregnancy drops of colostrum may flow from the nipples spontaneously. As term is approached, the colostrum takes on an opaque, whitish appearance, more resembling milk.

Nausea and Vomiting

Nausea and vomiting in pregnancy—"morning sickness," as they are so cheerfully termed in popular speech—are going out of fashion. Thirty years ago most pregnant women appeared to suffer from morning sick-ness. This is no longer true; if one eliminates slight cases of occasional, unimportant queasiness, far fewer than half of today's pregnant women are plagued by it. It is difficult to explain this. Perhaps the improvement is associated with better all-year-round diet, improved health, a higher incidence of planned conceptions, a changed attitude toward pregnancy and labor, or some unlisted factor. The last few decades have witnessed a marvelous revolution in the way the average woman regards childbirth. She was tense, fearful, apprehensive; but now she is relaxed, reassured, and confident. Multiple causes are responsible for the change in attitude. The pregnant woman realizes that obstetrics has improved vastly, so that pain, illness, and death for those bringing life are virtually relics of the past. Then, too, she is no longer kept in ignorance about the process of birth. Books like this one, government pamphlets, magazine articles, school lectures, maternity classes, and personal teaching by physicians, all have contributed to make the laity more knowledgeable regarding obstetrics.

Morning sickness usually begins when the pregnant woman's menstrual period is several days overdue, and then gradually disappears six to eight weeks later. In the beginning the patient awakens with a feeling of gastric instability, a little uncertain as to whether she is going to vomit or not. The uncertainty is replaced in a few days by the actuality, which usually occurs as soon as she lifts her head from the pillow. As the morning lengthens, the nausea and vomiting diminish, and by lunchtime she eats an ordinary meal. There are exceptions to this pattern; some women vomit only in the evening, and others at irregular times or all day long. Some are actively nauseated during early pregnancy by odors from the kitchen, and others by tobacco smoke.

It is not uncommon for the woman who vomits during pregnancy to observe that her vomitus is flecked or streaked with blood. This should not cause concern, as repeated vomiting from any source may rupture a tiny blood vessel in the throat or esophagus. Such a small vessel soon clots and heals spontaneously.

Many instances are recorded of particularly suggestible husbands who vomit with their pregnant wives; there are even cases in which the husband vomited though his wife did not.

Excessive salivation (ptyalism) to the amount of three or four quarts a day is sometimes a concomitant of pregnancy. It is likely to begin two or three weeks after the first missed period, persists throughout pregnancy, and disappears promptly after delivery. Treatment in the main is unsatisfactory. Mild sedatives, strong mouthwashes, and sucking peppermint candies may bring relief.

Changes in Appetite

It is not uncommon for the newly pregnant woman to note a temporary diminution in appetite, and ordinary amounts of food make her feel overfull and bloated; without the advice of a physician, she is likely to substitute frequent small feedings for scheduled meals. Some pregnant women develop a craving for one food to the point of mania. If allowed, they will eat the particular food to the exclusion of almost all else. In my own experience I have seen different women crave soup, pretzels, and dill pickles. Many years ago the wife of a young Johns Hopkins staff member with a very anemic academic salary selected, of all possible foods, lobster as the object of her craving. Two or three evenings a week the two would trudge downtown, and enviously he would watch her devour a lobster. Previously they had attended an occasional concert or theater, but these pleasures had to be foregone for lobster money. Today, happily, even very junior staff members are paid sufficiently well so that not only can both husband and wife afford lobster but also perhaps a show.

When one reads the obstetrical texts of a few centuries ago and observes the space and emphasis they gave to what they termed "pica," or aberrations of appetite, one gains the impression that the condition is probably only one-fiftieth as common today as it was then. Unquestionably diets are more diversified and better balanced today, and the opportunity to obtain milk, fruits, and vegetables at all seasons of the year is greater. Food cravings during pregnancy probably have their genesis in dietary omissions.

There is confirmatory data from observations on laboratory rodents. Cannibalism, the mother rat eating her newborn, is commonly practiced when the adult animal is on a deficient diet, but almost unknown if her diet is adequate and contains all food essentials in sufficient amounts. If laboratory rats have the various food essentials placed in separate trays so that the amount of each kind consumed can be accurately weighed, it is found that the appetite of the female changes almost as soon as pregnancy begins. She instinctively increases her protein and mineral intake as well as the total number of calories.

Excessive Need of Sleep

In some women one of the early symptoms of pregnancy is an overpowering sleepiness. Sleeping late in the morning and napping in the afternoon do not prevent the pregnant young wife from yawning in her husband's face and from dozing even at her own dinner parties. This excessive need for sleep disappears after the first few months.

Frequent Urination

Sometimes frequency of urination begins as early as the first missed period. This condition disappears about the tenth or twelfth week, often to recur a few weeks before delivery.

Abdominal Changes

As pregnancy progresses, the patient becomes conscious of the gradual enlargement of her abdomen. She first notices this about the twelfth week, when a small abdominal lump may be felt just above the pelvic bone. This lump, the pregnant uterus, grows upward, reaching the navel at about the twentieth week. The patient begins to "show" at some time between the sixteenth and twentieth weeks, and it is very unlikely that she can keep her secret much beyond this point. As the abdomen increases in size some curious, pinkish streaks appear in most pregnant women; the streaks are frayed-looking and slightly sunken beneath the surface of the skin. They run longitudinally on the lower abdomen and in a transverse semicircular fashion on the upper abdomen. The stretch marks increase up to term and fade after delivery, though they do not wholly vanish, assuming a shiny, pearl-white appearance.

There are other minor abdominal changes which the woman notices. Most develop a dark streak which runs down the center of the abdomen, its continuous course interrupted by the navel. This line pales after delivery, but never completely disappears. The navel itself, which is ordinarily a pit, becomes level with the rest of the abdominal wall and may even protrude, forced outward by increasing intra-abdominal pressure. After delivery the navel's previous pitlike state is restored. The end of the breastbone, the xiphoid, is attached to the middle of the ribs by a hinged joint. Ordinarily this dagger-shaped bone cannot be felt. However, in very late pregnancy the pressure within the upper abdomen may rotate it outward so that a bony bump may be felt in the "V" space between the two sets of ribs. Its presence is normal.

Quickening

Usually between the sixteenth and twenty-second weeks the patient first experiences "quickening"—that is, she first perceives the movements of the fetus. These movements have been poetically compared to the faint flutter of a bird's wings against an imprisoning cage. At the onset the motion is so gentle that the patient is uncertain what she feels, usually confusing the activity of the fetus with intestinal gas; she is sure only after the movements have been repeated several times. Later in pregnancy the movements of the child's arms and legs feel like powerful thrusts from within, and at this stage every woman is convinced she carries a centipede—if not a centipede, at least twins or triplets. These vigorous movements can be seen with the eye; the abdomen bulges momentarily under the impact of the thrust. Usually the movements are noticed earlier by those who have already borne children, for they have learned to interpret the first faint impulses, and in exceptional cases movements may be felt as early as the twelfth week. In the beginning the perception of fetal movements is not continuous, and at first days may pass when they are not felt at all. In later pregnancy, however, they are felt daily, but even then there are hours when they are absent; the supposition is that at this time the fetus is asleep.

All these evidences of pregnancy noticed by the patient—failure to menstruate, breast growth, morning sickness, changes in appetite, excessive need of sleep, urinary frequency, abdominal enlargement, and quickening—can be simulated by other real or imagined conditions.

Therefore a positive diagnosis of pregnancy cannot be made solely on the basis of the patient's observations. The observations of the physician and the laboratory are the only trustworthy means of making the diagnosis.

Physician's Findings on Physical Examination

Virtually every organ and tissue of the body is affected in some measure by the physiologic changes induced by pregnancy. These changes result, directly or indirectly, from the action of the chemicals produced by the afterbirth, the placenta (from the Latin, meaning a flat cake). Considering the fact that the placenta's primary function is to strain out food essentials from the mother's bloodstream for the baby and to excrete the baby's waste products, it is amazing that it is also such an efficient chemical factory.

The most striking pregnancy changes occur in the generative organs. Therefore, in order to diagnose pregnancy, the doctor examines the reproductive organs to determine whether any of the anticipated physiologic alterations have occurred.

Examination of Breasts

He ordinarily begins by examining the breasts. First he inspects them to see if they appear to have enlarged or if there is any change in nipple and areola pigmentation. He looks for Montgomery's glands as well. Then he palpates (explores with the tips of his fingers) the breast to determine if the glandular tissue has begun to spurt in growth. At the same time his trained and sensitive fingers feel for tumors or cysts which should not be there. The last step in his examination is to strip the gland in an attempt to milk colostrum from the nipple. If several of these observations are positive, there is presumptive though not absolute evidence of pregnancy.

Abdominal Examination

Ordinarily a doctor is a very thorough man; his training has made him so. Whenever he performs an abdominal examination he carries it out in a routine manner, no matter what the cause of the examination. First he palpates the liver and gall-bladder regions in the upper right abdomen. He then feels for the spleen in the left upper abdomen. This is followed by an attempt to locate the lower pole of each kidney in either flank. Next he turns his attention to the mid-abdomen, the region beneath and surrounding the navel or umbilicus. Next he examines the lower abdomen to determine whether he can feel a mass in an area which normally would be occupied by an enlarging uterus. At about the tenth or twelfth week the pregnant uterus begins to rise up out of the pelvis, forming at first a small, discrete midline swelling, globular and soft, which the experienced examiner can differentiate from firmer and less rounded tumors, such as fibroids of the uterus or cysts of the ovary, which may occupy the same area. The palpation of the typical softish, midline lower-abdominal mass is also presumptive, but not conclusive, evidence of pregnancy.

At varying periods after the twentieth week the fetal outline can first be discerned by palpating through the full thickness of the abdominal wall plus that of the uterus. The fetus can be felt as a firm, irregular mass within the relatively soft uterus which surrounds it. It is much like feeling a doll through several thicknesses of blanket: the larger the doll, the easier it is to be certain of its outline; the thinner the blanket, the surer the result. On abdominal palpation the head of a fetus feels like an apple and the buttocks—the breech—like a stuffed, slightly irregular cushion. The back feels quite firm and straight, while the hands, feet, arms, and legs are like irregular bumps or knobs. The palpation of such a fetal outline is almost 100 per cent proof of pregnancy, but occasionally it can be so closely simulated by a nodular, intra-abdominal, nonpregnant growth that confusion results.

Pelvic Examination

After completing his examination of the abdomen, the physician examines the vagina and pelvic organs for indications of pregnancy. In preparation for the pelvic examination the patient had previously been instructed by the nurse to empty her bladder completely before entering the examining room. She continues to lie on her back but with the buttocks brought down to the edge of the examining table, the knees wide apart, and each heel in a footrest.

The principal changes in the vagina during pregnancy are threefold: increased blood supply, softening of the tissues, and augmented secretions. Pelvic circulatory changes appear early in pregnancy, usually before the second missed period, and often serve as a valuable aid for the establishment of the diagnosis. The tissues about the entrance of the vagina and within it take on a purplish, dusky color instead of the normal pink (Chadwick's sign). The color deepens as pregnancy advances, and is likely to be more striking in those who have already borne children.

As pregnancy advances, the vagina becomes increasingly elastic and distensible because of the softening of the tissues which form its walls. This change facilitates the performance of a vaginal examination.

The increase in vaginal discharge which is usually concomitant with pregnancy is in large part due to the normal excess in activity of the mucus-secreting glands of the cervix.

To perform a pelvic examination the physician inserts the first and second fingers of his lubricated gloved hand into the vagina. He first feels for the mouth of the womb, the cervix, which protrudes down into the upper vagina like the tip of a finger. In the nonpregnant woman it is firm, but it softens considerably under the influence of the increased blood supply and hormonal changes of pregnancy. This softening begins at about the eighth week and increases as pregnancy advances. A week or two earlier, Hegar's sign may have appeared—it consists of an apparent diminution in thickness of the uppermost portion of the cervix, where it merges with the uterus. This reduction is only apparent; actually there is a localized zone of softening which renders the tissues at this point more compressible. It gives the examining physician the feeling that the uterus and cervix are separate organs instead of a continuous tract.

To conclude the examination the physician maps out the size of the uterus by grasping it between his two fingers in the vagina, pressing upward, while the fingers of his other hand exert an inward, downward pressure on the lower abdomen. This brings the uterus between the fingers of the examiner's two hands. Not until the seventh or eighth week after the last menstrual period can growth changes in the uterus itself be appreciated—now for the first time the uterus seems a little broader and softer. The increase in size and softness proceeds rapidly, and by the twelfth week the uterus is twice as large as the nonpregnant organ.

The changes noted on vaginal examination—bluing of the tissues, softening of the cervix, the feeling that the upper cervix and the body of the uterus are separate, enlargement and softening of the uterus— are only presumptive signs, since conditions other than pregnancy can cause them.

Indisputable Evidence of Pregnancy

Ordinarily, between the twelfth and twentieth weeks the physician is able to establish pregnancy on an absolute basis. Five important and definite signs develop; on the strength of any one of them the physician can be certain that his patient is pregnant. These signs are considered indisputable, since no other condition save pregnancy causes them. The five are: the examiner's perception of the movements of the fetus, his hearing the fetal heartbeat, detection of the skeleton by X-ray, an electrical tracing of the fetal heart, and mapping the fetal outline by means of special ultrasonic equipment. The latter two have only been added within the past few years and require specialized, complicated apparatus.

Movements of the Fetus Felt by the Physician

Fetal movements are divided into active and passive. The active movements can be elicited when the examiner places the flat of his hand over the lower abdomen. If the fetus moves, it feels to him as if something were squirming under a cover; in more advanced pregnancy there are soft, well-defined blows against the examiner's palm. The quiescent fetus may be stimulated to move if the examiner suddenly indents the abdomen with his fingertips; the jolted fetus reacts to this indignity by squirming. It is said that active fetal movements can also be elicited by placing a piece of ice on the abdomen; I have never made the experiment. Some of the early nineteenth-century obstetricians asserted that fetal movements could be more sensitively appreciated by the cheek than by the hand.

The passive movements of the fetus depend on the fact that the fetus floats about the cavity of the uterus in a small sea of fluid, the amniotic fluid. This fluid is actually present in the very first few days of pregnancy, even before the fetus is formed, and, as the fetus grows, the fluid increases in quantity. When the examiner gives the abdomen a sudden thrust with his fingers, the fetus recoils like a piece of ice in a glass, which, pressed upon, sinks and then slowly rises to the surface— or like an apple when one is bobbing for it on Halloween. The passive movements of the fetus are known as ballottement. Both ballottement and active fetal movements can sometimes be made out on vaginal as well as abdominal examination.

The Fetal Heart

Contractions of the heart muscle of the fetus begin within a month following conception, but the heart sounds remain inaudible through the mother's abdominal wall before mid-pregnancy. When first heard, the baby's heart sounds are found just below the mother's navel; later they are more readily auscultated (heard) toward one side or the other. When the fetus is large enough for the doctor to outline exactly its form and position, he listens for the fetal heart tones in the area overlying the baby's back, in the region between the shoulder blades. The fetal heart can be heard with the naked ear, but it sounds much louder through a stethoscope, particularly if the stethoscope is of the special obstetrical variety and is held in place by a metal headband which allows not only air conduction of sound waves but also bone conduction. The fetal heart has a double beat like the tick of a watch, but its rate is more rapid and it has a soft, nonmetallic pitch. The fact that the mother's heart beats much more slowly allows differentiation of the fetal heart from the maternal arterial pulse also heard through the mother's abdomen as her blood courses through the large arteries of the uterus.

A common and curious misconception is that a pregnant woman can occasionally feel the baby's heart pulsate as she lies on her back. She actually senses the pulsations of her own aorta, the largest artery in the body, as the pregnant uterus overlies and slightly compresses it. Finding the pulsation relatively slow and synchronous with her own pulse should convince the most ardent skeptic.

In addition to its value in the diagnosis of pregnancy, the fetal heart gives another important information. Normally it beats at the rate of 120 to 160 per minute; the average in 600 cases was 136. If during pregnancy or labor the rate slows drastically and at the same time becomes irregular, it is evident that something is wrong with the fetus, and appropriate remedial measures must be undertaken at once. Then, too, it is helpful in the diagnosis of twins, for in that case two separate heartbeats are often heard. In the middle of the nineteenth century it was believed that the rate of the fetal heart differed markedly in the two sexes. A rate of 124 or less was supposed to indicate a boy, and a rate of 144 or more a girl. Unfortunately, this, like most other simple methods of detecting the sex of the unborn, does not work.

By fixing or holding a special sound recorder to the mother's abdomen over the area where the baby's heart is loudest and feeding the impulse into a special machine, its heart sounds can be amplified many times. They can be broadcast so loudly that a mother in the hospital can successfully listen to her baby's heartbeat even months before birth. During labor, amplified fetal heartbeat sounds of several different fetuses can be monitored separately at a central nursing station by throwing an appropriate switch. In some instances the sound of the fetal heartbeat is relayed to the laboring woman's bedside to reassure her.

X-Rays

Ordinary X-rays penetrate the soft tissues of the body and cast no shadow; it is only when they are arrested by a radio-opaque substance that a shadow is produced on the film. The chief mineral in bone is calcium, which is opaque to X-rays, and, because of this, bone can be clearly and sharply outlined. The fetal skeleton is at first a framework of cartilage, or gristle, that is not detectable by X-rays. The cartilaginous skeleton is gradually converted into bone (ossification) by the cumulative deposit of calcium, and when this occurs the skeleton can be demonstrated radiographically. The process of ossification begins first in the collarbone during the sixth week of pregnancy and by the twelfth week centers of ossification have appeared in most bones. The visibility of bones by X-rays depends upon the amount of calcium they contain, and in the fetus this amount is too little until about the twelfth week. If conditions are ideal—very modern technical equipment, and a thin patient—parts of the fetal skeleton can be seen this early; however, in the average case it is unusual to get a positive result until the sixteenth or eighteenth week. A positive X-ray picture of the fetus is as irrefutable evidence of pregnancy as is the physician's detection of movements of the fetus or the baby's heartbeat.

Previous to 1955 X-ray during pregnancy was used extensively without restraint. In 1954 the medical world was shocked by a thoughtful paper by Dr. Alice Stewart at Oxford University, suggesting that diagnostic X-rays applied to the pregnant uterus might very occasionally harm the fetus. Until then X-ray had been used frequently not only to substantiate the existence of pregnancy but also to verify the physician's impression of the size and position of the fetus in the uterus or to determine the dimensions and configuration of the opening in the mother's bony pelvis, through which the child must pass to be born. X-ray was frequently used to investigate the skeletal normalcy of the fetus before its birth and sometimes in case of uncertainty to help determine whether it was alive or dead. Then too, if twins or triplets were suspected, the suspicion was confirmed or refuted by an abdominal X-ray, the number of fetuses determined by the number of heads or backs visible. There were other obstetrics uses for X-ray, for example, attempting by a special soft-tissue technique to locate the position of the placenta in patients who bleed late in pregnancy. If it was found to be low in the uterus, a condition called placenta praevia (Latin, "before the way"), a position ahead of the baby could be anticipated and proper steps taken.

However, during the past decade and a half the abdominal X-ray of pregnant women and even of nonpregnant women of reproductive age is being used far less, one might even say sparingly. That does not mean it is never used, because in many medical situations during pregnancy abdominal X-ray is essential and wise.

Why this radical change in medical attitude and practice? Scientific studies have shown that theoretically there is potential danger from exposure of the gonads (ovaries and testes) of parents-to-be or of the gonads of the fetus in utero to X-rays and also from exposure of the body of the unborn fetus. I should like to underline the words "theoretically" and "potential" because it has not been proved that the small amount of X radiation employed in diagnostic procedures, using modern machines with high-speed films, does actual damage. Yet it is unreasonable to assume even a theoretical risk unless circumstances make it justifiable.

Let us examine the three theoretical dangers.

First, the production of genetic mutations, alterations in the smallest known genetic unit, the gene, or the larger unit, the chromosome. Gene mutations, that is, physical or chemical changes in the genes, have been produced experimentally by beaming X-rays at the gonads of drosophila, the fruit fly, and other animals, such as mice, later causing anatomical or physiological changes in their immediate progeny or the offspring of subsequent generations. Mutations of the genetic structure of sperm or egg occasionally may cause improvement in the stock, but far more often they damage it. If the mutant gene is dominant the first generation demonstrates the mutant effect of alteration, and if recessive it is likely to be expressed only in subsequent generations.

In terms of medical practice the ovaries and testicles are protected at the time of X-ray by a thick lead shield placed over the lower abdomen or scrotum whenever possible if nearby areas of the body are X-rayed. A physician is more hesitant to take a series of pelvic X-rays or carry out fluoroscopy of the lower abdomen in a female who has not yet completed her family than one who has.

The second potential danger is the production of a congenital abnormality in the newborn, by submitting it to X-rays *in utero*. Since the neuroblast, the precursor of cells which form the nervous system, is the most vulnerable type of embryonic cell to X-ray damage, if damage occurs it would most likely involve structures of the central nervous system. Fetuses have been severely damaged when a pregnant mother inadvertently received an immense amount of high-energy radiation in the course of treatment for a pelvic tumor. Treatment by X-ray or radium is termed therapeutic radiation, in contradistinction to diagnostic X-ray, the taking of an X-ray film to establish a diagnosis. The difference in amount of X radiation which reaches the fetus in the two procedures is vast, pelvic therapeutic radiation submitting a fetus to several hundred or even several thousand times the dose that it receives with diagnostic X-ray. The earlier in pregnancy pelvic therapeutic radiation is administered the greater the damage. Therefore, if it must be given or is given through error—not knowing the patient is pregnant—before the baby has become viable, therapeutic abortion is usually performed, or if pregnancy is far advanced when the need for therapeutic radiation is decided upon, it is often postponed until after delivery.

The third potential danger is increased incidence of leukemia or cancer before the age of ten in children whose mothers received diagnostic abdominal X-ray during pregnancy. In 1962, Dr. Brian MacMahon of Harvard University did an excellent study of children born in the Northeastern United States between 1947 and 1957. He found an increased risk of 40 per cent of childhood death from leukemia or cancer if the mother had had diagnostic abdominal X-ray during pregnancy. According to the earlier Oxford study the incidence is double that of children of women not having abdominal X-ray or fluoroscopy during pregnancy. Abdominal X-ray is most dangerous in this regard during the first three months, and there is some correlation between the number of films made and the degree of hazard. It must be pointed out that the many studies all over the world which followed the original Oxford study show great disagreement, some confirming it and others refuting it.

What does all this add up to as far as you are concerned? Admittedly there is uncertainty, yet prudence bespeaks certain safeguards, such as shielding the gonads from X-rays whenever possible in nonpregnant individuals. Furthermore, it is safer in women who are being exposed to a chance of impregnation to carry out diagnostic abdominal X-ray or fluoroscopy during or just after the menses to avoid X-ray exposure of a very early and as yet undetected conception. During pregnancy, especially in the first several months, diagnostic X-ray and fluoroscopy should be avoided if possible. However, there are many medical situations which completely justify the assumption of this potential risk, and I stress the word "potential." The risk is so slight, if there is a risk, that even extensive diagnostic X-rays during early pregnancy, such as those in a gastrointestinal or kidney series, never dictate therapeutic abortion. Then, too, the more modern the equipment and the more expert the X-ray technique used, the less the potential risk. For example, fluoroscopy using a TV monitor for the doctor to make his observations yields far less radiation to a patient than the old and more standard type of fluoroscopy. Incidentally, dental, sinus, and chest X-ray, as well as X-ray of the extremities, pose no possible potential risk during pregnancy. There is no scatter of rays to a distant area of the body, and they cannot be transmitted by the bloodstream. The matter of gain and risk of X-rays during pregnancy is always carefully weighed by your physician, who knows all this, and he alone can make the final and correct judgment for you. The two newer techniques to be considered under the next two headings, fetal electrocardiogram and the Doppler ultrasonic technique, especially the latter, are gradually replacing X-ray for obstetrical purposes.

The Fetal Electrocardiogram (FECG)

The electrocardiogram has been used in medicine since the beginning of the century. An electrocardiographic tracing records the electrical activity of the heart muscle. Its unique pattern with the characteristic configuration of its "Q" and "T" waves cannot be confused with any other electrical activity of the body. With the heightened sensitivity of the recording apparatus, the recording of the fetal electrocardiogram in the uterus became possible more than a decade ago. This useful tool is now used in obstetrics for several purposes: diagnosing pregnancy, diagnosing twins, determining whether an unborn fetus is still alive, and monitoring the fetus during labor, one of the two electrodes is attached to the fetus vaginally through a partially dilated cervix after rupture of the membranes (bag of waters). This permits not only an accurate determination of the baby's heart rate but to some degree the normalcy of its heart action. Except when assessing the baby's condition during labor the FECG is taken with the pickup electrodes both placed on the mother's abdomen—neither of them intravaginally.

The FECG becomes positive in rare cases as early as the twelfth week of pregnancy, before the fetal heart becomes audible by stethoscope. However, a negative FECG up to the twentieth week does not argue seriously against the existence of pregnancy. After the twentieth week a positive FECG can be elicited in more than 95 per cent of cases. A fetal ECG can be distinguished from a maternal ECG by its much faster rate.

If fetal heart tracings are recorded with different rates in separate areas of the mother's abdomen, a positive diagnosis of twins can be made. In forty cases of twins studied at the Chicago Lying-In Hospital thirty-six showed positive twin FECG tracings. One may conclude that if the fetal electrocardiogram is positive for the twin pattern it means twins in every case; a negative twin recording rules out twins in 90 per cent of the cases. In the Chicago series the FECG diagnosis of twins was made in some instances before the obstetrician even suspected their presence.

In the Chicago study, when there was uncertainty as to whether a fetus was alive or dead, the FECG gave correct information in 95 per cent of the cases studied. A positive FECG always proves that the fetus is alive.

The Ultrasonic Technique

The ultrasonic technique of detecting fetal heart action is of recent origin. Ultrasonic waves are transmitted to and from the maternal abdomen by means of quartz crystals in a transducer applied to the skin of the abdomen and moved an inch at a time until the lower abdomen is completely monitored. Unless the waves strike a moving object they are reflected back at the same frequency at which they are sent, but if they strike a beating fetal heart they return with an altered frequency that can be audibly detected or graphically depicted. The fetal heart has been detected by ultrasonics as early as the tenth week of pregnancy and consistently by the twelfth week. In 97 per cent of 600 cases in which the patients were more than twenty weeks pregnant, a correct diagnosis of fetal life or death was made by the ultrasonic technique.

In some modern hospital facilities the fetal heart of each laboring woman can be separately monitored by this technique at the nurses' station during labor.

Modifications of the Doppler ultrasonic principle (ultrasonography) using more complex and sophisticated apparatus than is used in monitoring the fetal heart are employed in obstetrics for many reasons. It has been demonstrated that through its use accurate mapping before birth of the location of the placenta and reliable measurements of the fetal skull and chest can be made. Location of the placenta was made correctly in 96 per cent of 154 patients in one study reported. To determine fetal maturity, measurements are made of the width of the fetal skull just above the ears (biparietal diameter, BIP), and also of the width of the fetal chest. From many observations and tables constructed on the basis of the observations, it is now known that 91 per cent of infants with a BIP of 8.5 cm. or more and 97 per cent, with a BIP of 9.0 cm. or more, weigh more than five and one half pounds. Similar tables have been constructed for different chest diameters.

Since ultrasonography does not depend on the density of calcified bone as does fetal X-ray, but simply on the presence of a mass which reflects sound waves, the presence of a fetus within the uterus has been detected by this technique as early as the eighth week of pregnancy. To map out intra-abdominal objects the transducer is slid over the abdominal skin previously lubricated with mineral oil. The transmitted impulses are fed into a scanning machine which prints them. A signal of very high frequency and low intensity is used which does no damage to the fetus. The picture produced requires experience and skill for accurate interpretation. The ultrasonography apparatus costs between twenty and thirty thousand dollars and is ordinarily run by a technician specifically trained for the task. The pictures are usually read by one member of the medical staff experienced in this new field.

Obstetrical ultrasonography is still so new, and in some measure so experimental, that unless your doctor is associated with one of the large teaching centers he is unlikely to have it available to him. Because of the absence of potential danger to the fetus or mother, it is safe to predict that ultrasonography will gradually largely replace the use of X-ray in obstetrics.

Pregnancy Tests

When early diagnosis of pregnancy is important, and when the physical findings are inconclusive or confirmation is needed, a pregnancy test may be performed. For convenience this is usually carried out with the patient's urine, but other body fluids such as blood and spinal fluid also give a positive pregnancy reaction. The positive reaction is due to the presence of a specific hormone produced by the placenta, which passes into the mother's blood and from her bloodstream into other body fluids. A test usually becomes positive about three weeks after impregnation, ordinarily toward the end of the first week your period is overdue.

The first satisfactory pregnancy test was devised by Aschheim and Zondek in 1928. Although modern biological tests for pregnancy are almost never carried out by the original technique described by these pioneer investigators, numerous modifications having been developed, the animal tests are generically referred to as A–Z tests.

A–Z Tests

The test animals in common use include the mouse, rat, rabbit, South African clawed toad (*Xenopus*), and American frog (*Rana pipiens*). Both the rat and mouse tests employ twenty-one- to thirty-day-old immature female animals and are based on the appearance of blood spots, or hemorrhagic follicles, in the ovaries of the test animal after injection of urine or blood serum from a pregnant woman. At first it took five days before the result could be read, but, by certain modifications, a yes or no can now be gotten in twelve to eighteen hours. The rabbit test, which required forty-eight hours, is rarely used any more because of the expense of the animals. In the frog test the test urine is injected beneath the skin of an adult female, and when the test is positive freshly extruded frog eggs are found at the bottom of the cage twenty-four hours later. When it is negative, the test animal fails to ovulate. If a toad is used, the test urine is injected into a male animal, the end point being the release of spermatozoa into the cloaca. Fluid is removed with a pipette from the cloaca and examined microscopically for sperm cells; if they are found, the test is positive. The test can be read in two to five hours.

Immunologic Office Tests

There are now at least seven office tests using biologic materials but not live animals. These have almost completely superseded the older animal tests. Four are slide tests and three test-tube tests. The pregnosticon slide test, which takes only a few minutes to perform, is regarded by some authorities as the over-all best. As with the animal tests, they depend on the fact that the hormone HCG (human chorionic gonadotrophin) is secreted by the early placenta and can be accurately detected in urine or blood. When HCG is injected into rabbits, they develop an immune response to the foreign protein—the so-called antibodies to HCG. If rabbit's serum containing HCG antibodies is mixed with a few drops of human urine or human blood serum containing HCG, there is one type of slide or test-tube reaction, and if the test specimen contains no HCG, a clearly different reaction. Slide tests can be read in two minutes, and test-tube tests, after two hours. When a patient's period is three to seven days overdue and she is pregnant, 77 per cent give a positive test and 23 per cent a false negative. When menses are two weeks overdue, the immunologic tests are virtually 100 per cent reliable either way, that is, a positive test establishing pregnancy and a negative test excluding it.

If your test does not agree with the physician's impression of your pregnant state, either yes or no, he is likely to repeat the test in a week, perhaps using another one of the seven tests. Furthermore, he may request you to bring him a few ounces of your first morning voiding since HCG is present in greater amounts in concentrated urine than in a dilute specimen. In rare instances he may request corroboration by an animal test.

Progesterone Test

This test is based on the fact that if a nonpregnant woman whose period is overdue is given the hormone progesterone for a few days, she will usually experience bleeding two to seven days after the last dose. The test material may be given by intramuscular injection on three consecutive days or by mouth four times a day for three days. Progesterone is used in the intramuscular injection and certain varieties of birth-control pills for the oral form of the test. The test is positive for pregnancy if no bleeding occurs and negative if it does. An accuracy of 95 per cent is claimed for the test.

Interpretation of Pregnancy Tests

A positive pregnancy test indicates only the presence of actively secreting placental tissue in the patient's body; it does not necessarily mean a living embryo. In rare cases the test is positive in conditions other than a normal uterine pregnancy, as in tubal pregnancy, in a condition called hydatidiform mole (a pregnancy, ordinarily without a fetus, which is so abnormal that the placenta resembles clusters of grapes more than the usual afterbirth, hence the term, derived from the Greek word for "grape"), or when, as occasionally happens, the placental tissue continues functioning even though the fetus has died. However, in 99 per cent of the cases a positive test means a normally developing conception.

False or Imaginary Pregnancy

Very rarely a nonpregnant woman may experience all the symptoms and many of the minor vicissitudes of pregnancy, including absence of menses, breast changes, nausea and vomiting, and swelling of the abdomen resulting from gaseous distention of the bowel. Supposed fetal movements may be simulated by excessive contractions of the intestines or involuntary tensing and relaxing of the abdominal muscles. Despite medical assurance to the contrary, the patient steadfastly insists that she is pregnant and at the end of ten lunar months may even feign the pangs of labor. This condition, known medically as pseudocyesis, or spurious pregnancy, occurs predominantly in young, childless women with an intense longing for a baby, or patients nearing or entering the menopause. Pelvic examination in cases of spurious pregnancy reveals a normal-sized uterus, and the pregnancy test, of course, is negative. Treatment consists of sympathetic but positive explanations. If obstetric measures fail, psychiatric help is necessary. Queen Mary I of England is said to have suffered from the malady.

4

Duration of Pregnancy

Calculating the Date of Birth

Dr. Brown bent back in his swivel chair, tapped together the ends of his fingers, and asked gravely, "When did your last menstrual period begin?"

Rustling unsuccessfully in her handbag for the forgotten memorandum, young Mrs. Smith replied, "Let's see. It was the day of the last concert, you know. Let me think, wasn't it Wednesday, March eighteenth?"

With telegraphic speed, and without the aid of either fingers or calendar—the use of these marks the neophyte—the wise man announced, "Your baby is due on Christmas Day." Mrs. Smith was impressed! It was barely the first of May, and yet this seer foresaw the birth of her child, seven and a half months distant. How did he do it?

The calculation of the expected date of confinement is very simple, absurdly simple. I hesitate to divulge the formula for fear of revealing a guild secret. The rule is: Add seven days to the first day of the last normal menstrual period. Count back three months. In the case of Mrs. Smith, Dr. Brown added seven to March 18, and then counted back—February, January, December. That made the expected date of confinement December 25. The mystic formula is now exposed. In reality, this formula affords a short cut for counting 280 days from any fixed date. In other words, a woman ordinarily delivers nine months and seven days from the beginning date of her last menstrual period.

It must be stressed that the 280 days is an average figure, which means that a vast number of pregnancies terminate before the 280th day, a vast number after it, and only relatively few on the exact day. At best the calculated or expected date of confinement is an approximate date. This is an important fact for the pregnant couple as well as relatives and other interested persons to remember. It is all too common for panic to become general when "B" day arrives, then passes, and yet there is no sign of labor. Telephones soon begin ringing, and on each occasion the patient is unhappily greeted by the salutation, "Haven't you gone to the hospital yet?"

What Are the Chances of Delivering on Time?

In over 17,000 cases of pregnancy carried beyond the twenty-seventh week, 54 percent delivered before 280 days, 4 per cent on the 280th day, and 42 per cent later. Forty-six per cent had their babies either the week before or the week after the calculated date, and 74 per cent within a two-week period before or after the anticipated day of birth.

On the basis of these data one can calculate the likelihood which the average woman faces when carrying a single infant, not twins, of having her baby, during each week after the twenty-seventh week from the first day of her last menstrual period.

Weeks	Days	Approximate Chance
28	189-196	1:625
29	196-203	1:625
30	203-210	1:525
31	210-217	1:240
32	217-224	1:240
33	224-231	1:135
34	231-238	1:115
35	238-245	1:58
36	245-252	1:39
37	252-259	1:22
38	259-266	1:11
39	266-273	1:5
40	273-280	1:3½
41	280-287	1:5⅔
42	287-294	1:12
43	294-301	1:34
44	301-308	1:74
45	308-315	1:140
46+	315+	1:140

Another reliable study has shown that 40 per cent of women go into labor within a ten-day period—five days before and five days after the calculated date, and nearly two-thirds within plus or minus ten days of the expected time.

Factors Affecting the Delivery Date

Ordinarily the woman with a consistent, regular menstrual cycle is more likely to have a baby at the 280th day than the woman who menstruates irregularly. Furthermore, a short menstrual interval, such as twenty-five days, is frequently associated with delivery a few days early, and a lengthy menstrual cycle with birth beyond the due date. The calculated date increases or decreases by about one day for each day the patient's average menstrual cycle exceeds or falls short of twenty-eight days. Neither age, race, size, nor the previous number of children seems to influence the length of pregnancy.

In a study of almost 15,000 first births of a single infant in Aberdeen, Scotland, 24 per cent of patients with a male infant delivered during the thirty-ninth week and 28 per cent in the fortieth week (total 52 per cent). Twenty-three per cent of mothers in a first labor who gave birth to daughters bore them during the thirty-ninth week and 30 percent in the fortieth week (total 53 per cent). This slight difference in delivery dates between boys and girls is not statistically significant.

A study of over 20,000 total births at the University of Chicago showed that babies weighing over ten pounds averaged pregnancies of 288 days instead of 280 days.

A twin conception shortens pregnancy by about three weeks; actually, the average woman who carries twins delivers them on the 258th day instead of the 280th day. Triplet and quadruplet pregnancies are usually briefer than this, triplets commonly arriving five weeks early and quadruplets six weeks before time. Mrs. Dionne delivered her famous quintuplets on the 219th day (thirty-one weeks).

A Prolonged Pregnancy

A pregnancy carried more than two weeks beyond the calculated date is considered prolonged, and the resulting infant designated as post-mature. Such a delivery occurred in 8 to 12 per cent of the pregnancies in the two studies previously cited.

There are apparently medically authentic cases in which pregnancy extended to 336 and 337 days, and one in which the duration was 343 days (forty-nine weeks). When pregnancy is excessively protracted there are three possibilities: an error in menstrual dates; ovulation several weeks later than the usual fourteenth day of the cycle, impregnation therefore not taking place until forty or fifty days after the onset of the last menses; or actually several extra weeks of pregnancy beyond the usual forty weeks before labor commences. In most cases the true answer is never known, but it is generally believed that in most instances error is at fault. It is believed that at the most 4 per cent of pregnancies are truly carried two weeks or more beyond the average time.

Evidence is accumulating that a baby in the uterus gains little weight after the term date of 280 days is reached, so that the birth of a baby of excessive size adds little proof of true postmaturity. As a matter of fact, babies may actually lose weight in the uterus after the due date is reached, and it is thought by some authorities that the typical postmature baby is thin, scrawny, and old-looking, with loose, baggy skin, long nails, abundance of scalp hair, and a singularly alert look. They may also show desquamation, or peeling, of the superficial skin of the palms and soles. After birth such infants gain back the weight they lost and soon appear normally chubby and well padded. In addition, in such cases the surface of the placenta often displays thick deposits of calcium, perhaps evidence of its relative senility.

Legal Problems Associated with Duration of Pregnancy

The legal problem of legitimacy frequently revolves about duration of pregnancy, its prolongation on one hand or its brevity on the other. In the first type of case, a husband is absent from his wife's bed for more than nine months before the birth and fears that the vacancy was fruitfully filled in the interval. In the second case, a living child arrives with inconsiderate haste after the marriage, leading the husband to suspect the conception was not initiated by him. The laws of different countries differ greatly regarding these issues. In Austria the law recognizes the uncontested legitimacy of a living child born after 240 days of marriage or 307 days after the death of the husband. On the other hand the Scottish law fixes the minimum figure at 168 days (twenty-four weeks).

Both England and the United States have no such laws and each case is decided by court trial. In recent years pregnancies of 331 and 346 days were declared legitimate by English courts; and in the United States a New York Supreme Court found a 355-day (eleven months, twenty days) pregnancy legitimate (Lockwood vs. Lockwood). In the now famous 1949 Preston-Jones vs. Preston-Jones peerage case, conducted by the English House of Lords, the husband sought divorce on the grounds of adultery, since the date of last coitus preceded birth by 360 days. The divorce commissioner decided in favor of the wife, but the Courts of Appeals overthrew the verdict in favor of the husband, granting him a divorce.

Extremely brief pregnancies sometimes involve not only the reputation of the mother, but the father as well. In Scotland in 1835 the Reverend and Mrs. Jardine had a living baby born five months and three weeks after marriage (twenty-four and a half weeks). Charges of immorality against the reverend couple were brought by the Presbytery of Kirkcaldy, and after four years of investigation a doubtful verdict was rendered. Both sides appealed to the General Assembly of the Church of Scotland, which found the charge of immorality unproved, absolving the couple.

Calculating the Delivery Date from the Day of Insemination

In calculating the expected date of confinement from 425 cases in which a purported single, fruitful coitus led to impregnation, it was found that the average patient delivered 269.9 days after insemination. However, there was wide variation, extending from 231 to 329 days. A second study, involving fifteen cases of artificial insemination, yielded an average duration of pregnancy of 272 days from the day of treatment, with a span of 261 to 288 days. It is obvious that calculating the anticipated delivery date from coital data has little or no advantage over the more standard technique of utilizing the first day of the last menstruation.

Calculating the Delivery Date from Onset of Fetal Movements

Another method of computing the "due date" is to count eighteen or twenty weeks from the time the patient first feels fetal movements; however, this is even less exact than the calculations from menstrual and coital data.

After sifting all available modern scientific data, we come to the conclusion that the generalization first made decades ago about the duration of pregnancy is relatively correct. If the date is calculated from the onset of the last menses, almost 50 per cent will deliver within the week before or after the 280th day, and 75 per cent within two weeks of it.

The Effect of Prolonged Pregnancy on the Fetus

There is no clear-cut evidence one way or the other whether carrying the baby three or four extra weeks jeopardizes its safety. There are a number of studies which demonstrate an increased risk for the fetus, and an equal number which refute such hazard.

In the meantime, the important thing to do is not to panic and force your doctor into taking unjustified steps when he may rightly feel that the situation calls for no other treatment than the time-tested method of "letting nature take its course." On the other hand, if the cervix is "ripe" and ready for induction of labor, he may think it wise to take you into the hospital and simply rupture your membranes—the bag of waters—or initiate contractions through the administration of Oxytocin or sparteine (see page 225). It is difficult to justify Cesarean section for postmaturity unless there are complicating factors such as the rare occurrence of a baby of extraordinary size which appears too big for safe vaginal delivery, or the fetus has been observed to be growing very slowly near or after term is reached.

Determining the Duration of Pregnancy

The physician determines the duration of pregnancy in a given case from the patient's history and from his findings on physical examination. Usually they agree. From thousands of observations we know that a pregnant uterus of a certain size represents a conception of a certain number of weeks. For measurement, three abdominal points have been selected: the front of the pelvic bone (symphysis), the navel (umbilicus), and the tip of the breastbone (xiphoid). Sometime during the third month the uterus can be felt above the pelvic bone; it is felt midway between the pelvic bone and the navel at the end of the fourth month, at the navel in the fifth, and midway between the navel and the breastbone at the end of the seventh. At the beginning of the ninth month the top of the uterus is two and a half inches below the end of the breastbone. In most women pregnant for the first time, the top of the uterus is now lower in the abdomen because the child starts to descend into the pelvis. The layman calls this "lightening" or "dropping"; medically it is termed "engagement of the fetus." Frequently in those who have had previous pregnancies the uterus continues to grow upward until labor starts, virtually reaching the xiphoid, since the engagement of the fetus may not take place in them until labor has begun. The earlier engagement of the fetus in a first pregnancy is due to the greater pressure which surrounds it, since the uterus and the abdominal wall have not been stretched by previous childbirth.

If the menstrual history and the physical examination do not agree as to the duration of pregnancy, the doctor must investigate the cause of the discrepancy. Either there is an error in the menstrual history, or the uterus, because of some abnormality of pregnancy, does not correctly indicate the duration by its size. The uterus may be abnormally enlarged by tumors, a multiple pregnancy, excess of fluid (hydramnios), etc. It may be small because the fetus has died *in utero,* or the child's development is progressing slowly.

5

The Fetus

The origin and growth of the fetus was a simple thing to our medical forefathers. In 1548 all embryology could be put on a single page; today it cannot be crammed into a library of hundreds of volumes. I venture the guess that more pages have been written about the obscure fetus than about the illustrious Shakespeare.

The biological life of a fetus begins with fertilization, as stated in the first chapter. At that moment the precursor of the child is of almost microscopic size, a speck of tissue so very tiny that it is just barely visible to the naked eye of the expert—a mass so light that its weight cannot be expressed in even thousandths of an ounce. Within nine months this minute dot of tissue develops into a twenty-inch, seven-and-a-half-pound screaming infant. The initial ten days in the life of the future citizen are reported in Chapter 2. As described there, the ovum implants itself into the substance of the uterus, excavating the permanent home which it will occupy for more than eight months by digesting its way into the interior lining of the uterus. In the process it taps very, very small maternal blood vessels and soon finds itself surrounded by a veritable lake of its mother's blood, into which it dips vigorous, hungry cells. These cells, which grow like streamers from the surface of what is called the blastocyst at this state of development, absorb minerals, vitamins, carbohydrates, proteins, and fats essential to growth. With absorption of nourishment the fertilized ovum increases rapidly in size. At a certain region on the inside of the covering a thickened mass of cells now appears; this mass is called the inner cell mass or embryonic area, and it is from these cells that the embryo itself develops. The egg continues to grow, and the covering surface, which is most distant from the cavity of the uterus and deepest in the uterine lining, forms the placenta, or afterbirth.

Summary of Fetal Development for Each Period of Pregnancy

Let me now summarize the development of the fetus, always designating the weeks or months since the onset of the last menses. If one assumes that fertilization takes place on the fourteenth day of the cycle, then there is a constant difference of two weeks between the actual age of the conceptus and the duration of pregnancy, since the latter is calculated from the beginning of the last menses. To prevent confusion I shall discuss embryonic and fetal development in terms of duration of pregnancy, not in actual fetal age, for potential parents think in terms of weeks and months of pregnancy.

End of second week: Fertilization occurs. First day in the life of fertilized ovum.

End of third week of pregnancy; first week after conception: Fertilized ovum traveling down tube; on 17th day enters uterus as a round solid mulberry-like mass of cells; then transforms into blastocyst, an outside cover of hundreds of cells with fluid in the center, like a tiny hollow rubber ball filled with fluid instead of air. Floats in uterus (17th–22nd day). Blastocyst about 1/100 of an inch in diameter.

Beginning of fourth week: Implantation (23rd day), i.e., 9–10 days after fertilization. Egg still barely visible to naked eye. After implantation fertilized ovum begins to grow rapidly, doubling its size every 24 hours. Cells forming embryonic area (from which embryo will grow) appear on inner wall of blastocyst. Placenta begins to form on that part of outer wall of blastocyst deepest within maternal tissues.

Beginning of fifth week: The fertilized ovum is now termed an embryo. The embryo itself is a minute piece of uniform gray-white flesh. The primitive streak which will become the spine is laid down. The embryonic sac containing the embryo is ⅖ inch in diameter.

End of fifth week: Backbone forming, 5 to 8 vertebrae laid down. Nervous system and spinal canal forming. By end of fifth week the foundation for the child's brain, spinal cord, and entire nervous system will have been established, as well as rudiments of its eyes (20 days after conception). Tubular S-shaped primitive heart beginning to beat. Embryo 1/12 inch long and about ⅙ inch wide.

Beginning of sixth week: Head forming. Beating heart visible, located on outside of body, not yet within chest cavity. Intestinal tract forming; growth starts from mouth cavity downward. Mouth closed. Human embryo at this stage cannot be differentiated through its appearance from a pig, a rabbit, a chick, or an elephant embryo. Has a rudimentary tail, extension of its spinal column.

End of sixth week: All of backbone laid down and spinal canal closed over. Brain increasing conspicuously. Tail of embryo quite long. Be-

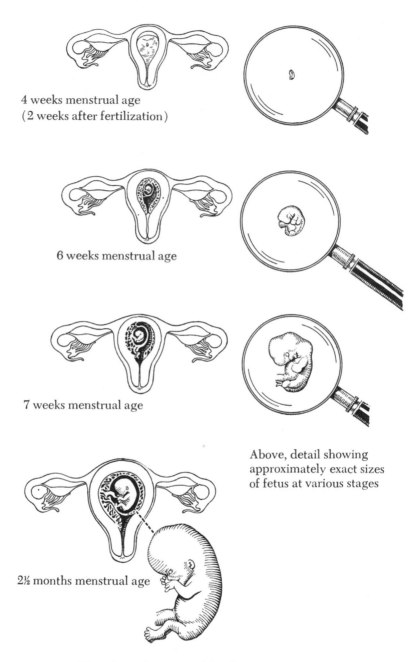

4 weeks menstrual age
(2 weeks after fertilization)

6 weeks menstrual age

7 weeks menstrual age

Above, detail showing
approximately exact sizes
of fetus at various stages

2½ months menstrual age

Fetus in early stages of development

ginnings of arms and legs visible. Depressions beneath skin where eyes and ears are to appear. Length, ¼ inch. Germ cells, to become either an ovary or testis, have appeared.

Seventh week: Chest and abdomen completely formed. Heart internal. Eye clearly perceptible through closed lids. Face flattening, shell-like external ears. Mouth opens. Lung buds appear. Big toes have appeared. Tail has almost disappeared. May begin to move body slightly. The great bulge of its brain predicts that this creature is destined to feel, think, and strive beyond the capacity of all other animals on this earth. Embryo is now termed a fetus and, small as it is, looks human. Length, ½ inch, weight 1/1000 of an ounce.

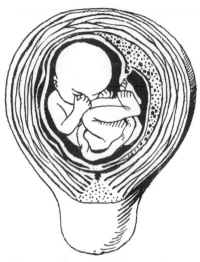

Fetus at 3½ months, placenta the stippled area above and to the right of the fetus

Eighth week: Face and features forming. Jaws are now well formed, and the teeth and facial muscles forming. Rudiments of fingers and then toes become evident. Ovaries or testicles taking form. In the male the penis begins to appear. Cartilage and bone may both be seen in the forming skeleton. Length, ⅞ inch. Weight, $\frac{1}{30}$ ounce (1 gram)—less than an aspirin tablet.

Ninth week (end of 2nd month): Face completely formed. Arms, legs, hands, and feet partially formed. Stubby toes and fingers. Abdominal-wall muscles of fetus, if removed from womb, will contract when touched. By microscopic examination of gonad sex can be determined. Clitoris of female appears. From this time on, looks very much like a miniature infant. Length, 1+ inch. Weight, $\frac{1}{15}$ ounce (2 grams).

Tenth week: The eyes, which were at side of head, moving to front. Face quite human except for jaws, not fully developed. Heart forming four chambers. Scrotum appearing. Palate to form roof of mouth closing. Major blood vessels assuming final form and muscle wall of intestinal tract forming. Fetal heart beating 117 to 157 per minute. Electrocardiogram of live born fetus of this age shows pattern of various waves similar to adult.

Fetus resembles miniature doll, slightly more than one inch in height with a very large head, which is almost half of the fetus, gracefully formed arms and legs, Oriental slitlike closed eyes, small ear lobes, protuberant abdomen. Fetus looks top heavy.

End of third month (13½ weeks): Arms, legs, hands, feet, fingers, and toes fully formed. Nails appear. Ears completely formed. External genital organs begin to show clear differences, and by 11th week trained observer can determine sex with naked eye. Now when the brain signals, muscles respond and the fetus kicks, even curling its toes. Arms bend at wrists and elbows, and fingers close to form tiny fist. The face with its tightly shut eyes squints, purses its lips, and opens its mouth. It may swallow amniotic fluid, excreting it back into the amniotic fluid as urine. All movements reflex from spinal cord. Brain not yet sufficiently organized to control them and will not be until after birth. Length, 3 inches. Weight, 1 ounce (30 grams).

End of fourth month (18 weeks): Casual observer could now distinguish sex in infants delivered at this phase of development. By end of month fetal movements felt by mother and heart can be heard with stethoscope. Fine, downlike hair all over, skin less transparent and pinker. Eyebrows and eyelashes appear. Length, 8½ inches. Weight, 6 ounces (180 grams).

End of fifth month (22½ weeks): Hair appears on head. Fat being deposited under skin, although fetus very lean. If born, may live a few minutes, in rarest of instances reported to have survived. Length, 12 inches. Weight, 1 pound (453 grams).

End of sixth month (27 weeks): Fetus covered with cheeselike secretion, vernix caseosa. Skin wrinkled. Hair on head fairly well developed. Eyes open. If born, most live for several hours or even days. When given expert premature-infant care, approximately one in ten born in the 27th week survives. Length, 14 inches. Weight, 2 pounds (906 grams).

End of seventh month (31½ weeks): In male fetus, testicles usually descend into scrotum. Child born alive during this month has slightly better than a 50 per cent chance for survival. The age-old superstition that a baby born in the seventh will do better than one born in the eighth is entirely fallacious. Each day nearer term makes the child's chances for survival that much better. Length, 16 inches. Weight, 3 pounds, 12 ounces (1700 grams).

End of eighth month (35¾ weeks): Child has better than 90 per cent likelihood for survival. Length, 18 inches. Weight, 5¼ pounds (2735 grams).

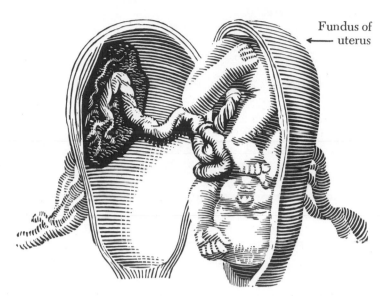

Fundus of
← uterus

Fetus in the seventh month. Placenta is usually on rear wall; umbilical cord is about 20 inches long

End of ninth month (40 weeks): Full term. Skin smooth, polished-looking, and still covered by cheeselike secretion. No downlike hair except over shoulders and arms. Head hair 1 inch long. Nails protrude beyond ends of fingers and toes. Eyes usually a slate color; impossible to predict their final tone. Average circumference of head equals circumference of shoulders (13 inches). Length, 20 inches. Weight, 7 pounds, 6 ounces (3350 grams). When born alive, 99 out of 100 survive.

At birth the various body systems of the newborn human are sufficiently organized to carry on the necessary activities for its survival outside of the uterus, provided it is protected and nourished. But the baby is far from being an independent individual. The complicated muscular coordination necessary for sitting must wait six months and for walking a year or more, until the nerves and brain have developed sufficiently. This is in bold contrast to lower animals. A newly born chick trots off almost at once in search of food. The newborn wildebeest on the plains of Africa is delivered during herd migrations and five minutes after its birth must trudge after its mother if it is to survive. In truth human parents have the privilege and duty to watch with their own eyes the final stages of fetal development in the nursery.

Life in the Uterus

The Amniotic Fluid

The colorless amniotic fluid by which the fetus is surrounded serves many purposes. It prevents the walls of the uterus from cramping the fetus and allows it unhampered growth and movement. It encompasses the fetus with a fluid of constant temperature which is a marvelous insulator against cold and heat. Above all it acts as an excellent shock absorber. A blow on the mother's abdomen merely jolts the fetus, and it floats away.

It is easy to appreciate a pregnant woman's special concern if she falls violently, is struck a hard blow on the abdomen, or is badly shaken in an accident. Of course pregnancy does not lessen her chance for injury, but external trauma rarely harms the unborn child. If there is no vaginal bleeding within an hour after the accident, it is almost an infallible rule that no damage has resulted to the pregnancy. Very rarely an accident may initiate premature labor, usually by an associated rupture of the membranes. One may state unequivocally that accidents occurring during pregnancy never cause birthmarks, malformations, or (save in the rare cases in which they cause miscarriage) any other ill effects to the child itself. The exception is an object which penetrates the abdomen and uterus, such as a bullet.

Amniotic fluid is by no means stagnant, about one-third being replenished every hour. It is constantly being reabsorbed back into the mother's blood system and excreted into the sac by the cells of the amniotic membrane, the inner of the two membranes forming the fetal sac. The chorion is the outer membrane. During intrauterine existence the fetus swallows amniotic fluid and voids fetal urine into it. It has been determined that the fetus swallows about one pint a day, and it is assumed voids a similar quantity. The fetus does not defecate under normal conditions before birth. At the twelfth week of pregnancy the volume of amniotic fluid in the uterus measures two ounces, in midpregnancy one pint, and at term (the end of nine months) a little less than a quart, though amounts up to eight gallons have been observed. When the amount of fluid exceeds two quarts the abnormal condition is called hydramnios. The amniotic fluid contains skin cells shed by the fetus, fetal hairs, specks of vernix, the oily, cheeselike material that covers much of the fetal skin, various minerals and sugar in weak solution, and products of fetal urine, such as uric acid and creatinine.

The Navel Cord

The umbilical cord runs from the navel of the fetus to the inner or fetal surface of the placenta. It is the lifeline of the fetus, in reality a vital cable circulating fetal blood low in oxygen and high in waste products through its two umbilical arteries to the placenta, where the blood is purified and takes up oxygen and food stuffs. The cleansed, well-oxygenated, placental blood, rich in nutrients, then returns to the fetus through the one umbilical vein. The umbilical cord, a moist, dull white, semitransparent, jellylike rope, averages twenty-two inches in length at term, although cords from a half-inch to fifty inches have been reported. Some are straight, others twisted, and some, in rare instances, are even knotted by fetal gymnastics *in utero*. The diameter of the cord is about three-quarters of an inch.

The Placenta and Its Function in Fetal Nutrition

The placenta is a complex organ, through which the fetus absorbs food and eliminates its waste products. The blood of the mother and the blood of the fetus come in close proximity in the substance of the placenta, and materials pass over from one blood system to the other. If, for example, the mother's blood contains more sugar than that of the fetus, the excess passes over into the fetal blood until relative equality between the two is reached. In this way sugar that the mother eats is fed to her baby. On the other hand, the excess carbon dioxide of the fetal blood goes over to the mother's blood and is exhaled by her lungs. Thus, the mother breathes for her child. Other waste products of the fetus are likewise absorbed by the mother's blood and voided by her kidneys. It is to be noted that not all vitamins, minerals, and hormones are in exact equality in the two circulations. For example, the amount of vitamin C in the fetal blood is several times that in the maternal blood. As another example calcium to build fetal bones passes to the fetus from the mother at twenty times the rate it passes back from the fetus to the mother. This delicate interchange between mother and fetus is further illustrated by the observation that cigarette-smoking by the mother temporarily increases the rate of the fetal heart. The maximum effect occurs from seven to twelve minutes after the cigarette is first lighted.

Intrauterine growth is largely governed by the development and functioning of the placenta. The placenta stops growing completely between thirty-four and thirty-eight weeks, and with cessation of placental growth fetal growth slows but nevertheless continues. It has been observed that women with relatively large placentas are usually delivered later than women with smaller ones. In some abnormal situations the placenta performs poorly, causing a condition termed placental insufficiency, which may adversely affect the growth and well-being of the fetus.

The bloodstreams of the mother and fetus are ordinarily quite separate, and the interchange of materials is carried on through a multicelled membranous partition. Some of the smaller molecules pass intact back and forth through the separating membrane; the larger ones, such as fats, have to be broken down on one side of the barrier, and then pass through to be reconstituted on the other side. This all sounds quite remarkable, and it is. To feed a rapidly growing organism, to keep it supplied with oxygen, and to excrete its waste products is a huge, complex task. The placenta, a relatively small organ, weighing one-fifth to one-sixth as much as the fetus, does this with unmatched efficiency.

Does the Blood of the Mother and of the Fetus Mix?

Before the end of the eighteenth century it was held that the blood cells of the mother intermingled freely with those of the fetus. However, at this time a famous English obstetrician injected a dye into the blood vessels of a woman who had died undelivered, and the dye did not appear in the blood vessels of her fetus. This was thought to prove the independent integrity of the two vascular systems, and the scientific world believed that mother and fetus never interchanged blood.

In the 1940s, when the disease erythroblastosis was first described, some doubt was thrown on this concept, for in order to cause erythroblastosis an immune response has to be produced in the mother to some factor present in the fetal red-blood cells—a factor which she would ordinarily lack. Theoretically, this required the passage of fetal red-blood cells into the maternal circulation.

We now have proof that this happens because fetal hemoglobin (the coloring matter of red-blood cells), which is readily distinguishable from adult hemoglobin, is found in the circulating blood of pregnant women. We also know that blood cells of the mother enter the blood of her fetus. Two types of experiments have been done which prove this. In one study, doctors transfused mothers at varying short intervals before birth with compatible red cells tagged with radioactive atoms. After delivery they checked the baby with a Geiger counter and got a positive response. In another series of experiments they transfused the mother before birth from donors whose blood contained some rare, abnormal cells that could be searched for later in the infant. The blood chosen had the property of sickling—the red-blood cells became sickle-shaped, instead of remaining round—when placed in an incubator at 37.5 degrees centigrade. The "sickle" cells were found in the baby's blood in more than 80 per cent of the experiments.

The pendulum has now swung back to the eighteenth-century opinion —not a complete swing, for it is not felt that the blood of the mother and the fetus intermix without restraint; it is more likely that during pregnancy there is occasional leakage of cells between the two circulations. However, after the birth of the baby before the placenta has been completely extruded there is commonly a shower of fetal blood cells from the placenta into the mother's blood. Less frequently, this occurs after abortion, particularly if the abortion has to be completed by a scraping of the interior of the uterus to remove retained placental fragments.

Most Drugs Cross the Placenta to the Baby

Almost all drugs taken by the mother cross, via the placenta, from her circulation to that of the fetus. The majority, such as aspirin and the digitalis family of heart drugs, neither benefit nor harm the baby. On the other hand, some drugs administered to the mother actually treat the fetus as well. A conspicuous example is penicillin for the cure of maternal syphilis (see the discussion in Chapter 11). Another example of treating the baby by treating the mother is the inhalation of oxygen. If from some complication of labor the baby's heart rate becomes slow and irregular, demonstrating that there is insufficient oxygen in the fetal tissues, pure oxygen breathed by the mother through an anesthetic mask will raise the level of oxygen in her blood and similarly elevate the baby's level. Oxygen administered to the mother may normalize a depressed, irregular fetal heart rate.

Drugs Harmful to the Fetus

Some drugs taken by a mother during pregnancy can be deleterious to the fetus. An outstanding example is that of morphine or heroin. When the mother is an addict, the fetus may become habituated to the drug *in utero*. Addicted women perhaps unfortunately show no reduction in fertility. I say "unfortunately," for a study has shown that relatively few babies born to addicted women are still with their mothers by the age of eight months. There is a high infant mortality and many are either taken away by court order or voluntarily surrendered to relatives or agencies.

The child's withdrawal symptoms will appear within twenty-four hours of delivery. It becomes irritable and overactive, develops tremors, and cries with a peculiar high-pitched note. Later, convulsions appear and sometimes, if untreated, the infant dies.

The addicted newborn must be given an opiate, usually paragoric, at regular intervals in gradually decreasing doses over the first several days of life. Some of the less severely addicted can be successfully treated with phenobarbital. About 20 per cent of babies born to mothers on methadone show mild withdrawal symptoms for which phenobarbital therapy suffices. The babies of heroin-addicted or methadone-treated mothers show a marked tendency to be underweight at birth, many falling below the 5½- pound birth weight that is used to separate premature from full-term infants. In these cases, however, the babies are not born prematurely, but are carried to term. There is no increase in congenital malformations in the babies of addicted women.

It has been known for years that some drugs taken during pregnancy are teratogenic (cause malformations in the embryo), but the whole subject was highlighted when in 1961–1962, 5000 armless and/or legless children were born in West Germany. This condition is known as phocomelia (from the Latin *phoca*, for "seal") because often the associated stunted extremities resemble a seal's flippers. Two-thirds of the children survived and showed no evidence of brain damage. Through thorough medical detective work it was determined that virtually all the mothers had taken Thalidomide, a mild tranquilizer for nausea or insomnia, during early pregnancy, almost invariably between thirty-seven and fifty days after the onset of the last menses.

The only other drugs with proved teratogenicity are antimetabolites, such as aminopterin, and other antitumor drugs, and drugs used to treat an overactive thyroid gland. If during pregnancy a woman takes the male hormone, testosterone, or the female hormone progesterone, which is broken down in the body of the mother into the testosterone-like substance, the chemical appears in the blood of the fetus and a small proportion of female infants born to these women will have abnormal external genitals—a greatly oversized clitoris with the lips of the vagina fused in front, both conditions correctable by surgery. Then, too, the antibiotic, aureomycin, taken by the mother during pregnancy may later cause yellow teeth in the offspring.

LSD is under suspicion as a fetal teratogen. If it has an effect, the effect may be not on the conceptus itself, but on the germ cells of the potential parent, causing a preconceptional chromosomal abnormality of sperm or egg. In several reported cases, either or both parents who gave a history of having taken LSD within a month to four years before conception had children with multiple malformations and with a discernible abnormality of its chromosomes as well. However, isolated case reports do not prove causal connection. If it were possible to collect incidence data on birth abnormalities associated with chromosomal abnormalities from a significant sample of parents who have used LSD and compare the figure with incidence data from a well-matched sample of parents who have never used LSD, we would have the answer, yes or no.

Let us see what we do know. The risk of teratogenicity causing a fetal abnormality during pregnancy is greatest between the third and eighth weeks of gestation, the period when the organs and skeleton of the fetus are being formed. Danger of an agent causing an abnormality decreases progressively thereafter, as fetal development becomes more and more completely established. The few facts we know and the immense amount we do not know have combined to make obstetricians therapeutic nihilists, particularly during the first half of pregnancy.

In making such a declaration to the lay reader an author makes himself liable to misinterpretation. I advise that you do not indulge in self-medication during pregnancy, but by all means take any drug which your doctor prescribes. He will not prescribe a drug for you unless in his judgment it is necessary for your health and well-being.

The second point I would like to make is that before young people take LSD they should consider the fact that there are serious gaps in scientific knowledge and one cannot assure them, at this point in time, it will not penalize their future progeny.

The Effect of Smoking during Pregnancy

It has been shown by several investigators that babies born to smokers of one pack of cigarettes or more a day average three-quarters of a pound less at birth than the babies of nonsmokers. This lesser weight does not seem to prejudice the baby's chance for survival, unless it is also born prematurely. The infants of heavy smokers have no tendency to be born prematurely; they simply weigh less at term. There is evidence that the size of the deficit in birth weight is in proportion to the daily consumption of cigarettes. Heavy smokers do not show an increase in births associated with fetal abnormalities.

In Britain the children of 3000 heavy smokers (ten or more cigarettes daily after the fourth month) were compared at the age of seven years to 14,000 children of nonsmokers or light smokers. The sample comprised all the children born in the United Kingdom the week of March 3, 1958, who could be traced for the follow-up study. The children of heavy smokers averaged four months behind in reading ability and were one centimeter shorter (0.4 inch) in height compared to the controls. The findings that as a group the smoking women were poorer and older and had more children than the nonsmokers must be taken into account. The report admits these factors may have been contributory but nevertheless concludes that the cigarette smoking was of greater importance.

In summary, for the protection of your own health in respect to lung cancer, emphysema, bronchitis, and heart disease, as well as possible benefit to the baby, give up cigarettes not only during pregnancy, but for keeps. If you can't, cut down as much as possible and use a brand with a low-tar and low-nicotine content.

The Effect of Alcohol on the Fetus

There is no logical reason to prohibit the moderate use of alcohol during pregnancy to the patient who enjoys and tolerates it. Alcohol diffuses rapidly across the placenta and soon attains equilibrium in the two circulations. This knowledge may dissuade the pregnant woman from taking just one more, since she cannot know and never will know whether her fetus will enjoy the additional drink as much as she thinks she will. It is to be remembered that alcohol is rich in calories, so that the pregnant woman who is gaining too rapidly had best omit, or strictly limit, its consumption. Such patients should be cognizant of the fact that straight liquor ordinarily has fewer calories than cocktails or several beers. If a patient develops any tendency to high blood pressure during pregnancy, her doctor is likely to put her strictly on the water wagon.

When it comes to heavy drinking it is a different story. A study of twelve babies born to chronic-alcoholic mothers at the University of Washington showed ten to have "intrauterine growth failure," and the postnatal growth and development of these infants did not proceed at a normal rate. Dietary histories obtained from the chronic-alcoholic mothers showed moderate to severe nutritional deficiencies which may be an important causative factor of the poor condition of the infant. A few cases of delirium tremens have been reported in newborn babies born to severely alcoholic mothers. The condition is an acute withdrawal effect similar to that seen in adults.

Factors Affecting Birth Weight

Do you want a small baby? Your chance is best if you are a Chinese peasant girl of seventeen or less, in your first pregnancy. Do you want a large baby? You are more likely to have one if you are a white woman of the upper social stratum, thirty-five years old or more, with your tenth or eleventh child.

Many factors affect the baby's size. Boys are usually three ounces heavier than girls. The average weight at birth of a Chinese baby is 6½ pounds (2958 grams); of a black baby, 7 pounds (3150 grams); and of a white baby, 7½ pounds (3350 grams). A white girl pregnant for the first time at age sixteen years or younger will have a baby weighing 5 ounces less than the baby of her sister who postpones her first childbearing until she is thirty-five.

Socioeconomic and Nutritional Factors

In addition, socioeconomic and nutritional factors affect the weight of the newborn. Babies born to patients in the economically privileged groups average a half pound more than those born to a less favored population sample. As brought forth in a study in Scotland, babies weighing less than 5½ pounds are far less common among the former. Their incidence in the most affluent tenth of the population was 4 per cent, in contrast to 8 per cent among the remaining nine-tenths. The affluent woman has relatively more rest and a superior diet, both of which probably contribute to fewer early-terminating pregnancies and fewer babies that weigh less than 5½ pounds at birth. For statistical purposes the convention is to categorize all babies weighing less than 5½ pounds at birth as premature, and those weighing more than 5½ pounds, mature, irrespective of the duration of pregnancy. This has come about because it is usually so difficult to determine exactly the date when pregnancy was initiated.

Modern studies, as we shall discuss in Chapter 6, have shown that a baby's chances of being born small are increased if the mother is underweight for her height, if she shows a low weight gain during pregnancy, or if her nutrition during pregnancy has been deficient.

The Role of Heredity

Heredity plays a role in fetal size. Ordinarily, parents descended from a lineage of big people breed infants of large size and those with small parents and grandparents produce babies of less than average birth weight. In my experience the size of members of the paternal line is at least as important as of those of the maternal line. Perhaps I was overly impressed of this fact by the case of a couple whose three children I delivered. The mother was of average size, but the father was a huge fellow who had been virtually the entire right side of the scrimmage line on his college football team. His brothers also were big and powerful. Each of the three babies was over nine pounds, which made the labor difficult for the mother and me. I was very relieved when my suggestion of sterilization after the third birth was enthusiastically accepted. A mother of short stature is especially likely to have a baby of relatively low birth weight.

Factor of Maternal Disease

Maternal illness may affect birth weight. Chronic diseases in mothers usually eventuate in small babies, as for example chronic high blood pressure and/or chronic kidney disease. The only illness associated with babies of excessive size is diabetes. The tendency of diabetics to deliver very large infants is independent of the severity of the diabetes or the degree of control of the diabetic condition. However, the woman whose diabetes is of recent origin is more likely to have a baby of excessive size than the woman whose diabetes is long-standing. All the factors listed here which affect birth weight apply to the average patient in a large series of cases; in this matter the individual is often an exception, so that the couple who, according to all rules, ought to produce a large baby may produce a small one, and vice versa. It may be said, however, that couples usually have a standard-sized term baby, so that if the first baby is large, subsequent babies are usually large, or, if the first is small, the second and third tend to be small.

Weight Range at Term

The only certain fact in this realm is the marked variation in the birth weight of nine-month children; any figure between five and eleven pounds is likely, and between three and a half and fifteen pounds, possible.

Excessive Size

How common are very large babies, and what is the most a newborn infant can weigh?

One frequently hears of babies with birth weights over eleven pounds, and sometimes one hears of newborns much larger. Most of the latter reports must be considered apocryphal; in such cases careful investigation will usually show that the weight had been estimated by hefting the child with one hand, not by weighing it.

In 23,500 consecutive deliveries at the Johns Hopkins Hospital, 251 babies weighed over 10 pounds (1 in 93.6); 35 (1 in 542) weighed over 11 pounds; 8 (1 in 2937) weighed over 12 pounds; and 2 (1 in 11,750) weighed over 13 pounds. These two were males, the smaller, who weighed 13 pounds, 7 ounces, was the ninth child of a thirty-four-year-old patient; and the larger—14 pounds, 4 ounces—was the seventh child of a woman of forty-four. During 1967 and 1968, Brooklyn's Kings County Hospital, which serves an economically depressed population, reported 3232 single births. Twelve infants, nine boys, and three girls, weighed over 10 pounds, 1 in 269 births. Among 30,000 deliveries in Munich, no baby weighed over 13 pounds, 4 ounces, and the largest infant in 100,000 cases born at the New York Lying-In Hospital weighed 15 pounds.

Despite the actual rarity of such phenomena I am sure that one-third of American mothers claim the distinction of having borne twelve-, fourteen-, or even sixteen-pound babies. The first question after each birth is, "How is she?"; the second, "What is it?" If to the third—"How much does it weigh?"—the doctor replies, "Seven pounds," jaws drop and joy is remote, but if he answers, "Twelve pounds," everyone beams. Physicians realized this long before the days of obstetrical hospitals, and since at the usual home delivery the only scale was the doctor's hands, he found it tactful to err by three or four additional pounds.

World's Biggest Newborn

The world's record for the largest baby is claimed by Sale City, Georgia, where in February 1916 Dr. D. P. Belcher attended Mrs. Rowe when she bore a stillborn female weighing 25 pounds. The physician failed to stipulate the type of scale or its condition. The largest baby with carefully verified weight was delivered at a hospital in Aldershot, England, and reported in 1933 by Dr. Moss in the *British Medical Journal*. The woman, twenty-two years old, had had one previous baby, which weighed 10 pounds. Both she and her husband were six feet tall. In this pregnancy, five days before the calculated confinement date, she gave birth to a baby weighing 24 pounds, 2 ounces. The newborn was thirty-five inches long—heavier and taller than the average child at one year. It was born dead. According to medical literature, no child has ever been born alive weighing more than 15.5 pounds, although the modern free usage of Cesarean section should make such a live birth not only possible but likely.

The Sex of the Fetus

Whether the baby will be a boy or girl is determined approximately eight and one half months before birth, at the critical second of fertilization. The mother's egg has nothing whatever to do with determining the sex of her offspring. The father ejaculates two types of spermatozoa in apparently equal numbers. The two types differ from each other to a minor degree, yet this small variation makes a major difference—the sex of the individual. Every spermatozoon contains the same twenty-two chromosomes (autosomes) which affect the inheritance of all bodily structures and functions except the sex of the fetus and some associated characteristics. The twenty-third chromosome, the sex chromosome, is very different in the two kinds of spermatozoa. In half, the sex chromosome of the sperm cell is relatively large, a replica of the twenty-third or sex chromosome of the egg, and is called the "X chromosome." In half of the sperm cells the sex chromosome is much smaller and very different in appearance; it is called the "Y chromosome." When an ovum is fertilized by an X-bearing sperm cell, a female fetus is created; when it is fertilized by a Y-bearing sperm cell, a male results.

Is Sex Inherited?

There is a popular fallacy that the tendency to produce a preponderance of males runs in some families and an equally strong tendency toward the creation of girls in other families. This concept has been repeatedly investigated by geneticists and statisticians, and each study leaves no doubt that the production of a child of one sex or the other is not affected by heredity; the sex of an infant is purely a matter of chance. The problem goes back to the old coin-tossing experiment. Once in 128 tosses there will be seven tails or seven heads in succession.

Your chances for having a boy in the next pregnancy are precisely the same whether you have already had five daughters in five pregnancies, or five sons.

Can We Control the Sex?

As I have just stated, apparently chance determines sex, and we cannot affect chance. The multiple prescriptions recommended at one time or another work correctly half the time and incorrectly half the time.

We shall not be able to control the sex of the offspring until some practical means becomes available either for sorting the X-bearing from the Y-bearing spermatozoa, or for rendering the ovum refractory to fertilization by one variety or the other of sperm cell.

To be sure, in this era of overpopulation if there were a simple, fool-proof method of calling one's shots, ordering either a boy or a girl, many more families would have just two or three children rather than the five or six they now have in seeking a child of the sex which thus far has eluded them. And with abortion on demand becoming more widespread, early diagnosis of the sex of an unborn might make the decision to abort or to continue pregnancy much easier.

Dr. Landrum Shettles of Columbia Medical School states that in both fresh and fixed preparations of all ejaculations he has observed two distinct varieties of sperm cells, androsperms with relatively round small heads, and gynosperms with relatively large oval heads. The former he assumes are Y-bearing cells, the Y chromosome being much smaller than the X which gynosperms carry. Shettles has also resurrected two previously rejected theories concerning determination of sex. The first is that sperm cells producing females are hardier than cells producing males, and therefore an acid environment created by a precoital dilute vinegar douche weeds out androsperms, leaving the field to the hardier gynosperms and hence daughters. On the other hand a precoital alkaline douche protects the weaker androsperms and enhances the likelihood of a male heir, since in the absence of hostile acids, androsperms are able to use their advantageous speed and agility because of the smaller heads and longer tails with which nature endows them. The second basic concept of Shettles's theory is that female secretions are more alkaline at the time of ovulation and therefore intercourse at this time favors androsperms, but intercourse two or three days before ovulation, when the female tract is more acid, favors gynosperms, as those that would produce males have fallen by the wayside two days later when an egg becomes available. Female orgasm, Shettles postulates, increases the flow of alkaline mucus favoring androsperms, while its absence gives gynosperms a better chance.

On the basis of these theories, to me as yet unproved, Dr. Shettles has created two coital programs; one, he claims, is more likely to engender sons and the other, daughters. Involved is precoital douching with acid or alkali, stimulating or inhibiting orgasm, supine or posterior coital positioning, and timing coitus to avoid or coincide with ovulation. Before one takes such advice seriously and transforms making love into a chemical reaction, Shettles's theories require more basis of fact and his own results in a small patient series unprejudiced corroboration.

I am not certain we have gotten any further than Aristotle did 2300 years ago when he advised farmers who wanted a bull calf to have the cow's right flank sloping downhill as she was being served, and her left flank sloping downward if a heifer was desired.

Can the Sex Be Diagnosed before Birth?

Since the time of the Pharaohs men have promulgated first this method and then that for predicting the sex of the unborn. They have used urine, blood, and saliva as test substances; they have depended on the color of the mother's skin, the relative size of the right and left breasts, or the way the infant was "carried," to uncover the answer. Each method in its time and place was hailed as the key to the solution and brought temporary fame and sometimes fortune to its innovator. Each in turn was soon challenged, and each was soon discarded.

Since 1949 Dr. M. L. Barr, a Canadian anatomist, and his associates have published a series of articles demonstrating that if cells from any part of the body are properly prepared, stained, and magnified under the microscope, a recognizable difference exists between the cells obtained from a female and a male. The cells from a female show a dark-staining, bean-shaped body, one micron in diameter, lying along the inner surface of the nuclear membrane. The cells from a male lack this specific body, named a Barr body, thought to be derived from one of the two X chromosomes in each female cell. Early in the embryonic development of the normal female fetus, probably about the twelfth day after fertilization, before gonadal cells of the ovary appear, one member of the X-chromosome pair within each cell becomes inactivated. This inactive X chromosome then becomes applied to the nuclear membrane as a Barr body. The single X chromosome of male cells does not become similarly inactivated. Epithelial, or skin-type, cells show the difference particularly well. About 65 per cent of the cells of the female, fetus or adult, show Barr bodies. It is believed that they are not absent in the remaining 35 per cent but that their Barr body lies in a plane turned away from the microscopist and therefore not visible.

While the fetus occupies the uterus it constantly sheds skin cells into the amniotic fluid surrounding it. Making use of this fact, Israeli investigators put a fine hollow needle through the abdominal wall and uterus of a pregnant woman and aspirated a small amount of fluid from the amniotic sac (amniocentesis). They recovered fetal skin cells from it by centrifuging the amniotic fluid and were able by the Barr technique to prediagnose accurately the sex of the unborn, and in their small series of cases each pregnancy progressed undisturbed.

Amniocentesis can be done at any time after the thirteenth week. It is a simple procedure. After injection of a little anesthetic into the abdominal wall a three-inch, hollow needle of moderate bore is inserted through the anesthetized abdominal wall into the uterus lying just beneath. A syringe is attached, a fluid sample aspirated, and the needle withdrawn.

Amniocentesis is being used more and more extensively. It not only enables one to diagnose fetal sex but is used to recover fetal cells for chromosomal studies of the unborn, a new field called cytogenetics, and for the presence and amount of certain chemical constituents in the amniotic fluid. Cytogenetics and chemical tests of amniotic fluid both are discussed later in the book. No doubt amniocentesis will have many more uses in the future; perhaps it will become a vehicle for medicating the fetus directly. In the rare disorder hydramnios, when the uterus is overdistended by an excessive amount of fluid, a tap, or repeated taps, may be performed to reduce the distention. Quarts, or even gallons, of amniotic fluid may be removed. This degree of hydramnios is often associated with a multiple pregnancy, twins or triplets, and also certain varieties of congenitally malformed fetuses. Hydramnios is also occasionally encountered in pregnancies with a normal single infant.

A study to determine the sex of the unborn can be performed on fluid leaking from the vagina after premature rupture of the membranes before the onset of labor or early in its course. The Barr technique, as would be expected, again foretells the sex.

In breech presentations a vaginal examination late in labor will occasionally permit the doctor to determine the sex before birth by feeling the genitals. Also in most breech cases the genitals are visible through the vaginal orifice in the last minutes before actual birth.

Sex Ratio

Sex ratio, by definition, is the number of males to every hundred females. There are several types of sex ratio: primary, the number of males conceived per hundred females conceived; secondary, the number of males born per hundred females; and tertiary, the number of males living at any given postnatal period per hundred females.

The sex ratio at birth, the secondary sex ratio, is uniformly between 105 and 106 throughout the world. What accounts for this universal and consistent preponderance of male births? The first assumption would be that there are more male-producing sperms than female-producing sperms. But this is not the case. As we stated before, X- and Y-bearing spermatozoa theoretically are in equal numbers. One might suspect, then, that more female fetuses die before birth. Actually, the reverse is true. More male fetuses die than female; in every five miscarriages, and in every five babies born dead, there are approximately three males and two females. The primary, or conception, sex ratio is postulated to be 130, twenty-five higher than the sex ratio at birth. Perhaps this high conception sex ratio is due to some inherent advantage that Y-bearing sperms possess over X-bearing sperms. It could be that Y-bearing sperm cells are more active and vigorous; or it may be that a greater chemical affinity exists between the unfertilized egg and the Y sperm. Whatever the reason, man in his ignorance cannot as yet wrest the secret from nature.

Certain small ethnic groups are reported to have a higher (more males per 100 females than 106) or lower (fewer males than 106 per 100 females) secondary sex ratio than the general population. In this country the Jews are said to have a high sex ratio and the blacks a low sex ratio. Also, the sex ratio is said to rise a point or two after wars which involve most of the population. The variable is the incidence of miscarriage in a given sample; when its frequency rises the sex ratio declines, and when it falls the sex ratio is elevated. It is believed that among Jews there is a lower miscarriage frequency than among blacks. After a war impregnation occurs in a population whose women have had enforced reproductive rest, which may reduce the incidence of miscarriage.

The Fetal Position in the Uterus

In the earlier works on obstetrics it was taught that the fetus might assume any position in the uterus, the number of positions being limited solely by an author's imagination. Accurate observations gradually eliminated the more fanciful.

The positions which the child assumes *in utero* may be divided into two general classes—longitudinal and transverse. In the longitudinal the spinal column of the child is parallel to the spinal column of the mother; in the transverse it is at right angles to that of the mother, forming a cross with it. The former is normal, accounting for more than 99 per cent; while the transverse position is rare, occurring in less than 0.5 per cent.

These two general classifications of fetal positions may be subdivided into more exact groups. We term these more specific positions presentations; this refers to the precise part of the fetus which presents over the bone-surrounded birth passage, the pelvis. At term, 96 percent of fetuses present by the head (cephalic presentation); 3.5 per cent by the buttocks (breech presentation); and in less than 0.5 per cent the child lies transversely with a shoulder presenting.

Cephalic Presentations

If, during labor, the head presents, it ordinarily flexes, so that the infant's chin rests on its breastbone. When this occurs, the crown of the head first enters the mother's pelvis and is the part of the fetus earliest visible as the birth takes place. This is the common variety of cephalic presentation, accounting for almost 99 per cent of the cases in which the head presents. Such babies frequently are born with a temporary swelling over the area which the hair whorl will later occupy; the swelling is caused by pressure, since this area is the lead point in the birth process.

Occasionally, instead of being flexed, the head of the fetus is extended during labor, and the infant delivers with the face presenting. Under such conditions the features may appear as swollen as those of a badly mauled prizefighter, but within forty-eight hours the contusions and swellings have disappeared. If the head is only partially extended, the baby's brow is the lead point.

In a cephalic presentation, the back is convex, the thighs flexed over the abdomen, the legs bent at the knee joints, and the feet crossed so that the toes point toward the opposite armpit. The arms are either crossed over the chest or straight and parallel to the sides. The umbilical cord nestles looped in the adbdominal space between the arms and legs.

Breech Presentations

A breech presentation, relatively rare at term, is common during the earlier months. Nearly 50 per cent of babies present by the breech before the seventh month, but all except a few revolve through 180 degrees to present by the head at some time before the end of the ninth month.

There are three types of breech presentation—frank, footling, and full. In a frank breech, much the commonest, the legs of the baby are flexed up over the abdomen, with the knees straight so that the toes touch the shoulders and the two buttocks present over the pelvis. If it were not for the very loose joints of the fetus, this position would be almost unattainable and, to say the least, uncomfortable. After delivery it is not uncommon for the baby who delivered as a frank breech to keep his legs flexed at the hip and straight at the knee for several hours. Since the buttocks and genital area are the lead points in the birth of a frank breech, they are often swollen and discolored black and blue at delivery. This clears up rapidly without permanent damage. In a footling breech one or both legs are held straight, as in the standing position, and act as the lead point in labor and delivery. The full breech is rare; in it the fetus sits cross-legged in the mother's pelvis, like a tailor on his sewing bench. Breech presentations have a slight tendency to recur in subsequent labors.

As is discussed later in this book, a fetus presenting by the breech is sometimes manipulated by the doctor to a cephalic presentation late in pregnancy before labor begins; this procedure is termed external version.

Transverse Presentation

Once in two hundred or more pregnancies the fetus lies transversely and a shoulder, or occasionally an arm and hand, enters the pelvis. Natural delivery is impossible and either a Cesarean section must be performed or the infant turned in late labor, after the mother is deeply anesthetized.

Presentation of Twins

In twins the ordinary proportion of the various presentations is greatly altered. Both children present by the head in 39 per cent of the cases, one by the head and the other by the breech in 36 per cent, both by the breech in 11 per cent, and one or both transversely in 14 percent.

Determination of Fetal Position

The position of the fetus is usually determined by feeling or palpating the abdomen. From the thirtieth week on, the physician can usually identify the fetal head, back, and extremities without great difficulty.

Activities of the Fetus in the Uterus

Obviously we lack subjective observations of intrauterine life, but many objective data have been obtained. I have already mentioned the fact that the fetal kidneys function *in utero* and the fetus voids into the amniotic fluid. The fetus also swallows amniotic fluid, whether or not to quench its thirst will never be known. The intestines are also active, and a thick, viscid, tarlike excrement (meconium) is found in the lower bowel. Under normal conditions meconium is not excreted until after delivery. The fetal heart and some phases of fetal movements have

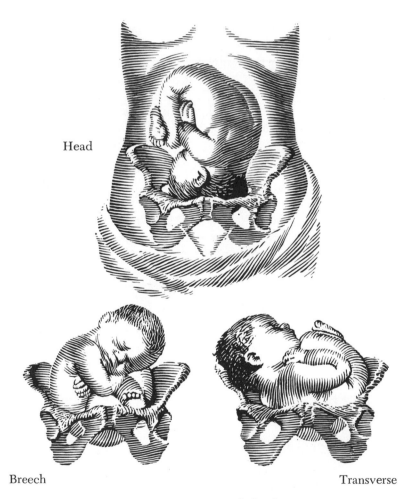

Head

Breech   Transverse

Three common positions of the fetus

already been discussed; there are several additional facts about intrauterine activity which merit discussion.

The fetal movements felt by patient and doctor are usually the
thrusting and bending of arms and legs. The motion of the legs is
more extensive than that of the arms, and therefore if movements appear
most active in the upper abdomen it is likely that the fetus presents by
the head. If late in labor, in a breech presentation with membranes
ruptured, a foot protrudes from the vagina its movements can be seen
some time before birth. If the foot is pinched the child attempts to
withdraw it, and if the sole is scratched the toes bend wildly. Occasionally a hand may present along with the head (compound presentation) during labor, and if on vaginal examination the obstetrician should
shake hands with his unborn patient, the baby's fingers squirm in a
most unpleasant fashion. In face presentations sucking movements are
produced if the examiner inserts a finger into the child's mouth.

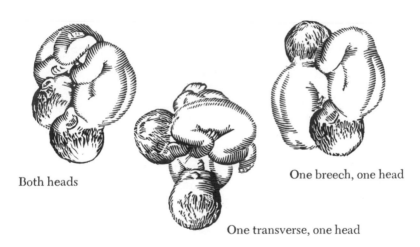

Both heads

One breech, one head

One transverse, one head

Common ways that twins present

Ahlfeld, a German scientist, was the first to claim that the fetus sucks
its fingers *in utero*. He reported the case of a child born with a swollen
thumb; immediately after birth it put the swollen member into its
mouth and sucked. Recent X-ray pictures have shown fetuses with a
thumb or even a hand in the mouth.

Fetal hiccups have been repeatedly observed by both physician and
patient. The movements are short, quick regular jerks of the child's
shoulders and trunk, fifteen to twenty a minute. They can be seen, as
well as felt, by movements of the mother's abdomen. They resemble
ordinary hiccups except for the absence of the stridor, the harsh noise.

An attack of intrauterine hiccups usually lasts about fifteen minutes and may recur several times before delivery.

As stated earlier in this chapter, the fetus does not breathe *in utero*; the work of the lungs is carried on by cooperation between the placenta and the mother's blood. However, there is much evidence that the chest of the fetus moves rhythmically with a rapid, shallow respiratory pattern during the last part of pregnancy. The observation of prenatal respiratory movements was first made in 1888 and has been corroborated several times since. These observers noted a slight rising and falling of the abdominal wall of the mother near the navel; it occurred sixty to eighty times a minute and was most marked in the region which overlay the child's chest. The series of movements were intermittent, ceasing after several minutes and recurring later.

In more recent investigations the abdomen of a pregnant rabbit at term was immersed in a large bath of special fluid (Ringer's Solution) kept constantly at body temperature. The abdominal cavity of the living animal was opened under spinal anesthesia, and the intact uterus exposed. Several minutes later, when the fetuses had become acclimated to the change in environment, respiratory-like movements could be distinctly observed through the semitransparent, thin-walled uterus. Such movements can be clearly differentiated from other movements of the fetus.

It is hard to believe, but nevertheless true, that occasionally the human fetus cries while still *in utero*. Many cases have been reported by reliable observers, so that even the most skeptical must accept this bizarre occurrence. In every instance some operative procedure had allowed air to enter the cavity of the uterus before birth, usually either a version (turning of the child) or a forceps operation. The cry is clearly audible and sounds as though it came from an infant hidden under the covers. This phenomenon is termed *vagitus* (Latin: "the crying of an infant") *uterinus*.

Another precocious trick has been discovered in the repertoire of the fetus. The reaction of the fetus to vibratory stimuli applied to the mother's abdomen has been tested. The stimulus used was an ordinary tuning-fork with a frequency of 120 oscillations per second. No response was noted until the twenty-ninth week, but from this time on all the fetuses responded by an acceleration in the rate of heartbeat, and some by an increase in fetal movements. The speeding of the fetal heart became progressively greater as term was approached; in the seventh month there was an average increase of eight beats, in the eighth month thirteen, and during the last month fourteen. The explanation for this interesting response is uncertain. It probably represents relayed tactile stimulation rather than true hearing. Other observers have reported isolated instances of fetal reaction to vibratory sounds. A patient noted that her fetus stirred vigorously whenever the audience applauded at a concert.

Almost every woman near term attests to the fact that the fetus alternately sleeps and wakes. An hour or several hours of quiet will be replaced by a period of obvious fetal activity. Some scientists believe that there is correlation between the extent and degree of prenatal activity and the later make-up of the individual. The tense, hyperkinetic child leads a restless life even *in utero*, while the placid, even-dispositioned youngster is quiet in the womb.

There is no evidence, of course, that any of this fetal activity is accompanied by consciousness. Every instance cited seems to be a matter of involuntary response to various stimuli. Even at birth the newborn seems to have very little, if any, use of the upper brain, the cerebral hemispheres.

6

Medical Care during Pregnancy

Before discussing prenatal care—medical care of the woman already pregnant—it would be well to mention the need for anteconceptional care—medical care before pregnancy has been initiated. A prize cow or thoroughbred mare is not mated until it is determined the animal is in optimal condition. In theory and in fact, a woman should consult her doctor and not attempt pregnancy until he gives her the green light. If any abnormality is found, such as anemia, undetected diabetes, underweight or overweight, high blood pressure, or a pelvic tumor, remedial measures can be instituted before pregnancy is allowed. Then, too, if a woman has never had German measles (rubella) and shows no immunity to it, prophylactic vaccine should be given several months in advance.

Predelivery medical care has greatly changed in the last half century. Until the late 1920s or early 1930s physicians felt their task to be wholly a technical one. Their goal was simple, to conduct pregnancy so that it ended with a healthy mother and a perfect infant. The concept that the process of having a baby in itself could and should be a full, happy experience, bereft of fear and anxiety, was virtually nonexistent. In their attitude toward pregnancy and labor doctors were as well starched intellectually as they were externally. They conducted prenatal care with the viewpoint, "Don't bother your pretty young head about pregnancy and labor; expunge them from your thoughts; this is an area of my concern, not yours. And as for my answering your questions, a little knowledge is a dangerous thing." Obstetric hospitals thought along the same lines; the concept of giving patients emotional support or confidence through antenatal instruction was foreign to their responsibilities.

Today both physician and hospital have executed an about-face. Recognizing the immense value of knowledge in the eradication of fear, they are attempting to deprive reproduction of its mystery through instruction in the facts of conception, pregnancy, labor, and infant care. This effort to replace ignorance with understanding has been waged with the help of the printed page, motion pictures, mothers' classes, radio, television, lay tours of hospital obstetric facilities, and discussions between the doctor and his patient. The discussions have become so frank that physicians feel there is no question which the pregnant woman and her husband may not ask.

Classes for Expectant Parents

The great number of classes for expectant parents in all communities, given under such varied auspices as the Red Cross, Visiting Nurse Service, churches, hospitals, and even private physicians is the tangible expression of this change in attitude.

When I was Chief of Service at the Mount Sinai Hospital in New York we offered two courses for our pregnant patients, a day course of nine classes and an evening course of seven classes. The day course had seven classes in the afternoon which the woman attended alone, and two evening sessions for husband and wife. The evening course was an example of complete togetherness—husband and wife went to each meeting. Instruction was under the direction and supervision of a public-health obstetric nurse, but additional faculty consisted of obstetricians, dietitians, physiotherapists, psychiatrists, and pediatricians. At one of the sessions key personnel with whom the patient was to have contact during her hospital stay, such as residents, anesthesiologists, and head nurses were introduced. This was to make her feel at home and secure when it was time for her confinement. For the same reason, one of the classes for husbands and wives included a tour of the labor and postpartum floors. The delivery room and its equipment were demonstrated, including the complex-looking anesthetic machine. Nurseries and postpartum accommodations were inspected. A trial run was made of the proper door to enter and where to go if the stork started landing by the light of the moon. The resolution of such simple doubts may dispel the insomnia of some expectant parent.

The content of the course included a thorough discussion of sex anatomy, conception, pregnancy, prenatal care, signs of labor, labor, and delivery. The matters of rooming in, natural childbirth, pain relief, breast feeding, demand feeding, and early ambulation were considered.

The baby's layette, formula preparation, and infant bathing were demonstrated. The psychiatrist explained the normal mood swings of pregnancy and the early postpartum period, and offered a program of early infant training. The pediatrician talked about the care of the baby: feeding, bathing, circumcision, diaper-changing, stools, crying, rashes, and other happenings in the life of a newborn child. The dietician offered sample menus of the normal pregnancy diet and low-calorie meals, as well as listing the foods safe to consume when salt must be restricted. The physiotherapist conducted exercises for muscle-strengthening and showed the patients how to relax, which is particularly useful for those who plan "natural childbirth."

As Chief I assigned myself several sessions because I enjoyed it and also wanted to underline my appraisal of the importance of the courses. My involvement paid unexpected dividends. One of the couples attending, patients of another staff member, were a team of celebrated movie stars. And today when the charming lady and I meet on an occasional TV interview show she warmly greets me as her "teacher." Then, too, if I impose on her by asking her to aid Planned Parenthood by filming a TV spot, she graciously consents.

This is a far cry from the medical care and guidance given the pregnant woman half a century ago. What happened then?

Prenatal Care Is Relatively New

In 1912 Tom Smith stopped Dr. Jones on Main Street. "Hey, Doc, Emily's expecting, and we're wondering whether you wouldn't look out for her."

"Why, I'd be pleased and honored, Tom. When is it coming off?"

"Well, as near as we can reckon, the week after Easter."

"Good, my boy. Just send for me when things get started. I'll be there. You know my slogan—'Doc Jones hasn't missed a baby yet.' So long, boy. I'll be seeing you after Easter." They parted, Tom happy in the knowledge that Emily was being watched over by Providence and Doc Jones, and Dr. Jones happy in the knowledge that Mrs. Jones was assured of a new Easter dress. Even less than sixty years ago such a conversation between the expectant father and his doctor might have happened anywhere in the civilized world. That a physician could protect the woman's life by carefully examining and advising her at frequent intervals during pregnancy (prenatal care) was a brand-new idea in the first years of the twentieth century. Prenatal care was first given to the well-to-do and the very poor by a handful of specialists, obstetricians (Latin: "One who stands in front of or near the laboring woman"). The very poor were poor enough to attend the great university clinics, where these newfangled specialists studied and taught, while the wealthy were rich enough to pay the extra tariff. This expert medical supervision of the woman throughout pregnancy, America's main contribution to the safety of childbirth, has gradually spread so that now most gravid women in industrialized countries receive it.

In a recent trip to India and Nepal I observed that the concept of the importance of prenatal care, especially dietary supervision, is widely accepted. In some regions the care is given by physicians and in other places by trained nurse-midwives or even paramedical personnel. However, the scarcity of physicians or any trained personnel makes the delivery of adequate prenatal care very difficult, especially in rural areas. In India there is one physician to every 4800 people; in the United States the ratio is 1 to 700. As in the United States, Indian physicians are concentrated in the cities, but 80 per cent of the Indian population is rural, compared to less than 30 per cent of the United States population.

Unsolicited Unprofessional Advice

Almost any woman who has had a baby feels specially qualified to give managerial advice to pregnant relatives, friends, and even strangers. A parallel exists in the male's relationship to our national pastime. As long as the spectator has worn a baseball mitt at some time in his life, no matter how transient or inglorious his career as player, he feels similarly qualified to advise. The shouts of "Take him out," "Leave him in," or "Bunt, you dope," attest this. However, the difference between pregnancy and baseball is a real one; the pregnant woman pays attention to her advisers, often to her detriment. It is not so with either baseball player or manager. As the result of the pregnant woman's low resistance to advice from anybody at any time, the doctor frequently has to correct all manner of false notions and ideas.

From several decades' experience in obstetric practice, I could give pages of examples. I shall content myself by citing a few. A very intelligent patient, the wife of a physician, asked me if it was dangerous to raise her arms above her head. I was startled to hear so primitive a question from so sophisticated a person. On inquiry I discovered that one of her mother's friends had gratuitously warned her that the child might be strangled in the loops of its cord should she stretch her arms aloft. Another patient asked me if a friend's contention was correct, that coitus during pregnancy would make the child oversexed. A third told me that her mother-in-law had warned her against high heels because they would make the child cross-eyed. All sorts of bizarre dietary restrictions are imposed by these lay boards of strategy with their notions passed on by one gullible generation to the next.

Maternal Impressions

It is hardly necessary to inform the modern reader that no experience or thought which the pregnant woman has could possibly influence the body form, intelligence, or character of her unborn child. There is no shred of scientific evidence that any component of a baby's make-up is influenced *in utero* by factors other than heredity, maternal diet, intra-uterine conditions, and maternal health. All the hours spent by our pregnant forebears in attempts favorably to influence unborn children by classical music to which they were antipathetic, by famous art for which they had no liking, or by serious literature for which they had no relish, were wasted. Both fortunate and unfortunate fetal outcomes must be attributed to sources other than maternal impressions.

I cannot refrain from inserting an anecdote which happened many years ago. At that time we had on the faculty of the Johns Hopkins a famous, *gemütlich*, jolly German-born professor of Medical Art, Max Brödel, and an equally famous, serious-minded German savant, Isidro Hofbauer. One day as the savant and I entered the Women's Clinic Max stopped us. He said to my companion, "Isidro, what do you think of maternal impressions?"

My companion replied, "Ach, that's monkey business, not science."

The professor said, "I wouldn't be so sure it's monkey business. I'll tell you what happened to a friend of mine. When seven months pregnant, she went to the zoo and as she stood before the bear's cage the huge animal growled and made a lunge at her with his paw. She fainted, and two months later her baby was born with bare feet."

"That's impossible, that cannot be, that's foolishness," refuted the savant.

Who Is Qualified to Supervise Pregnancy?

The only person fitted to give modern prenatal care is a specially trained physician or an expertly trained nurse-midwife who has the services of a qualified obstetrical consultant readily available.

When the word "midwife" is mentioned in the United States, one immediately conjures up a decrepit, kindly, illiterate, often not too clean old "granny" type of woman, a creature whose only professional claim was the number of children she herself had had, plus a desire to be an obstetrix (female obstetrician). This variety of midwife, except for her sex, has nothing in common with nurse-midwives. These remarkable women are graduate nurses who have invested one year or longer in the special postgraduate study of obstetrics. They are relatively plentiful in Europe, especially in the British Isles, Scandinavia, and the Low Countries. In some areas of Europe nurse-midwives conduct almost all of the vaginal deliveries, receiving help from a physician only when a complication arises. Nurse-midwives are so well instructed that they can recognize both a complication and their own limitations in handling it.

The latter phase of their work is quite clearly spelled out in governmental or local regulations under which they operate.

Here in the United States, even in much of the Deep South, the granny type of midwife is becoming an extinct species. In most states none are being newly licensed and the old licensees are dying off. On the other hand, we are beginning to amass a small group of well-trained nurse-midwives. They are being taught in several places: the Maternity Center, New York City; the Frontier Nurses Association in Kentucky; the Catholic Maternity Center, Santa Fe, New Mexico; and in the obstetrical departments of many university clinics, such as the Kings County Hospital in Brooklyn, the Columbia-Presbyterian in Manhattan, and the Johns Hopkins in Baltimore. These schools are presided over by highly motivated, competent faculties and are graduating very superior pupils, who are then distributed all over the world, largely in administrative posts in public-health agencies. A half-dozen are giving expert prenatal and delivery care to a large indigent rural population on the Eastern Shore of Maryland under the aegis of the State Health Department.

The future of the nurse-midwife in this country is unclear. There is desperate need for her in rural areas which are too sparsely populated to attract the settlement of qualified physicians. It is likely she will play an increasingly important role in the urban practice of obstetrics as well. In the ideal situation a well-trained nurse-midwife could be usefully integrated into private obstetrical practice. She could do most of the patient education in the office setting; answering questions and becoming informally acquainted with patients. When the patient comes to the hospital in labor she could enter with her and remain throughout labor, carrying out appropriate examinations and informing the physician of labor's progress. Most of all, she could give the laboring woman immense emotional support and confidence. With the great demands made on a busy practitioner's time it is virtually impossible for the doctor to remain with a patient throughout the labor, and having a competent substitute present, well known to the laboring woman, would be a great boon. Perhaps this will be the way of future American obstetrics.

How to Choose an Obstetrician

Almost half the births in this country are still conducted by a general practitioner, though the proportion of deliveries he performs is gradually decreasing. In some geographic areas obstetric specialists are unavailable. However, it is a good rule that whenever possible the patient should place herself under the care of a competent, well-trained specialist. Today a specialist is a physician who has had at least three years of postgraduate training in his specialty in a hospital accredited to offer such training. This qualifies him to take the rigorous written and oral examinations of his specialty board. If he passes them he becomes a diplomate, in this instance in Obstetrics and Gynecology. There are 8000 Diplomates in Obstetrics and Gynecology scattered all over the country. The selection of a doctor should not be guided by the fee he is reported to charge, for almost every doctor is humane and will adjust his price to the limited means of a frank and honest patient. Happily the cost of obstetrical services is not fixed like that of a government bond.

The only criterion of a doctor should be his ability, in the broadest sense of the word. The following two questions are worth serious consideration. First, if he graduated from medical school six or more years ago, has he passed his Ob-Gyn boards and become a diplomate? One must be out of school six years before being permitted to take Board examinations. Or if he is a more recent graduate, is he qualified to take the examinations? If in doubt consult the *Directory of Medical Specialists* in a library or call his office and make inquiry. Second, is he a member of the staff of a good hospital in your community; in other words, is he considered a first-class doctor by the superior members of his own profession? (If you are planning to attempt psychoprophylactic childbirth, see also page 188.)

If you move into a new community and need the services of any physician, either have the doctor at your previous home refer you to a trusted colleague, or, if no such opportunity exists, call up the best hospital, not just any hospital, in the area and ask for a list of the staff in the particular field in which you need medical help. The competence of every physician on such a list is virtually guaranteed. In almost every instance they are already diplomates.

Once the patient has carefully selected her doctor, she should let him shoulder the full responsibility of her pregnancy and labor, with the comforting knowledge that, no matter what develops, he has had similar cases and her health will be safeguarded by this background of experience.

The First Prenatal Visit

Most obstetricians prefer to see their patients early in pregnancy, two or three weeks after the first menstrual period is missed. Many women look forward to this first interview with unnecessary dread. Perhaps a friend with previous experience has told them that it is a most embarrassing examination, and such questions! The patient is apt to forget that the doctor has examined literally thousands of women, and in the course of this experience has learned to impersonalize his attitude toward his patients.

Your Medical History

Realizing that this first session is likely to be awkward for his patient, the doctor tries to put her at ease by social pleasantries before taking a careful and thorough history. His questions are designed to construct a complete surgical and medical background of the patient from birth to the present, with emphasis on any diseases which may have left aftereffects. Age, length of marriage, and work record are sought. The date of the last menses and the previous use of contraceptives are noted. The months or years it took to achieve the current pregnancy are recorded. The questions now turn to the family and the possible presence of any disease with familial tendencies such as diabetes and also the existence of twins in the family tree—alarming suggestion! The husband then shares the limelight for one brief, casual moment while his health, height, weight, and occupation are noted. Each previous pregnancy, if there were any, is successively reviewed: its date, duration, length of labor, and type of delivery, the size of infant, and several other facts, including abortions. Finally the data concerning the present pregnancy are recorded— symptoms and complaints, or their absence. The patient's nonpregnant weight is asked and the history brought to a close, much to the relief of the patient, who has become very confused trying to remember whether she was five or seven when stricken with measles, or if old age was really the cause of her grandmother's demise.

The Physical Examination

By now the patient and doctor are well acquainted and on friendly terms. The tension has lessened; the ordeal is not proving so dreadful as expected; and the stiffly starched nurse or office attendant, who is summoned to conduct the patient to the dressing room, is pleasant and reassuring. The patient undresses completely and, after voiding a specimen of urine, is initiated by the nurse into the art of wrapping herself in a sheet. After being weighed and then covered by a breast towel and the unfurled sheet, she lies on the hard, uncomfortable examining table. The doctor enters, and after a few words the examination begins.

At the first visit the obstetrician examines the woman completely from top to toe. It is essential that he determine the exact physical condition of his patient, so that he may judge her ability to withstand the strain of pregnancy and labor. In addition to a general physical examination, including height, weight, and blood pressure, several laboratory procedures are included: tests of urine and hemoglobin, and serology. In most states a test for syphilis is obligatory for all pregnant women, even though the premarital one was negative. The blood is drawn by needle and syringe from a vein on the inner aspect of the arm where the forearm and upper arm join. The Rh of the blood is determined from part of the same specimen—that is, whether the blood is Rh positive or Rh negative (the importance of which will be taken up in detail in Chapter 20). At the same time the blood is grouped into one of the four blood groups, A, B, AB, or O, in anticipation of possible transfusion at delivery. After the general physical survey, the obstetrician performs a vaginal examination to map out the form, size, and consistency of the uterus; to determine the condition of the ovaries and Fallopian tubes; and to make certain that the pregnancy is situated in the uterus and not in the tube (tubal pregnancy). For the pelvic examination the physician may insert a metal or plastic two-bladed speculum in the vagina to expose the cervix, the mouth of the womb. If so he almost certainly takes a "Pap" smear to be certain no cancerous or precancerous condition exists, and perhaps also a bacterial culture of the cervix to make sure no gonorrhea-producing bacteria are present. Neither test hurts. Assessment of the size of the pelvis, the bony canal through which the baby must pass, is part of this first examination. It is an obvious rule in mechanics that in order to determine if a rigid body can pass through a rigid tube, the size of the body and the tube must be compared. The physician feels carefully the bony architecture of the pelvis and may take one or two standard measurements; from these data and the general roominess or lack of roominess he senses of the bony pelvis he approximates its normalcy.

Subsequent Prenatal Visits

During the first five months the obstetrician sees his patient at monthly intervals, during the next two months every three weeks, and during the final two months at least every week or two. Naturally, if any complication arises, he may see her more often.

At these subsequent visits the physician discusses any new symptoms which the patient has reported, and he takes the blood pressure, weighs her, and examines the urine. He then gives directions for the ensuing few weeks and prescribes drugs when necessary. At almost every visit, in addition, the doctor palpates the abdomen to find out if the fetus is growing at a normal rate. He determines this by measuring the height to which the top of the uterus (fundus) has risen in the abdomen and compares his findings to those recorded at the previous visit and to the expected height for the number of weeks of pregnancy. If there is growth of the fundus and no discrepancy between uterine size and dates, he can assume all is progressing normally. When the pregnancy is far enough advanced he listens to the fetal heart and determines the fetus's position. In later pregnancy his experienced hands can estimate the weight of the baby. To be sure, such estimates by even very experienced hands are approximations.

The Obstetrician's Fee

In most communities an obstetrician's fee includes all charges and covers prenatal supervision, delivery, and aftercare for the six weeks following childbirth, including contraceptive advice. An inclusive fee rather than a per visit charge is advantageous to both patient and doctor; the obstetrician can see his patient whenever necessary without the deterrent of expense to her. In general, obstetric fees are disproportionately low considering the great amount of time the doctor invests in each case. A surgeon can charge a goodly amount for a simple appendectomy, or the same obstetrician-gynecologist can make a considerably higher charge for the removal of an ovary or a uterus than for a delivery, and the bill is cheerfully paid. Surgeons spend half an hour making the diagnosis and three-quarters of an hour operating, and then make six postoperative calls of ten minutes each, giving a total of a little more than two hours of their time. If the obstetrician attempts to charge an equal amount for his months of care he may meet resistance. Yet the obstetrician spends three-quarters of an hour at the first visit, fifteen minutes at each of the ten prenatal visits, and at least five hours on the average during labor; afterward he calls daily at the hospital, and he gives the final office examination a month after delivery. This makes a total of eleven or more hours. It is difficult to know why this attitude exists toward obstetrical fees. Perhaps since the general practitioner still does a significant share of the deliveries, the layman feels that the obstetric specialist is not entitled to a pay scale commensurate with other specialized surgical modalities. Blue Cross and Blue Shield have been far from generous in coverage of maternity benefits. In most instances their contributions turn out to be partial payment of the total financial obligation.

7

The Pregnant Months

I wish to make the clear-cut, unqualified statement that the directions included here are intended in no way to displace or alter those of the reader's physician. There are great differences of informed opinion on the lesser details of the conduct of normal pregnancy. Further, every obstetrician's treatment will vary in detail to suit variations in individual patients. No matter how carefully a pregnant woman may study this or any other book, she will not obviate the necessity of paying an early visit to her physician.

It is remarkable how life during pregnancy has been simplified in recent years. With the observation of large numbers of healthy women —previous to the eighteenth century midwives cared for all normal cases, and doctors had the opportunity to see only ill pregnant women—the medical attitude toward pregnancy has changed. Since in the premodern era pregnancy was treated as an illness (from its very inception) it was deemed imperative to employ the most complicated measures to prevent dangerous complications. We now realize that pregnancy is a normal, simple physiologic state, and ordinarily all that need be done is to maintain the woman in good physical condition by the enforcement of an uncomplicated, common-sense regimen. If an abnormality develops, then of course the doctor must step in and aid nature to correct it.

The Declining Risk

Until 1930 the maternal mortality in the United States (all deaths occurring during pregnancy, delivery, and the first six weeks following delivery, in which the state of being pregnant or having been pregnant plays the primary role, conditions such as hemorrhage, or infection arising from the reproductive tract) was high and stationary. Maternal mortality is expressed in terms of the number of women who die per 100,000 babies born alive. In 1930 the rate was 670; then it began to decline, slowly at first, later swiftly. It dropped to 620 in 1933, 370 in 1959, and in 1967, the last year for which complete data from the National Center for Health Statistics are currently available, to 280. The number of women who died as the direct result of pregnancy and childbearing was 987 in the course of 3,512,000 live births. In 1930 one woman died from obstetric causes for every 149 live births; in 1967 one for 3570. In other words, in four decades, childbirth in the United States has become twenty-four times as safe.

This achievement in obstetrics has few, if any, parallels in the whole field of modern medicine.

Factors Affecting the Risk

The risk of childbirth is not uniform; it is sensitive to various factors. If one examines the matter superficially he will come up with the conclusion that the most important factor in this country is the race to which one is born, because modern statistics show a maternal mortality for United States whites of 19.5 per 100,000 live births and for non-whites of 69.5. Therefore one may assume that the nonwhite woman is less sturdy and has some inborn defect which makes cihldbirth less safe. This is not true. The difference in mortality rate results from social and economic factors, such as lack of availability of facilities for prenatal care or reluctance to make use of them, the absence of a physician or nurse-midwife at delivery, scarcity of hospital beds in certain areas, malnutrition, poor hygiene, inadequate contraceptive services resulting in unsafe abortion or excessive childbearing, and poor health education. Virtually every white baby born in the United States is delivered in a hospital, but only 93 per cent of the nonwhite babies. Hospitals not only provide better obstetric facilities but guarantee the presence of a trained accoucheur. In three of the states with the worst maternal and newborn records, Mississippi, Alabama, and Arkansas, nearly one quarter of the births take place outside of the hospital. The Children's Bureau of The Department of Health, Education, and Welfare has taken cognizance of these disturbing realities and has persuaded Congress to appropriate almost $50 million annually over the past few years to support and expand maternity- and infant-care centers.

The recent improvement in the over-all maternal mortality rate in the United States is shared by the other industrially developed nations. In the period 1963-1965, the United States with a rate of 33.6 per 100,000 ranked eleventh among developed nations. Sweden was first with the lowest rate of 20.0. The United States white rate was 22.4, and if non-white births were excluded from the mortality figures the United States would rank fourth, just behind Norway with 21.7.

The vital statistics of the developing nations are far less accurate than those of the Western developed nations. Nonetheless they offer an interesting comparison. The figures published by the World Health Organization for 1966 show that Sweden's maternal mortality had dropped to 11.3 per 100,000 live births. Among the nations reporting in 1966, Chile's rate was the highest—271.8 per 100,000. No doubt the extraordinarily high prevalence of illegal abortion in Chile—reported to be one out of three pregnancies—is an important contributory factor, especially since illegal abortions usually are not performed by medical personnel.

Among other factors associated with maternal mortality is the age of the mother. The lowest figure for mothers in the United States in 1967 was 16.6 per 100,000 between the ages of twenty to twenty-four; for teen-agers it was 22.1, but for mothers older than forty-four the rate rose to 312.7. First births carry a slightly higher mortality risk than second and third deliveries, but appreciably less than sixth and higher birth orders.

The three chief causes of maternal mortality in 1967 were, in the order of their importance, infection, toxemia (high blood pressure with kidney or liver complications), and hemorrhage. Infection accounted for one-quarter of the deaths, about half of which occurred after delivery and the remainder after abortion. It is fair to assume that most of the abortion deaths were associated with illegal operations.

Factors Which Have Made Childbirth Safer

What specific factors are chiefly responsible for making childbirth so safe in the United States?

1. As previously stressed, the greater use of hospitals.

2. The elimination of the "granny" midwife except in the Deep South, and the increased attendance of obstetrical cases by physicians who are obstetrical specialists. We remind the reader of the difference between "midwife" and "nurse-midwife"; the latter are still so few that their excellent work has made little impact on our vital statistics.

3. The availability and the acceptance of good prenatal care by a huge preponderance of the population. In addition to careful medical surveillance good prenatal care includes lay education in dietetics, and the creation of faith and confidence in the safety of childbirth.

4. Widespread use of antibiotics and chemotherapeutics to overcome or prevent infection.

5. Availability and use of blood for transfusion to correct anemia, especially when it is due to hemorrhage.

6. The wider use of anesthesiologists and the consequent improvement of obstetrical anesthesia.

7. Application of the progress in medicine and surgery which has distinguished the past three decades.

8. Improved teaching in obstetrics to medical students, nurses, and residents.

9. Better facilities for the postgraduate medical education of practicing obstetricians through national societies such as the American College of Obstetrics and Gynecology, and the local County Medical Societies. Most of the latter have "maternal mortality committees" who investigate every maternal death. Each case is presented and discussed at a meeting open to all physicians; some committees frankly fix responsibility for the death on the shoulders of the physician, the hospital, or the patient, or if the cause cannot be assigned to one of the three it is categorized as nonpreventable. In about one-third to one-half the cases, the maternal death is judged nonpreventable.

The Birth Rate

The crude birth rate is expressed in terms of the number of children born per 1000 population, and annual rates are available since 1915. At that time the rate was relatively high, 25 per 1000. From then on it declined steadily, with minor interruptions, to a low of 16.6 in 1933, resulting in 2,307,000 live births. The chief factor for the decline was economic, for the birth rate is sensitive to national prosperity. The low birth rate remained relatively stationary from 1933 to 1940, when, because of economic and psychological factors mainly of war origin, it began to rise sharply. An accelerated marriage rate is followed by an accelerated birth rate, and the marriage rate during the war years soared majestically. Then, too, couples contemplating an additional child ceased postponing the blessed event lest the separation of war make it temporarily or permanently impossible. It is also rumored that during the first war years some couples initiated a projected pregnancy earlier than they otherwise might have, because of the decorative value the stork or even part of it might have on a draft card. The steep upsurge of the birth rate in 1947—it reached a modern high of 25.8—was the result of the demobilization of 1945 and 1946 with its aftermath of previously postponed marriages and postponed pregnancies. The crude birth rate hovered around 25 per 1000 for a full decade, being 25.3 in 1957, when it began to fall each year reaching 17.4 in 1968. Even though the birth rates in 1933 and 1968 were within one point of each other, 1.2 million more babies were born in 1968 because of the growth of population in the interval.

Recent fluctuations in the crude birth rate show how impossible it is to forecast it. In 1969 and 1970 it rose slightly to 18.3, but then fell to less than 17.0 in the first eight months of 1971. Several trends seem to have contributed to this drop in the birth rate. The National Fertility Study, a survey of a meaningful sample of married women conducted every five years, reports that in 1970 women in their late twenties who married early expect to have an average of 2.53 children, while five years earlier the expectation in the same group was 3.03 children. Furthermore, the median age of first marriages for women has been slowly rising and is now 20.8 years. According to the Census Bureau, there is a marked increase in the proportion of young women who are single. In 1960 about a third of women aged twenty-one were single, but by 1970 the proportion had risen to almost one-half. There were 3 per cent fewer births in August 1971 than in August 1970, despite the fact that the number of women of childbearing age had increased 3 per cent during the same period. In 1957 the figure for family size was 3.8 children, but in August 1971 births had declined sufficiently to yield an achieved family size of 2.2 children, just barely above the figure of 2.1 children that would eventually establish an equilibrium between births and deaths in the United States.

No one has the temerity to forecast that the low birth rate of the first eight months of 1971 will be permanent, since we do not know the causes of the decline. Among the factors that may have been operative are the economic recession; greater availability of effective contraceptives and of safe, legal abortion; and a new sense of responsibility that persuades couples to limit progeny so that they do not contribute excessively to an increase in population and pollution. However, by the end of 1971 the Census Bureau was projecting a slightly increased estimate for the United States population in the year 2000—between 271 million and 322 million—based on the finding that American women are having children at an earlier age.

A more sensitive barometer of births than the crude birth rate is the fertility rate, the number of children born in a given year per 1000 women in the population between the ages of fifteen to forty-four. The fertility rate removes the modifying effect of age alterations in the general population. In 1957 the United States fertility rate was 123 and by 1967 it had decreased to 88, a decline of 28 per cent. The declining rate was evident in both white and nonwhite populations, although rates for nonwhites remain above those for whites in each age group. The fertility rate appeared to level off, for it was 87.6 in 1970. However, it too seems to have plunged in 1971. In May, June, and July, it dropped to 77.5. If it drops to 70 and remains there the United States will have reached population equilibrium. The key question is where is our fertility rate headed?

Persons born in the baby-boom years between 1947 and 1957 were twenty-five to fifteen years old in 1972. Therefore, the pool of females in the twenty to twenty-nine age group—the interval during which most Americans become mothers—has been rapidly increasing in size each year, and will continue to do so for several years to come.

The United States Bureau of the Census in a 1968 publication projected the increase in the numbers of women of childbearing age, from fifteen to forty-four for the twenty-year period 1965–1985:

1965—39 million
1970—42 million
1975—47 million
1980—52 million
1985—56 million

Therefore, with 17 million more women of childbearing age over the next two decades, almost one million being added per year, one could anticipate an annual increase in the crude birth rate, as well as an increased crop of babies each year. But who knows whether this will happen?

Today in the United States about 10,000 babies are born daily and 5000 people die. In addition, 1000 more foreigners each day immigrate into the United States than the Americans who emigrate. This 6000 daily increase adds up to an annual population growth of slightly more than 2 million persons, or roughly 1 per cent—0.8 per cent representing the average excess of births over deaths and 0.2 per cent from excess immigration over emigration. The U.S. population in mid-1971 was 207 million.

Because of the very large number of women entering the reproductive pool over the next several decades and the youthful age profile of today's United States population, one can anticipate a long latent period, from fifty to seventy years, after the United States maintains a completed family size of 2.1 children, before the total number of annual births will equal the total number of annual deaths. In the spring of 1970 President Nixon appointed a commission on "Population Growth and America's Future," chaired by John D. Rockefeller III. The preliminary report issued in 1971 largely states the problem. If United States citizenry would suddenly and miraculously accept the two-child family, and if the current rate of immigration continues at 400,000 persons per year, at the end of the twentieth century there would be 266 million Americans, but if between now and the year 2000 the completed family size averages three children, United States population will be 321 million. To achieve rapid and relatively immediate population equilibrium, Americans would have to be satisfied with one child per marriage for the next few decades—a wholly improbable prospect, and furthermore, not necessarily a desirable one. The impact of suddenly arrested population growth on education, economics, and several social parameters would be damaging. Further discussion of the population problem will appear in Chapter 18.

Exercise

Before offering advice about activities during pregnancy, I once again stress the point that if the words printed here are at variance with those given you by your physician, pay heed only to his instructions, not mine.

The long-held conviction of yesteryear that practically anything except lying alone in bed might bring on abortion or premature labor must have been devastating to both mind and conscience. Until very recently, whenever a woman miscarried she searched her life for the cause and with no difficulty discovered it either in some minor accident or in the simple exertions of her everyday existence. With advance in knowledge concerning the real causes of abortion, our attitude toward exercise during pregnancy has changed. We realize that the majority of miscarriages are blessed acts on the part of nature to terminate further development of an abnormal ovum.

Many physicians allow their patients any form of exercise throughout pregnancy: swimming, tennis, dancing, golf, bike-riding, hiking, and horseback riding. Others, adopting the more conservative course, allow only milder forms of exercise, especially during the first three months, when miscarriage is most common.

I belong to the former group, the any-exercise-within-moderation school. I was converted through two incidents early in my obstetric career. The first occurred just after I started practice. One morning more than four decades ago my revered mentor, the great obstetrician Whitridge Williams, and I were peering through microscopes side by side in the laboratory when suddenly he asked, "Guttmacher, what do you tell your patients about exercise during pregnancy?"

Startled that he cared what such a neophyte thought, I replied, "I let them do anything except ride horseback."

He snorted. "That's queer. I tell them to do everything except play tennis." On comparing notes, it turned out that Dr. Williams was one of the world's worst tennis players, and, without possibility of contradiction, I was and still am the world's least talented equestrian.

My conversion was completed by a ballerina. One of my earliest private patients was a dancer at a night club. She first consulted me when she had successfully completed three months of pregnancy. In taking the history and discovering her occupation, I was curious to see just how much dancing she did. I went to watch. Not only did she twirl, pirouette, and leap in the air, but two strong-muscled gentlemen tossed her back and forth between them like football ends warming up before a game. She continued her career and pregnancy for yet another month, unharmed.

All physicians warn the pregnant woman against overfatigue, no matter whether the source is horseback riding or housecleaning. She lacks a certain resiliency in recovery; whereas the nonpregnant woman is restored to normal vigor by lying down for half an hour, the pregnant woman requires half a day.

A pregnant woman often asks if there is any minimum requirement of exercise. This must vary with each patient, depending on how much she is accustomed to do, and, above all, how much she enjoys. Walking or some form of mildly vigorous outdoor activity is advisable, but not essential, to a healthful pregnancy.

As mentioned earlier, there are special exercises for the pregnant woman to strengthen certain muscles used in childbirth (the abdominal muscles), and to learn how to relax others (the vaginal and perineal muscles). These exercises will be discussed in the section on psycho-prophylactic pain relief in Chapter 13.

Employment

There is no reason to stop work because of pregnancy. I have observed that if a pregnant woman finds her work enjoyable she is better off physically and psychically if she continues working. During the last three months I advise shortening the workday by going in late and leaving early. This not only avoids the buffeting one is subjected to by rush-hour transportation, but it gives additional time to rest and relax. Discomfort or fatigue should be the key as to when to stop working altogether. In Russia, China, and some other socialist countries pregnant women are given six weeks leave with pay before and six weeks after delivery. One of my residents worked until she went into labor and returned to partial medical duties when the baby was one week old. I do not cite her case as one to follow, though for her it worked splendidly.

Travel

There are only two arguments against travel during pregnancy:

1. Abortion or labor can happen at any hour on any day, and it is nearly always impossible to predict the occurrence. If the pregnant woman happens to be traveling at the time of such an emergency, or is residing in a community other than her own, it is both inconvenient and frightening. One way to lessen the difficulty is to ask your doctor to furnish you with the name of an obstetric colleague living in the area you plan to visit. Put the memorandum in your handbag and expect not to need it—almost certainly you will not.

2. Traveling can be fatiguing and uncomfortable, especially in late pregnancy. This is particularly true of automobile travel. The only antidote is to break up the trip every one hundred to a hundred and fifty miles, get out of the car, void, and walk about for a few minutes. It is probably unwise for a pregnant woman to motor more than three hundred miles a day.

There is no qualified evidence that traveling by any means of locomotion brings on labor, abortion, or any complication of pregnancy. Naturally, if a thousand women travel who are eight to twelve weeks pregnant, a certain small percentage will miscarry; or if a thousand are thirty-four to thirty-five weeks pregnant a certain proportion will go into premature labor. However, the same thing is almost certain to happen to the same women if they stay home in bed. Carefully balanced studies of the pregnant wives of armed-service personnel in World War II, those who traveled about with their husbands and those who remained at one post, showed no significant difference in the incidence of abortion, premature labor, or any other obstetric complication.

Contraindications to travel at any time in the last half of pregnancy because of the naturally increased likelihood of premature labor are a previous history of premature labor or the diagnosis of twins. For the same reason a patient who has had several spontaneous abortions is ill advised to travel in the earlier months. An excellent rule, which should have but few exceptions, is that during the last six weeks of gestation the pregnant woman should give up all travel except within a radius of fifty miles of her home base.

Decisions as to mode of travel during pregnancy should be governed mainly by common-sense considerations. For example, if the woman is prone to motion sickness, the train is probably best. Long distances are usually accomplished with least fatigue and discomfort by air. Air travel during the first three months has been subjected to discussion on the basis that lessened oxygen at this critical, formative period of the fetus's development might in rare cases cause a fetal abnormality. There is no grounds for such apprehension if the cabin is pressurized as it always is in commercial planes.

Automobile Driving

It is not injurious for the pregnant woman to drive a car herself, and she may continue to do so as long as she can sit comfortably behind the wheel. During the last trimester it is inadvisable that she drive alone at night, or on little-frequented roads, because of the potential problems that might arise from a flat tire or other automotive emergencies. Unless a car is equipped with power steering, urban parking may be very exhausting, and this should be taken into account during the late months of pregnancy.

Pregnancy is a poor time to learn to drive because of the clumsiness sometimes associated with it and the possible slowing of reactions from lessened powers of concentration. Also, the seriousness of an accident may be compounded by the pregnant state, for occasionally it involves the fetus as well as the mother.

Sleep and Rest

In early pregnancy the average woman requires an unusually large amount of sleep; this need disappears between the twelfth and sixteenth weeks. The last months are marked by sleeplessness, mainly due to difficulty in finding a comfortable position. Frequently I am asked if it is harmful to sleep on the back or stomach. No possible harm can result from any position, since the fetus is so well protected that pressure on the pregnant woman's body does not affect it. Pregnant women are often convinced that the fetus is nocturnal in its habits and with studied malice chooses nighttime to cut capers. The doctor disagrees, for he thinks that the woman simply has a greater opportunity to appreciate the movements at this time since nothing diverts her attention. As there is no way to diminish fetal movements, the only remedy is a hypnotic (but only if prescribed by your doctor) that will make the woman sleep despite them. The amount of sleep should be governed by habit and desire, the safest rule being to sleep enough to awake well rested. The best health insurance during pregnancy is an hour's bed rest in a darkened room late each afternoon; with this rest before dinner food tastes better, life appears rosier, and late evening hours are more happily tolerated. If frequency of urination disturbs your rest, see the advice given on page 120.

To Breast Feed or Not to Breast Feed: That Is the Question

Whether to breast or bottle feed your baby is a personal decision which you must make. You may wish your husband's advice, and it may be helpful to discuss it with your obstetrician and the pediatrician whom you plan to use. There is neither right nor wrong in this matter. However, the decision rests mainly on your attitude toward nursing and this in turn rests on your background, personality, emotional make-up, life situation, and careful weighing of advantages and disadvantages.

Before you make your decision let me point out that the size of the breast is no indication of how much milk a breast will produce. Some women with small breasts produce copious quantities and some with large breasts insufficient amounts.

I shall list the advantages of each method to help you decide.

Advantages of Breast Feeding

1. Mother's milk is usually easier for a baby to digest. The protein, fatty acids, and other essential constituents of milk are similar but not identical in the cow and human.

2. Human milk contains antibodies, not present in cow's milk, which protect the newborn against some infections. However, the exposure risk to these infectious agents is least in a hygienic home environment. Dr. John Gordon, the Harvard nutritionist, wrote, "In many preindustrial areas of the world the fate of newborn infants came close to being a choice between nurse or die." This is not true in America.

3. Breast feeding requires more intimate contact between the baby and mother. Some believe that the warmth of her body, its pleasant texture and familiar odors, create a sense of security in the tiny baby which leaves a permanent, favorable impact on its later character.

4. Unless a mother is prejudiced against breast feeding and thinks it is messy and vulgar, nursing may be a pleasurable experience for her. It gives most women a feeling of satisfaction, as well as a sense of purpose and fulfillment. For many the physical act of nursing is sensually pleasant.

5. Breast milk is always ready and at the right temperature. This is especially convenient if one's baby is on a demand-feeding schedule.

6. Breast feeding is cheaper.

7. The act of suckling sends a reflex nervous impulse to the mother's pituitary gland which causes it to release the hormone pituitrin. Pituitrin not only causes the milk ducts and glands to discharge their milk, but it also causes the newly emptied uterus to contract firmly. This aids and speeds involution, the process of returning the uterus to its nonpregnant condition. The uterus involutes in those who bottle feed but at a slower pace.

In the first few days a nursing mother is often puzzled by the fact that every time she puts the babe to breast she develops uterine cramps. Release of pituitrin through suckling is the answer.

In premodern obstetrics, before there were effective chemicals such as syntocinon and ergotrate to control hemorrhage from a uterus that failed to contract well after delivery, a standard technique was to borrow a sturdy, hard-sucking neighbor's infant and put him to breast. Obviously, the pituitary gland is an impersonal chemical factory and cannot differentiate between nursing infants.

Advantages of Bottle Feeding

1. It creates more certainty for the mother; she knows exactly how much milk the baby is getting with each bottle.

2. The mother may get more rest, as her husband or a helper can give the bottle in her stead.

3. Formula feeding may fill the baby up more so that he may go longer between feedings.

4. The mother will escape the discomfort many women experience from milk leakage during the period of lactation.

5. The pain of a cracked nipple which some nursing mothers experience will be wholly avoided, and the slim chance of a breast abscess becomes even slimmer.

6. The mother is much less tied down and if she has a job she can return to work sooner.

7. Not nursing preserves the shape of the breast better. Pregnancy itself softens the firm breast, irrespective of nursing. However, sagging of the breast is more common in those who have nursed, but is by no means present in all, or even most, who have nursed. It can be prevented, or at least minimized, by wearing a proper nursing bra, by not nursing for too long a period (more than six months), and by limiting the number of children nursed.

La Leche League

With the introduction of optional rooming-in in many hospitals and the popularity of demand feeding, feeding a baby on the basis of its own hunger needs rather than by the clock, a resurgence of interest in breast feeding has come about. The first meeting of La Leche ("the milk" in Spanish) League International was held in Illinois in 1956. Today La Leche has more than 250 chapters all over the world. The purpose of the League is to promote breast feeding by helping mothers become successful breast feeders. They do this through publications and assistance on request by telephone or personal visit, if necessary, by a member, a woman in the same community who has nursed successfully. The League tries to avoid giving medical advice which might interfere with the doctor-patient relationship. If you are seriously interested in breast feeding and feel insecure in your knowledge and ability, you may want to contact your local La Leche chapter either before or immediately after delivery. You can discover if there is a chapter in your area by writing to: La Leche League International, 9616 Minneapolis Avenue, Franklin Park, Illinois, 60131.

Care of the Breast

Whether you intend to nurse or not, wearing a good bra during pregnancy is wise. It should be well fitting, made of sturdy cotton, and without being tight should offer good support to your breasts by coming high up over the sides of the breasts, toward the underarm. Occasionally a patient, finding that pull from the weight of the breasts as she turns disturbs sleep, asks to be allowed to wear the bra all night. There is no objection, unless it is too tight. If you do not nurse, continue to wear your maternity bra until the breasts shrink to normal size.

If you plan to nurse you may want to take a nursing bra to the hospital. The best have fastenings in front which allow each side to open separately. Do not buy a nursing bra which has a plastic liner because the plastic prevents air from circulating around the nipples and keeps them constantly moist.

The breast itself requires no special care during pregnancy. Massaging it with or without an ointment and attempting to milk secretion from the nipple is valueless.

On the other hand if you plan to nurse, your nipples may require special care. Nipples which project normally require no preparation. To test this, pinch the areola, the pigmented circular zone around the nipple, between your fingers and see what happens. If the nipple projects you have no problem. If the nipple appears to remain flat or even turns inward, you may have permanently inverted nipples. In four out of five cases, however, the condition corrects itself during pregnancy, and by term the nipple can be erected. Recalcitrant inverted nipples may be made erect by a process called nipple rolling, which should be started two months before term and done twice daily. Support the breast with one hand and grasp the nipple at its base between the thumb and first finger of the other hand. Pull the nipple out gently and roll it between the fingers. Even if this fails to cure inversion there still may be a chance that you can nurse successfully. Many a strong, hungry baby has made an inverted nipple erect by sucking.

There is no approved technique for toughening nipples to prevent the development of cracks or soreness while nursing. Scrubbing them with a nail brush or applying alcohol has been proven harmful.

Normal nipple secretion helps prepare them for sucking and should not be washed off with soap. During the last six weeks wash the breasts with plain water if you plan to nurse.

Breast Asymmetry

It is not unusual to observe that one breast is larger than the other; this difference in size may become accentuated as pregnancy progresses.

Some asymmetry between two identical anatomic structures on opposite sides of the body is common and normal.

The Abdomen: The Maternity Girdle

The retention of youthful shapeliness has been one of the main concerns of womankind probably since the days of Eve. Therefore, in all ages remedies have been employed to prevent the belly from sagging after delivery. The preventives were most elaborate and consisted of two types: the wearing of an abdominal support and the anointment of the abdomen with some greasy medicament. The supports were of two varieties: either a specially treated animal skin, or a broad linen swath "made fit for the purpose to support her Belly." The rubbing ointments were legion, and each author seems to have had several of his own special concoction; the very number leads one to suspect their efficacy.

Today some people still retain this partiality for rubbing the abdomen. Most physicians are skeptical of its value; however, if the patient strongly desires to do it, we permit her to use a noninjurious substance like cocoa butter or cold cream.

We have abandoned dogskins and swaths in favor of nothing or a well-fitting special maternity corset. As a rule, the athletic woman who through tennis, golf, dancing, or swimming has developed such good abdominal muscle tone that she never had to wear a supporting girdle when not pregnant does not require one when pregnant. As a matter of fact, a maternity girdle usually subtracts from such a woman's comfort rather than adding to it; it makes her feel as though her abdomen were encased in a straight jacket. There is no inherent value in a maternity girdle except personal comfort; it neither prevents the muscles from stretching nor prevents the abdominal skin from developing pregnancy marks—striae. Nor does it aid in the disguise of the pregnant silhouette, since it lifts the abdomen through its support and does not flatten it.

I do not imply that the maternity girdle has no place in obstetrics, for it clearly has. Its use is almost obligatory for the woman who has been accustomed to wearing a girdle all her adult life, and a maternity girdle may give comforting support to the pregnant patient whose abdominal wall is lax and stretched from previous childbearing. Occasionally bachache or just a tired feeling across the small of the back is relieved in the last third of pregnancy by a maternity girdle. Also, the woman who is going to deliver twins with a resulting overfull abdomen usually feels less uncomfortable in a girdle.

Neither wear nor be fitted with a maternity girdle until the fourth or fifth month of pregnancy. If you buy one at this time, be sure it has a six- to eight-inch let-out. The saleswoman should measure you for the correct size, and the measuring should be done at the heaviest part of your hips. While you are being fitted, always test the girdle for its comfortable quality by sitting down in it for a few minutes. This is very important, for the garment may bind and be too tight when you are in this position.

Do not buy the cheapest or the most expensive girdle. I know of a *corsetière* who decorates her more expensive garments with embroidered forget-me-nots to give them the desired custom-made look. A medium-priced garment will be well made and of good quality.

Lie down when you put your girdle on; preferably, adjust it before arising in the morning. Hook it from the bottom up.

No method is known for preserving the tone and integrity of the skin and abdominal musculature during pregnancy. Their preservation depends on the sinewy strength of the abdominal wall before pregnancy, the relative length of the abdomen, its capacity, and the degree of distention during pregnancy. The latter is increased by multiple pregnancy, excessive amniotic fluid, or a single oversized fetus.

Even if the abdominal wall bulges and sags immediately after delivery, it will spontaneously regain much of the tone it previously possessed within the first six to ten postpartum weeks.

Bathing

Today both showers and tub baths are permitted throughout pregnancy. The previous ban on the latter during the late months or weeks has been rescinded. The only time that tub baths are strictly taboo is after the membranes have ruptured. Pregnancy makes no special requirements as far as the temperature of the bath or shower is concerned.

Care of the Genitals

No special hygiene of the genitals is recommended. They should be carefully cleansed with a soft washcloth and soap and water as usual.

In the normal woman, douching is not necessary during pregnancy or at any other time. However, some American women feel unclean unless they douche, and since in moderation it does no harm, douching is permitted during pregnancy up to the last four weeks; obviously, this does not include the patient whose membranes have ruptured or who has had any vaginal bleeding. A douche can or bag must be used, not a bulb syringe, and the source of water should be kept low, lower than two feet. The nozzle is inserted no more than a distance of two or three inches within the vaginal entrance, and the lips of the vagina are not held closed by the fingers, so that the water may flow in and out freely. Most physicians feel that douching should not be performed more than two or three times a week. Plain water is not advised. Three tablespoons of white vinegar or table salt to two quarts of water in the douche bag make a satisfactory mixture. If the patient feels the need for a deodorant in her douche, she may use one of the many standard douche powders that her pharmacist stocks. My reaction to the new vogue of perfumed vaginal sprays is similar to my reaction to a douche during pregnancy. I am neither for nor against, but see no necessity for them with frequent showers or baths. Since medical opinion is divided about the safety of the douche or "feminine spray" during pregnancy, be sure to consult your own doctor beforehand.

Clothing

We have already considered the matter of brassières and maternity corsets. Clothing should in general be loose, comfortable, attractive, and gay, and, if possible, hung from the shoulders to prevent constriction of the waist. The weight of clothing and underclothing should be the same as usual. Circular garters should not be worn; they act as tourniquets and serve to increase the likelihood of varicose veins, which are common in pregnancy because of the normally increased pressure in the veins of the pelvis and legs. Suspensory garters are therefore to be worn instead. Shoes with broad toes and low, flat rubber heels are usually more comfortable at this time. The extra weight that the woman carries in front tends to disturb her sense of balance, and she is liable to trip and fall forward; low heels help to prevent this. However, if balance remains undisturbed and ordinary shoes with ordinary heels are comfortable, continue to use them.

Teeth

"Each child a tooth" is one of the commonest aphorisms about pregnancy; its author remains anonymous.

But it is no longer necessary to use teeth as coin for babies. Early in pregnancy the woman should go to the dentist and reveal her secret; strict attention to small cavities at this time and throughout pregnancy will save many a tooth. In addition, the calcium content of the diet must be adequate to take care of her own needs as well as those of the fetus.

The gums in some patients have a tendency of overgrowth during pregnancy; they become spongy in texture and bleed consistently when the teeth are brushed. Try massaging the gums vigorously twice a day with dry sodium perborate liberally sprinkled on the index finger. If this does not control the bleeding, consult your dentist.

Unless it is essential dental X-ray is postponed during pregnancy. However, if essential it should be done. The scatter is minimal and almost certainly cannot reach the distant fetus.

Sexual Intercourse

Desire for intercourse is variable during pregnancy. In most women it is unaffected, while in some, particularly those for whom contraception was a burdensome chore, both sex interest and response are greatly heightened. Occasionally a pregnant woman may develop total aversion to intercourse—usually a temporary reaction almost always disappearing after delivery. If it does not disappear, either a physician well oriented in this field or a professional marriage counselor should be consulted. It is in no way harmful for a woman to experience orgasm during pregnancy; actually, its achievement is just as beneficial and important as at any other time.

There is still division of medical opinion about the safety of sexual intercourse during pregnancy. A small segment of physicians forbid it throughout the nine months—an unnecessary and impractical recommendation, in my view. Others urge that it be omitted during the days of the month when the first few menstrual periods would be due. In the absence of vaginal bleeding or a history of repeated miscarriages, sexual intercourse is permissible, desirable, and safe at any time during pregnancy until three or four weeks before the expected delivery date—unless, of course, there has been premature rupture of the membranes. Coital frequency during gestation is wholly a matter of the desire of the two marital partners, which naturally varies markedly from couple to couple. Position during coitus may have to be modified as pregnancy progresses; many women find it more comfortable astride the man or lying on the side. If there is vaginal discomfort preliminary lubrication by one or both with petroleum jelly or cold cream may be helpful. When there is any staining or bleeding after sexual intercourse, abandon complete sex relations until you see your doctor. Under such circumstances intercourse between the thighs may be temporarily substituted.

Obviously, contraceptives need not be used during pregnancy. Douching after intercourse is unnecessary, but the fact that a woman is pregnant does not make it unsafe.

Immunization

Pregnancy does not interfere with the safety of any immunization procedures except for rubella—immunization against German measles. At this time it still remains unclear whether rubella vaccine will cause abnormalities in the fetus, and therefore the vaccine is not given during pregnancy and should not be taken by anyone who could be pregnant or who contemplates the initiation of pregnancy within the subsequent sixty days. (For further information, see the section on German measles on page 158.)

In view of the increased susceptibility to polio during pregnancy and its greater hazard to the pregnant woman, all pregnant women who have not already been immunized against it should be promptly vaccinated. Whenever an epidemic of influenza is anticipated, pregnant women should receive suitable preventive vaccines, since pregnancy heightens the likelihood and gravity of lung complications. Typhoid inoculation and vaccination against smallpox are also safe during pregnancy. No increase in the rate of abortions or in the incidence of congenital malformations among the infants of mothers immunized during any stage of pregnancy has yet been demonstrated except from rubella vaccine.

Drugs

The safest rule to follow is: *Don't self-medicate during pregnancy*; if in doubt about safety just ask your doctor. On the other hand the four common self-medicating situations—desire for pain relief, indigestion and heartburn, constipation, and insomnia—permit standard remedies during pregnancy. Each of these complaints will be discussed in Chapter 9.

8

Weight Gain and Diet during Pregnancy

Increase in weight occurring in pregnancy stems from several sources: first, fetal tissues—the baby, placenta, and amniotic fluid; second, the physiologic growth of specific maternal organs, particularly the uterus, the breasts, and the blood circulating in the body. Finally, there is the tendency of a pregnant woman to retain within her tissues an additional quantity of fluid and also to accumulate fat.

Normal weight gain during pregnancy is about twenty-four pounds. The increase is usually distributed as follows:

	No. lbs.
Fetal tissues—baby	7½
Placenta	1
Amniotic fluid	2
Organ growth—uterus	2
Growth of breasts	1½
Increase in blood	3½
Total	17½

The additional six and a half pounds come from retained tissue fluid and stored body fat.

Change in Attitude toward Weight Gain

Until five years ago the obstetrician did double duty—he was his patient's friendly counselor and tough "cop." His assignment as policeman was simple and straightforward—to prevent a gain of more than fifteen to twenty pounds during the course of pregnancy. At each prenatal visit the scales were meticulously balanced and the sheet-enshrouded patient solemnly weighed. The result was read as breathlessly as a Dow-Jones average by doctor and patient. A gain beyond the slender allotment produced a wrathful lecture, garnished by severe dietary penalties and restrictions.

Early in the century, a German obstetrician, Ludwig Prochownick, contended that semistarvation was warranted to keep the baby small for an easier delivery. Then, other specialists here and abroad advanced the premise without sound data that low maternal weight gain reduced the incidence of certain complications, particularly high blood pressure, termed toxemia. I confess freely that I accepted the wisdom of my peers and went along with the herd. During my tenure at Mt. Sinai Hospital a joint study was made by the departments of Psychiatry and Obstetrics to discover the chief anxiety of patients attending the prenatal clinic. It was not fear of illness or pain but of gaining too much weight. Many patients told of repeated nightmares in which a resident always gave them hell for excessive weight gain.

As early as 1949 some scientists suggested that the quality of the diet, particularly the protein content, was more important than the total calories. More recently, Dr. Nicholson J. Eastman showed the correlation between maternal weight and the incidence of prematurity, babies weighing less than five and a half pounds at birth. He found that when the mother's weight gain was less than twenty pounds, regardless of her prepregnant weight, the incidence of prematurity was more than doubled. Prematurity, calculated on the baby's birthweight, carries with it a greater risk to fetal survival and increased incidence of cerebral palsy and mental retardation. And other studies have exposed the fallacy that toxemia is associated with weight gain in pregnancy. On the other hand, its association with socioeconomic conditions has been established, toxemia being more prevalent among the poor, who are likely to have insufficient protein-intake, particularly animal protein.

The pendulum concerning weight gain in pregnancy has swung, I like to believe, to dead-center. It is clear that insufficient weight gain is deleterious, particularly to the baby, and evidence further shows that nothing constructive is achieved by a weight gain beyond twenty-five or thirty pounds. It does not help the baby, and it penalizes the course of pregnancy. Excessive gain places a burden on the pregnant woman, making her breathless and awkward, and when pregnancy is over it makes the task of returning to prepregnant weight more onerous.

It was formerly believed that pregnancy was the ideal time for an obese woman to lose weight. She simply held her weight stationary by strenuous diet, and when pregnancy was over she was twenty pounds lighter. Now this is strongly advised against. Pregnancy is the wrong time to diet *strenuously*. A weight-losing diet can be safely begun when a baby is two weeks old unless the mother is nursing.

Weekly Distribution of Weight Gain

In the 1970 publication *Maternal Nutrition and the Course of Human Pregnancy*, the Food and Nutrition Board of the National Academy of Sciences recommends that 1.5 to 3 pounds be gained during the first three months and 0.8 pounds per week during the remaining six months, a total of 23 to 24.5 pounds. They follow their recommendations with this sentence, "There is no scientific justification for routine limitation of gain in weight to lesser amounts." A normal weight curve will almost certainly not be smooth during the last six months. Undoubtedly some weeks the weight gain will be more than 0.8 pound, and other weeks less. If during any week the gain is two pounds or more, the increase probably represents abnormal retention of tissue fluids, and your obstetrician should be promptly notified.

If you weigh yourself at home, do so consistently in the morning, after voiding and before breakfast, while still unclothed. Weighing just after a meal may frighten you unnecessarily. It is confusing to weigh daily; once a week is often enough. When you go to your doctor for prenatal visits try to wear clothing of the same weight each time, unless he weighs you draped only in a sheet; also, be uniform about the relation of the visit to eating, so that you are weighed each time either before or after lunch.

Nutrition

It was once falsely believed that a fetus was a true parasite and that no matter how poor the maternal diet, it got enough for all its growth needs from the tissues of the host, in this case its mother. In experiments on animals this is true for some substances but not for others. This is probably equally true for the human. If the human mother's iron intake is insufficient during pregnancy to meet maternal plus fetal needs, the baby is born with a normal amount of iron in its blood (hemoglobin) but the mother has developed anemia. On the other hand evidence is accumulating that this is not the case with insufficient ingestion of protein, particularly animal protein. Rats on protein-deficient diets produced smaller young; fewer offspring survive and the survivors have been found to have defective intelligence when their performance in maze experiments is compared to that of control offspring from rat mothers fed proper quantities of protein. It appears that certain amounts of some amino acids, the ordinary constituents of animal protein, are particularly essential to the normal growth of the rapidly developing fetal brain. Confirmatory evidence in humans is difficult to accumulate. However, preliminary data from the National Institute of Neurological Diseases and Blindness in Washington on the long-term follow up of 50,000 children born to mothers whose pregnancies and labors were carefully studied and recorded, suggest that the ill effects of protein deficiency in human offspring parallel those in rats. Nineteen mothers on protein-deficient diets during pregnancy had children at age four whose IQs were sixteen points below the average of children born to women on normal diets. This suggests that the increased incidence of slow learning responses observed among children living in poverty could be accounted for in some instances by the malnourished state of the mothers during pregnancy.

All this adds up to the fact that not only sufficient weight gain is important, but the content of the diet is equally important. If the prenatal diet is proper, obstetricians and nutritionists see no need for special preparations containing vitamins and calcium. On the other hand, if for some reason there is doubt about the adequacy of the diet, such dietary supplements do no harm.

A healthy nonpregnant female averages 13.7 grams of hemoglobin per 100 cubic centimeters of blood. If the same young woman becomes pregnant she is likely to develop a temporary anemia during the second half of pregnancy unless an iron supplement is added to her daily diet. The iron available from her diet is usually not sufficient to supply both the fetus and the normal increase in her own volume of blood during gestation. It is a recommended routine that one of the simple, inexpensive ferrous salts (sulfate, gluconate or fumarate) be taken orally every day from mid-pregnancy until delivery. Your doctor will make the choice and prescribe the dosage.

The Daily Essentials of Your Diet

The United States Department of Agriculture has prepared a practical guide for well-balanced human nutrition. It involves a daily food plan that is fully applicable to good nutrition during pregnancy and lactation. There are four essential groups of foods. The four groups and the basic plan for each day's intake are as follows:

Milk Group. A *quart of milk daily is basic. Cheese and ice cream are readily available and are advised as additional foods.*

Meat Group. Two or more servings of meat are mandatory and should include beef, veal, pork, lamb, poultry, and fish. In addition, two eggs a day are obligatory. For variety dry beans, peas, and nuts may occasionally be substituted—or better yet, added to the meat group. One serving equals two or three ounces of boneless cooked meat, poultry, or fish; or one cup of cooked dry beans or peas.

Vegetable-Fruit Group. Four or more servings should include a dark-green leafy vegetable and a deep-yellow vegetable at least every other day; a citrus fruit or another fruit or vegetable high in vitamin C; other fruits and vegetables, including potatoes. One serving equals one-half cup of vegetables or fruit.

Bread-Cereal Group. Four or more servings in this category should include whole-grain, enriched, and restored products. One serving equals one slice of bread, or one-half to three-fourths cup of cooked cereal.

The above diet will supply one-half to two-thirds of your caloric requirements and all the vitamins needed.

Let me comment on some items.

1. *Milk.* One quart daily (four glasses)—or a lesser amount, with cheese supplying the deficit. If you gain too rapidly, your doctor may require that you drink skimmed milk or fat-free buttermilk. You get equal credit for the milk you drink or pour over cereal and for the milk used in the preparation of custards, pudding, cocoa, and milk soup. A one-and-one-quarter-inch cube of American cheese equals a glass of milk. It may be utilized plain or in recipes such as a Welsh rabbit. Cottage cheese is a less satisfactory substitute for milk since it is relatively low in calcium. Occasionally a cottage-cheese salad or a slice of cottage-cheese cake may replace a glass or two of milk.

2. *Leafy green and yellow vegetables.* As rich sources of vitamins A, B, and C, and iron, as well as other essential minerals, the green and yellow vegetables are second to none.

The more common green vegetables are asparagus, green beans, lima beans, broccoli, Brussels sprouts, green cabbage, chard, endive, kale, leaf lettuce, okra, green peas, peppers (green and red), spinach, turnip greens, watercress.

Broccoli, chard, kale, spinach, and turnip greens are specially healthful, since they are the richest in iron.

The best yellow vegetables are carrots, pumpkins, and yellow squash.

Vegetables should be used while fresh. If they are cooked, the cooking should be brief and as little water used as feasible. Protracted heating destroys vitamins, so that ten minutes in boiling water should be the maximum for most vegetables. The water may be saved and used as a stock for soups, since it contains abundant minerals and vitamins of value. Canned or frozen vegetables may be substituted for the fresh; their vitamin content is frequently higher than those home-cooked.

Salads are splendid food. In their preparation, use fresh vegetables. Also, prepare the salad just before it is eaten, since chopped and grated vegetables and fruits quickly lose their vitamin content on exposure to air.

3. *Citrus fruits, tomatoes, and other foods rich in vitamin C.* Among the fruits are cantaloupes, grapefruit, grapefruit juice, kumquats, lemons, limes, muskmelons, oranges, orange juice, pineapples, strawberries, tangerines, tomatoes, and tomato juice. Vegetables especially rich in vitamin C are cabbage (slaw), salad greens, green peppers, and turnips.

Both the fruits and vegetables must be eaten uncooked and unpreserved. Canned or frozen juices are satisfactory substitutes for the fresh juices.

4. *Meat, poultry, fish, and eggs.* Egg yolks are rich sources of iron, vitamins, and tissue-building proteins. Meat, especially beef, is a perfect food for the pregnant woman. It bestows more nutritive value when not overcooked; broiled or baked meats have less caloric value and are easier to digest than those fried.

Liver and oysters contain a particular blood-building substance, and one or the other should be eaten at least once a week.

Poultry, fish, and other sea foods are also good sources of animal protein, but not the equal of beef. Fatty meats such as pork and sausage should be eaten in moderation, if at all.

5. *Breads and cereals.* Use whole-wheat, dark rye, or enriched breads. Approved cereals for the pregnant woman are oatmeal, whole cornmeal, rye, barley, whole-wheat-enriched or restored cereals.

The germ and shell of the wheat kernel are rich in iron, protein, and two essential vitamins, B and E. Therefore, the ingestion of whole-wheat breads and cereals is given preference to products made of milled, unenriched flour.

6. *Potatoes, other vegetables, fruits, butter, and salt.*

The following vegetables and fruits also contain valuable minerals and vitamins, but have greater carbohydrate content, and therefore a higher caloric value, than the vegetables already listed. However, they introduce variety into the diet and because of their bulk appease the appetite.

Vegetables: Artichokes, cauliflower, corn, cucumbers, eggplant, head lettuce, mushrooms, onions, parsnips, potatoes, white and sweet, radishes, sauerkraut, summer squash, turnips.

Fruits: Apples, apricots, avocados, bananas, berries, cherries, dates, figs, grapes, peaches, pears, plums, prunes, watermelons.

Butter or fortified margarine. Butter is rich in vitamin A, but since this vitamin is amply supplied in several of the foods previously listed, butter is not essential to the well-rounded diet during pregnancy. If weight gain is normal, two pats of butter a day (one inch by one inch by one-fourth inch) should be spread on bread or toast or used in cooking.

Salt in moderation is permissible throughout pregnancy, unless your own doctor says no.

A Sample Daily Menu

Breakfast

Fresh fruit—½ grapefruit, 1 medium orange, ½ cup citrus juice, or 1 cup tomato juice

Cereal—½ to ¾ cup whole-grain cereal with milk and sugar

Eggs—two

Whole-grain or enriched bread or toast—1 slice, with 1 pat butter if weight gain is normal

Coffee—with 1 ounce cream if desired; sugar

Lunch

Main dish such as macaroni with cheese, or cream soup—¾ cup. A serving of meat may be substituted

Fresh salad, with dressing if desired

Whole-grain or enriched bread—2 slices with 1 pat butter

Milk—8-ounce glass

Fruit—½ cup

Afternoon Snack (4 p.m.)

Milk—8-ounce glass

Fruit, if desired

Dinner

Meat, fish, or poultry—¼ pound

Potatoes or equivalent (see under 6, page 109)

Green vegetable from list under 2 (page 108)

Whole-grain or enriched bread—1 slice, or 4 whole-wheat crackers

Salad with dressing if desired

Simple milk dessert such as custard, pudding, or ice cream—½ cup

or

Fruit—½ cup

or

Cheese—1¼-inch cube

Milk—8-ounce glass

Before Bedtime

Milk—8-ounce glass, or equivalent amount of cheese (or, if the day's calcium needs have been met with 1 quart milk or equivalent, you may substitute ½ cup orange or grapefruit juice or 1 cup tomato juice)

Fluid Intake

Adequate fluid intake is just as essential to health during pregnancy as adequate caloric intake. The minimum amount of fluid necessary is two quarts or eight full glasses a day. Anything which one can pour from glass to glass is counted as fluid, and equal credit is given for soup, coffee, fruit juice, milk, and water.

Special Dietary Problems

A common problem in pregnancy is gaining too much weight. What can be done about it?

First and foremost, exert your will power.

Second, examine your conscience for dietetic sins. What nonessential foods have you been eating or drinking, perhaps as snacks between meals? Eliminate all ginger ale, Coca-Cola, beer, cocktails, chocolate bars, doughnuts, pies, cakes, and all between-meal rations except milk.

If these remedial measures are insufficient, use skimmed milk for drinking and cooking, cut out all fried foods, substitute a salad dressing made of mineral oil for mayonnaise and conventionally prepared dressings, and use saccharin or sucrol for sweetening in place of sugar. Choose lean meats rather than fatty meats. Eat fresh fruits in place of canned or preserved fruits.

Low-Salt Diet

If and only if your doctor specifically places you on a low-salt diet, eliminate salt at the table and in cooking.

Under these conditions all soups are taboo, except unsalted, fat-free chicken or beef broth.

No smoked, pickled, cured, frozen, or canned meat, fish, or poultry is permitted. In addition, bacon, bologna, chipped beef, corned beef, frankfurters, pastrami, pork in every form, sausage, and tongue are put on the condemned list. The meats, poultry, and fish which may be eaten are: lean beef and lamb, liver, veal, chicken, turkey, codfish, flounder, halibut, oysters, salmon, scallops, sole, and whitefish.

Unsalted butter must replace salted butter, and skimmed milk should be used instead of whole milk. The only cheese allowed is unsalted cottage cheese. Both sweet and sour cream must be eliminated. The eating of unsalted bread is permissible—but no other breads or any crackers.

9

Complaints and Complications of Pregnancy

Minor Complaints

A pregnant woman is more prone to physical discomforts than the non-pregnant. Some of these are occasioned by pregnancy, others exaggerated by it.

Nausea and Vomiting

Since nausea and vomiting are usually mild, confined to the first few waking hours, and self-limited to five or six weeks, they rarely require specific medication. Nevertheless there are a few hints which may prove valuable even for those mildly affected.

Before going to bed place a couple of dry, crisp crackers in a tin box on the bedside table. Upon awakening, eat the crackers without raising your head from the pillow and continue lying on your back for twenty minutes, then get up.

If washing your teeth on arising induces or exaggerates the queasiness, postpone that ritual until later in the day when your stomach feels settled; in the interim simply rinse your mouth.

If the nausea persists after the dry-cracker routine, ignore temporarily the diet rules in Chapter 8 and eat the following:

1. A light breakfast—for example, oatmeal (or, if preferred, a poached, shirred, or boiled egg); unbuttered toast with marmalade, jelly, or honey; and a cup of coffee or tea.

2. At midmorning, crackers, cake, or toast with a glass of milk or a cup of cocoa.

3. Luncheon, some broth or soup with crackers or toast; rice or a baked potato sprinkled with salt (a baked potato is the nauseated girl's best friend); a salad without oily dressing; and a roll or slice of toast.

4. Midafternoon, crackers, zwieback, or toast with a glass of fruit juice.

5. Dinner, lean meat or sea food; a green vegetable; baked, mashed, or boiled potato; salad; a dessert of ice cream, sherbet, or any other sweet which you feel confident you can keep down; plus bread, toast, or crackers according to taste.

6. Before bed, crackers, cake, or toast with a glass of milk, a cup of cocoa, or a malted milkshake.

Additional fluids should be taken throughout the twenty-four hours. Over a short period fluids are more important to health than solids. Very often iced liquids are best tolerated. Many women in early pregnancy find plain water nauseating, but if a little lemon or orange juice is added it becomes drinkable. Almost all patients, no matter how nauseated, can take teaspoons of crushed ice flavored by fruit juice, which is a splendid source of fluids. The same may be said for sherbet or water ice, which makes an excellent midafternoon supplement; ginger ale and the non-diet Colas are valuable drinks since they are rich in carbohydrates.

There are other aids beside diet. Your physician may prescribe a sedative such as ½ grain phenobarbital three or four times a day, or 10 milligrams of Compazine with the same frequency. Some patients are helped by 50 milligrams of Dramamine every four hours, and others by Bonine or Bonadoxin. If cooking your husband's breakfast aggravates the condition, temporarily cease being domestic. Going out into the air frequently makes you feel better. Don't feel sorry for yourself, keep occupied, and remember the condition is self-limited in duration and almost always a memory by the twelfth week. Keep going; if you have a job, continue working if possible. Carry some crisp salt crackers, graham crackers, or zwieback to munch if a wave of nausea strikes you while on the bus or at the office. Eat small amounts often, not much at one time, to prevent your stomach from becoming empty.

The nausea and vomiting of pregnancy usually do not clear up dramatically. Improvement is gradual with the appearance of good days which soon gain the ascendancy over bad days, and then the bad days become fewer and fewer and finally disappear.

A cardinal rule in the control of nausea and vomiting of pregnancy is to avoid foods that you think you cannot keep down, no matter how nutritious and beneficial they are. Substitute any food you think you can retain, no matter whether it is crabmeat or pig's feet. While you are plagued with nausea and vomiting, all the rules of diet promulgated in the previous chapter are temporarily suspended; but should be in force as soon as the condition clears up.

If you lose ten pounds or more, or find yourself unable to retain any fluids or solids during a twelve-hour period, notify your doctor immediately.

One patient in several hundred vomits drastically enough during early pregnancy to require hospitalization. In such severe cases treatment is aimed at keeping the patient's body fluids at normal levels by administering glucose solution (sugar) into the vein. The glucose not only serves as food but also protects the liver from the changes of starvation. Vitamins, particularly C, B_1, B_6, and B_{12}, are given by injection or added to the intravenous fluids to prevent vitamin lack which may cause nerve inflammation, muscular weakness, etc. All foods and fluid by mouth are withheld for twenty-four to forty-eight hours, and then small feedings are begun every hour or two, particularly dry foods. Attempts are also made to correct the psychic factor, if any is present, through strictly isolating the patient from the stimuli of family, friends, newspapers, radio, and television. Sufficient sedation is given to keep the patient sleeping three-quarters of the twenty-four hours.

In particularly stubborn cases psychiatric help is useful.

In the early years of my practice some of those admitted to hospitals with this complaint defied treatment so utterly and completely that pregnancy had to be interrupted by abortion. This was done with only one goal, to save the patient's life. However, with the institution of modern therapy this is virtually never required.

Heartburn

Heartburn, a fiery burning sensation in the chest, is frequently associated with the belching of small amounts of bitter, sour fluid. The name given to the disorder is a partial misnomer because the condition has nothing to do with the heart but results from a reflux of acid stomach juices into the lower esophagus. It may occur in anyone but is more common during pregnancy because of the upward displacement and compression of the stomach by the enlarged uterus and decreased gastrointestinal action, causing the stomach to empty more slowly. It is a type of indigestion. The omission from the diet of rich, greasy foods—such as mayonnaise, cream, and fried foods—helps, as do smaller and less hurried meals. Relief from heartburn may be gotten by taking a level teaspoonful of milk of magnesia or a milk of magnesia tablet after each meal and again whenever heartburn occurs. If this should cause loose stools substitute other antacids such as Amphojel, Gelusil, Rolaids, Tums, or Maalox. Some are in tablet or liquid form, others in both. Do not take bicarbonate of soda, soda mints, or Alka-Seltzer because of their high sodium content, which may be injurious during pregnancy. Chewing gum after meals lessens heartburn for some.

Excessive Salivation

This uncommon complaint (called ptyalism) caused by excessive secretion of the salivary glands is very annoying and difficult to cure. The secretion of saliva virtually floods the mouth and is so profuse that the woman cannot manage to swallow all of it, so she must continually expectorate. Ptyalism is often accompanied by a foul taste, which some patients find can be relieved by sucking peppermints or chewing gum. Small daily doses of a mild sedative such as phenobarbital may diminish the ptyalism. The condition, which frequently persists throughout pregnancy, tends to diminish in its latter half and always disappears promptly with delivery. It is said that any foods containing starch aggravate ptyalism, so as the first step omit all of the many vegetable foods containing starch.

Constipation

Some women become constipated only when pregnant, and others prone to constipation find that pregnancy increases the difficulty. The condition results from physiologic changes occurring normally as the effect of pregnancy: decreased contractions of the intestinal tract, pressure from the enlarged uterus on the bowel, and diminished expulsive ability of the overstretched abdominal muscles. The hazards of constipation are greatly overrated in the public mind, probably in part from the emphasis on a daily bowel movement in pharmaceutical advertising in all popular media of communication. There is no evidence of harm resulting to the patient who does not have a daily movement, except the harm which her propaganda-fired mind imagines. However, an evacuation every twenty-four or forty-eight hours is preferable.

The following regimen will aid constipation.

1. Take a moderate amount of daily physical exercise.
2. Keep up your fluid intake.
3. Eat a coarse cereal such as oatmeal for breakfast, and have whole-wheat bread in place of white bread. Also eat freely of salads and leafy vegetables.
4. Take some fruit at night before going to bed. Certain fruits are especially efficacious, notably prunes, apples, figs, dates, and raisins.
5. Licorice candy has a mild cathartic action; take advantage of this property.
6. Try to develop the habit of a regular, unhurried visit to the bathroom at the same hour each day, preferably after breakfast. Incidentally, when you become a mother, institute a program of routine bowel training for your youngster, especially if she is a girl. This is the best preventative against constipation in pregnancy. A stool reflex should be

established on the basis of conditioning. A conditioning factor may be breakfast, a specific food, or some form of exercise.

7. Refrain from excessive straining while at stool.

When additional measures are necessary, one or two tablespoons of mineral oil nightly before retiring may be tried. This should not be taken during the day because of its interference with the absorption of vitamins and other nutrients. If necessary, a mild laxative such as milk of magnesia or cascara may be taken together with the mineral oil. A popular combination of mineral oil and milk of magnesia is Haley's M-O. Medicines such as Colace and Doxinate, which cause the stool to absorb water, can be taken daily. Rectal suppositories may be used with impunity if efficacious. Occasional small warm soapsuds enemas are ordinarily permitted, particularly if there is fecal impaction, unless there has been some complication such as vaginal bleeding or previous premature delivery. It is safest to consult your doctor before resorting to an enema.

Flatulence

Distention of the stomach and intestines by gas, resulting in a bloated feeling and the frequent desire to pass flatus, is a common complaint during pregnancy. Milk of magnesia after each meal to increase intestinal activity helps, also the avoidance of gas-producing foods such as beans, parsnips, corn, onions, cabbage, fried foods, and sweet desserts. Puréed vegetables may give additional relief.

Hemorrhoids (Piles)

As pregnancy advances, the veins at the rectal opening become enlarged by the gradually increasing pressure within the venous system of the lower half of the body. Hard bowel movements and straining at stool have a tendency to cause these veins to protrude through the rectal opening and to cause local pain, bleeding, and itching. The best treatment is prophylactic by the prevention of constipation through employment of the measures listed under that heading on a preceding page. If there is slight rectal bleeding without pain or a bulging lump, it is usually sufficient to apply carbolated Vaseline to the anus with the finger on arising, before bedtime, and after each defecation. If this does not cause the rectal bleeding to stop within forty-eight hours, notify your doctor.

If there is a tender, swollen mass protruding through the anus, you should attempt to reduce it with a well-lubricated finger after sitting for several minutes in a tub of comfortably warm water. When this is unsuccessful, lie on your back with the hips slightly elevated and apply to the rectal region a washcloth or piece of cotton which have been soaked in iced water—or, better yet, iced witch hazel. Change the dressing frequently so that it remains moist and cold. This may shrink the hemorrhoidal mass sufficiently to permit its reposition. If the pain does not subside with this regimen, an anesthetic ointment such as Nupercainal can be applied to the area, or medicated suppositories such as Anusol may be inserted.

Occasionally a painful clot occurs in one of the protruding small branches of the hemorrhoidal veins (thrombosed hemorrhoid). Immediate relief follows incision under local anesthesia and evacuation of the small clot. It is inadvisable to undergo a radical operation for hemorrhoids either during pregnancy or at the time of delivery, since even the severe ones may disappear soon after labor.

Varicose Veins

Varicose veins are common during pregnancy because of normal physiological effects, effects which cannot be controlled. Heredity also plays a role; there is a familial tendency toward the occurrence of varicosities that may be inherited from either parent. According to two different studies varicosities were present in 11 per cent of pregnant women in one group and 20 per cent in the other. Varicose veins first appeared as early as the second month in one-fourth of the cases and as late as the fifth month in one-fifth of those developing them.

In susceptible women varicosities are likely to be noted in a first or second pregnancy and tend to reappear earlier in the next pregnancy. Each succeeding pregnancy makes them worse. Fortunately the enlarged veins regress between pregnancies, with the first few pregnancies after their initial appearance almost completely, but only partially after later pregnancies. The vessels first involved are most frequently on the inner aspect of the calf, but the process may begin in the space behind the knee or on the thigh, and may involve one leg or both. In the early stages the veins may appear as a spidery network of superficial blood vessels, but when more advanced they stand out as straight, tortuous or knotted, soft blue cords just beneath the skin. A less common site is the outer vaginal region.

Varicose veins may cause either no symptoms or considerable discomfort. Once the veins become large, a feeling of "heaviness" and fatigue may occur. A dull ache is not infrequent. True pain is only met if the vein becomes inflamed.

If varicose veins develop during pregnancy, several measures may help:

1. Do not stand if you can sit and, when you sit, sit with your legs elevated so that your heels are above the level of the hips. Do not sit if you can lie and, when you lie, lie with your legs raised on a pillow.

2. Elastic ace bandages are used to compress all varices from the time they appear until several days after delivery. They are worn from the toe to the knee for varices involving the lower leg. With enlarged thigh veins a second elastic bandage is wound from the knee upward. If there is swelling of the leg the elastic bandage is applied in the morning before arising. This will necessitate bathing or showering the night before. If there is no swelling the bandage can be applied in the sitting position. The best type of bandage is the four-inch, rubber-reinforced elastic variety. Elastic stockings can be substituted, but they are prone to stretch. For varicose veins involving the lip of the vagina there is a special four-buckle, adjustable support, worn about the hips and over the buttocks, and fitted with a compression vulvar pad that has disposable inserts.

3. Every few hours the pregnant woman with leg varicosities should elevate her legs for several minutes while sitting or lying down, if possible. When standing she should encourage the blood flow by rising up on her tiptoes frequently. When sitting, if it is impossible to elevate the legs, the feet and toes should be flexed and extended frequently for the same reason.

Injections to obliterate varicose veins or surgery to eliminate them can be performed during pregnancy, but most authorities much prefer to wait for such treatment until several weeks after delivery because complications are less likely and many of the large veins fade away postpartum. A woman with several children and severe varicose veins should consider sterilization at the time of delivery. If she suggests it there is every likelihood her obstetrician will agree with enthusiasm to perform the operation.

Nosebleeds and Nasal Congestion

Nosebleeds are common during pregnancy, particularly during the winter months. Since ordinarily they are brief, they rarely present a serious problem. Usually they result from a drying and crusting of the membrane lining the nasal cavity, a membrane which temporarily has a greatly increased blood supply. If you have nosebleeds, lubricate the nasal cavity by instilling night and morning a few drops of a .25-per-cent solution of menthol in white oil, with an eyedropper, in both nostrils. Then tip your head back so the medicine runs into your throat, and spit it out. Almost certainly this will stop the nosebleeds; if not, notify your doctor.

Frequently throughout pregnancy the pregnant woman feels as though her nose is swollen by a perpetual cold which interferes with breathing. Doctors have a specific name for it, allergic rhinitis of pregnancy, but they do not have an equally specific cure. Vasoconstrictor nose drops such as Neosynephrine or Privine, sprays, and inhalers produce temporary relief but should be used seldom and sparingly; their excessive use succeeds in making the condition worse. As with almost all the evils mentioned in this chapter, there is a cheerful addendum: allergic rhinitis clears up with delivery.

Leg Cramps

Spasm of the calf muscles and muscles of the foot is a common and painful nuisance during pregnancy. The condition is likely to begin about mid-pregnancy, but is usually less frequent the last month. It comes unannounced; most often the patient is aroused from her sleep to find the calf muscles of one leg knotted into a painful, firm ball. The best treatment is local massage, a kneading of the muscle until it relaxes. The area may remain tender for several hours thereafter. Such muscle spasm is not damaging, nor does it denote any abnormality of health. Two remedies have been suggested: two tablets or two teaspoons of Gelusil or Amphojel three times a day with meals; and a 50-milligram capsule of an antihistamine, Benadryl, before bedtime. Before trying either, obtain your doctor's permission.

Swelling of the Ankles and Legs

About one-quarter of the normal weight gain during pregnancy results from an increase in the amount of water held by the tissues. This excess fluid tends to pool into the dependent part of the body, so that the feet and ankles first show evidence of it. Many normal pregnant patients complain of swelling of the ankles, the lower legs, and the feet toward the end of the day. This is aggravated by periods of standing and is materially worse in warm weather. A patient with these symptoms should elevate her feet whenever possible during the day—prop them on a chair or bench, or stretch out on the bed or sofa. Larger shoes may have to be worn in late pregnancy to allow for the swelling of the feet. If the feet have a tight feeling and burn, immersing them in cold water gives relief. Ordinarily the swelling of the leg and foot subsides during the night, and by morning the normal contours of the ankle are visible once again.

The fingers are the next commonest site of pregnancy tissue swelling, which causes them to feel stiff. Frequently the puffiness of the fingers makes rings uncomfortably tight, and they may be difficult to remove. If so, soak the hand in cold water; then hold the finger pointing upward and soap the finger and ring before attempting to remove it.

Swelling of the face may normally occur to a limited extent, causing features to look relatively thick and gross.

If the tissue swelling is moderate, particularly if it is confined to legs and fingers, and unassociated with either an excessive or very rapid weight gain, it has no special significance. On the other hand, if it is associated with either, especially when it involves the eyes, notify your doctor at once.

Frequency of Urination

The urge to urinate with increased frequency is commonly met at the beginning and end of pregnancy. The condition may be particularly annoying at night, interrupting sleep. The best way to handle the situation is to omit all fluids after six in the evening; then you will void most of the urine before bedtime. If omitting fluids after six does not give you a sufficiently undisturbed night, ask your doctor about a sedative.

Painful Contractions

The uterus, like all smooth muscle structures, is constantly alternating between a phase of contraction and a phase of relaxation. This begins before you are born, but is not noticeable to you until the middle of pregnancy, when you may feel a hard lump in your lower abdomen which remains for thirty seconds and disappears, to reappear ten or fifteen minutes later. Such contractions ordinarily are not painful. However, in some women—rarely in a first pregnancy—these contractions become painful at times during the late months. Such painful contractions, false pains, are difficult to differentiate from true labor. We have noted that a change of position often stops the false type of painful contractions, so, if you are lying down, stand and walk about; if you are standing or sitting, lie down. Also, true labor pains gradually get closer together and harder. Then, too, true labor pains may or may not be accompanied by a show of blood, whereas false pains never are. If a bout of painful contractions begins during the night and you think this may not be true labor, take a teaspoonful of paregoric; if the pains are false, you will probably soon drop back to sleep, but if they are the contractions of true labor, the teaspoon of paregoric will not stop them. In many states paregoric is a prescription drug and therefore if you don't have it in your medicine chest you will have to get your doctor to prescribe it.

Faintness

There is a tendency to faintness, even fainting, at any period of pregnancy. It is particularly likely to occur on suddenly standing from a sitting posture, or rapidly rising from a supine position. If such is the case, the best advice is to assume the new position gradually. Faintness is also likely to occur after prolonged standing in buses or on shopping tours, or when the woman is confined in a warm, close room. Recovery is rapid and without incident unless she falls and injures herself. If you have a tendency to faint during pregnancy, carry a bottle of smelling salts or aromatic spirits of ammonia in your handbag and, at the first suggestion of faintness, remove the stopper and inhale deeply.

Backache

Because of a special chemical produced by the placenta, there may be physiologic relaxation of the joints articulating together the large bones to form the pelvis. During pregnancy this frequently causes a sense of fatigue, backache, or occasionally pain low down in the front where the two large pelvic bones join. In the last trimester the latter symptom may cause difficulty in walking. A well-fitted maternity girdle should help both pain and walking. Massage and heat often provide welcome relief for the tired or aching back of pregnancy. Rubbing liniment applied with the palm of the hand to the back is particularly excellent, but one must be careful not to apply heat over freshly applied liniment lest it blister the skin. In stubborn cases of pregnancy backache, strapping by a physician with adhesive tape may be required or an orthopedic consultation. Pain from a herniated disc occurs in pregnant women with about the same frequency as in the nonpregnant.

Insomnia

Despite the increasing fatigue and the desire for additional rest that most women experience in the last trimester, sleep may be seriously disturbed by the nocturnal athletic pursuits of the fetus, plus inability of the mother to get into a comfortable position. This is particularly distressing in the heat of midsummer and may be aided by an air-conditioned bedroom. A relaxing bath before bed may be helpful. If the insomnia is severe and causes you concern, discuss it with your physician. He may prescribe a barbiturate capsule or some other sleep-producing medicine. We counsel our patients to take Seconal a half-hour before turning out the light, when falling asleep is the main problem. On the other hand if they go to sleep easily but wake after a few hours and then cannot go back to sleep, they are instructed to take a Seconal capsule on waking during the night, or a capsule of Nembutal or Carbital or a Doriden tablet just as they are ready to go to sleep for the night. We warn patients not to take a capsule more often than two nights in three, so that they do not become too dependent on hypnotic drugs. Obviously, do not take any sleeping drug before consulting your own doctor, and never more than a single dose in one night without his express permission.

Vaginal Discharge (Leukorrhea)

A certain amount of pale yellow, thin vaginal discharge is normal for pregnancy, resulting from the increased activity of the cervical glands. Usually bathing with the liberal use of a soft washcloth is sufficient to take care of the problem. If not, douching as outlined in Chapter 7 may be practiced with your doctor's consent. If the discharge becomes very profuse and thick and is associated with vaginal itching, consult your doctor promptly. Occasionally the leukorrhea is the result of a vaginal infection with a troublesome parasite called a trichomonad, or with a yeastlike fungus that has the poetic-sounding name of *Candida albicans*. No one knows how either comes about, except that the vagina is an open cavity in contact with the exterior and like the mouth, it is never free of harmless bacteria. The vagina of pregnancy offers an unusually hospitable environment, chemically, for *Candida*. Your physician can determine whether either infestation is present by vaginal smears and cultures. If he discovers that the trichomonad *Trichomonas vaginalis* is the villain, he will prescribe a miracle drug, Flagyl, to be taken by mouth and perhaps vaginally. It is not uncommon for the wife to pass the condition to her husband and vice versa. In the male it causes a sense of irritation, sometimes burning on urination. It is a very mild infection that never causes any systemic illness and is readily curable by Flagyl in both female and male. If the investigation shows *Candida* to be the cause of the leukorrhea, a fungicide in the form of Mycostatin tablets is usually prescribed for vaginal insertion, once or twice a day for several days. In resistant cases the physician may choose to paint the interior of the vagina with 1 per cent gentian violet, a purple dye which does a superior job in messing everything up, including panties. *Candidiasis* has the tendency to recur during pregnancy, thereby requiring resumption of treatment, but usually subsides with delivery.

Shortness of Breath

In part because of the raised diaphragm from heightened pressure within the abdomen, and in part because of increased weight, shortness of breath is common in pregnancy, especially during the last two months. In many, particularly in those with first pregnancies, decided relief may occur a few weeks before confinement, when the summit of the uterus drops two or three inches as the baby's head descends part way into the opening of the bony pelvis. If the shortness of breath interferes with sleep, the head and shoulders should be propped up by several pillows to a semisitting posture. To be safe, report to your doctor shortness of breath that seems more than slight, especially if you are winded by climbing a flight of stairs.

Skin Rash

Stout women with heavy breasts and fleshy thighs often develop an irritating skin rash either beneath the breast where it joins the chest wall, or in one or both groins. This is especially common in warm, humid climates and is caused by an accumulation of irritating perspiration. The best treatment is the application of a mixture of three parts of calomine lotion and one part of witch hazel in an amount sufficient to form a surface cover over the irritated area, then dusting with talcum powder.

Pregnancy Moods

Pregnancy is notorious for its mood swings. Previously stable women may find themselves going through periods of depression, with tears just beneath the surface—so near the surface that they well up for the most insignificant reason, or no reason at all. Other women find themselves irritable about nothing; trifles which ordinarily barely ruffle their aplomb become momentous and seriously upset them. The best therapy is to discuss the matter frankly with your understanding doctor. He, no doubt, will be able to tell you truthfully that he has seen many cases just like yours which got better as pregnancy progressed. After delivery, the stable, sweet, tranquil dispositions of the patients return untarnished.

A second therapeutic suggestion is to keep going. Don't become a stay-at-home introvert. If you are not working, see your friends; join education-for-childbirth courses at the Red Cross, your church, or hospital; work as a volunteer in some communal activity. It is possible that some of the women you meet at the prenatal visits to your doctor would wish to be friends. Pregnant women have a lot in common, and becoming pregnant is like joining a huge national sorority, your doctor's patients forming one local chapter.

A third possibility is the temporary use of tranquilizers, on your doctor's prescription. When indicated they may turn out to be excellent morale boosters.

What to Do in Case of a Fall or Accident

First discover whether you have injured yourself. Determining this does not differ from doing so when you are not pregnant. Do you hurt? Are you bleeding from any wound? Are your movements restricted? If these three questions are answered in the negative, you are probably uninjured

—yet if you are in doubt, see a doctor at once. Next, turn your attention to the pregnancy. If there is no vaginal bleeding and the fetus continues to move, pregnancy was unaffected. If you are too early in pregnancy to have felt fetal movements, the only criterion regarding the status of the pregnancy will be vaginal bleeding. The fetus is so perfectly protected by the cushioning fluid surrounding it and the veritable shock absorbers built in the uterus that only rarely does even the most direct blow disturb either the infant or the fortress in which it is ensconced. If there is vaginal bleeding, get in touch with your physician at once. If fetal movements appear absent, do not panic; wait an hour or two and, if they have not reappeared, call your doctor.

Occasional Complications

Complications may arise during pregnancy which are peculiar and specific to the pregnant state. They are uncommon, and your mathematical chances of developing any one are slim—in fact, so slim that the odds are better than you would get on a long shot at the race track. Be additionally reassured by the knowledge that obstetrics today is a modern miracle and virtually all of its problems can be safely and skillfully solved.

Pregnancy in the Tube (Ectopic)

Once in 300 pregnancies the fertilized ovum develops in a site other than the cavity of the uterus. Pregnancies implanted in an aberrant locale are termed ectopic pregnancies. An ectopic pregnancy may be situated in the ovary, abdomen, or cervix, but well over 95 per cent take place in the Fallopian tube. There are several reasons why the journey of the blastocyst from the ovary to the uterus may not be completed, terminating instead in the conduit (Fallopian tube) through which it is traveling. These include developmental abnormalities of the tube, previous inflammation causing obstructing scars, and also, no doubt, abnormalities in the rhythm of tubal contractions which propel the egg into the uterus. Not cognizant of its abnormal site, the egg burrows into the wall of the tube and begins to develop. The condition is ordinarily diagnosed by the occurrence of one-sided lower abdominal pain six to twelve weeks after a period is missed, frequently associated with vaginal bleeding, which causes the patient to seek medical help. Occasionally a symptomless tubal pregnancy is discovered by the doctor in the course of his pelvic exam at the initial visit. He may feel a tender mass alongside the uterus and by differential diagnostic procedures determines that it is a tubal pregnancy, and not an inflamed tube, ovarian cyst, or uterine fibroid. At other times no intimation of a tubal pregnancy appears until the tube ruptures. Then the patient is suddenly seized by a severe, stabbing, grinding lower abdominal pain frequently radiating to the shoulder, accompanied by faintness. The symptoms are often so typical that a doctor can diagnose it over the telephone with a 90 per cent chance of being right. When the diagnosis of tubal or ectopic pregnancy is established, abdominal operation is necessary at once; then either the entire tube is removed, or it is opened, the pregnancy evacuated, and the tube repaired. The ovary on the side of the tubal pregnancy may or may not be removed depending on findings at the operating table.

Frequently transfusion is necessary on the operating table to make up for the blood lost into the abdominal cavity. Mortality is very low, less than 1 in 800, and recovery is very rapid. Unfortunately about half the women operated upon for an ectopic do not conceive again. And of those who do, 15 per cent of the conceptions are ectopics in the remaining tube.

If one already has children it is probably wise not to take the 15 per cent risk by trying again. On the other hand, if one's family is incomplete by all means try again, probably beginning a few months later. However, as soon as there is evidence, or even suspicion, of pregnancy see a doctor so that he can determine whether it is an intrauterine or ectopic gestation.

Placenta Praevia and Premature Separation of the Placenta (Abruptio)

These conditions are relatively infrequent, and each happens about once in 200 pregnancies. They usually occur in the last trimester, and the predominant symptom in both is vaginal hemorrhage. In placenta praevia, the placenta, instead of being at the top of the uterus, is situated low down, and part of it overlaps the mouth of the womb (internal os). The uterus is shaped like a large inverted bottle, and ordinarily the placenta is implanted high up inside the bottle, usually on the back of the bottle, less often on the front. In the case of placenta praevia, however, it is situated so low down that part, or all, of the round opening from which the cervix arises is covered by it. Late in pregnancy, preparatory to the onset of labor, the cervix expands slightly and any placental tissue that overlies it is torn loose from that part of the uterine lining to which it is attached, leaving a raw area from which the patient bleeds. The more completely the cervix is covered, the earlier in pregnancy is the bleeding likely to commence. There are three types of placenta praevia depending on whether all of the cervical opening in the lowermost part of the uterus is covered by placenta (central), a part of it (partial), or only its edge (marginal). The relative frequency of the three is 20 per cent, 25 per cent, and 55 per cent respectively. Placenta praevia is uncommon in a first pregnancy and increasingly more common with additional gestations, the rate rising from 2.5 per 1000 first births to 8 per 1000 for eighth births. Advancing age is also an independent positive factor.

Every patient who bleeds (more than a simple stain) in the latter half of pregnancy warrants prompt hospitalization. Her hemoglobin is determined to estimate the amount of blood already lost and, after blood grouping and matching, she is transfused if necessary. If the baby is estimated to be less than five pounds and placenta praevia is thought to be the diagnosis, expectant therapy is likely to be employed. Since baby fatalities in placenta praevia are largely due to prematurity, expectant therapy means keeping the mother under observation in the hospital and transfusing her if necessary until the baby is judged to be five and a half pounds. She is then taken to the operating room, where the doctor carefully inserts his finger through the cervix to determine how much, if any, placental tissue can be felt covering the cervix. If none is felt or only a small sliver, he is likely to rupture the membranes and permit labor and vaginal delivery. If an appreciable amount of placenta is felt immediate Cesarean section is performed. About six in ten women with placenta praevia are delivered by Cesarean section and four in ten vaginally. From 80 per cent to 85 per cent of placenta praevia cases treated in this manner eventuate in surviving babies, and a maternal death occurs very rarely.

Premature separation of the placenta (frequently termed placental abruption), as the name suggests, is the separation of part or all of the placenta from its attachment to the uterus before the child is born. A localized hemorrhage begins in the maternal tissues underlying the placenta; blood accumulates and sheers loose the placenta from its delicate, spongelike fastenings. Premature separation occurs most frequently in those who have borne more than five children, being three times as common in such cases as in first pregnancies. Age seems to play no role. About 40 per cent of the cases show high blood pressure and albumin in the urine, suggesting the association with a generalized toxic process. Also very occasionally a placenta is jarred loose by a severe abdominal blow. Abruption has a tendency toward recurrence, repeating in 10 per cent of subsequent pregnancies.

In approximately one case in five the hemorrhage from the separated or partially separated placenta is concealed and there is no visible bleeding. Pain and faintness are variable, but in every instance the uterus, instead of being soft, is rigid on examination through the abdominal wall and tender to touch. Treatment of abruption requires prompt hospitalization with replacement by transfusions of the visible or concealed blood loss. Then either the membranes are ruptured and intravenous pituitrin given to promote prompt delivery, or a Cesarean section performed. The choice is dictated by many factors, such as whether or not a fetal heartbeat is detected and an estimate of how soon vaginal delivery can be effected. Premature separation was formerly associated with a high maternal mortality, but today the mortality rate in such cases is less than 1 per cent. However, the baby does not fare as well, its chance for survival being about fifty-fifty.

Toxemia

The development of high blood pressure—or the worsening of such a pre-existing condition—in the latter half of pregnancy, at times associated with the appearance of albumin in the urine and water-logging of tissues (edema), is termed toxemia of pregnancy. From the word's derivation (Creek: "poison" and "blood"), one would assume that a toxic substance entering the mother's blood, with its origin probably in the placenta or fetus, had created the illness. But after years of earnest search no such toxic substance has been identified. Toxemia is called "the disease of theories" because so many theories of what causes it have been advanced, each in turn discarded. When I was a student it was thought that too much protein in the diet was an important factor, and today, fifty years later, one prominent theory suggests the lack of protein in the diet as a cause of the disease.

There are two varieties of toxemia, one most likely to appear in a healthy woman during the last several weeks of a first pregnancy and the other affecting older women, usually already mothers, who have some evidence of elevated blood pressure before the onset of the present pregnancy. The first is called preeclampsia, in other words, the prelude to eclampsia. Decades ago, when preeclampsia was not recognized or was improperly treated, it frequently became eclampsia, a serious convulsive disorder. Today eclampsia has become a disease of neglect, usually the neglect of the patient in not seeking competent prenatal care. Believe it or not, in this enlightened country there are still a considerable number of women who simply walk into a hospital in labor, never having seen a doctor during the whole course of pregnancy. Eclampsia is a preventable disease because it can be eliminated by recognizing the illness in its pre-eclamptic phase and by instituting proper treatment at that stage. In 1928, at a time when most of the poor either did not seek or could not get prenatal care, on one November weekend, four patients were admitted to the clinic service of The Johns Hopkins Hospital with eclamptic convulsions. Now eclampsia is so uncommon that many large obstetrical services go a full year without admitting a single case. The second type of toxemia, the aggravation of pre-existing hypertension, usually in older women who have borne children, is called chronic hypertensive disease.

There is still a socioeconomic difference in the frequency and severity of pregnancy toxemia, the less affluent showing a higher incidence. Those with the greatest risk of preeclampsia and eclampsia are illegitimately pregnant teenagers. Most of them do not take seriously the need for prenatal care or prescribed diet. The following figures show how magnificently danger from eclampsia has receded, largely through its prevention. In New York City during 1920 there were 190 deaths from eclampsia, in 1967, 3, and in 1968, none.

The incidence of toxemia in private practice is less than half the number encountered in the usual clinic population. Furthermore, the private practitioner virtually never has a case of eclampsia in his own practice, since he can arrest the condition in its pre-eclamptic stage by prompt and vigorous treatment.

To prevent serious toxemia every patient should be examined by her obstetrician every week during the last month of pregnancy and every two weeks during the two previous months. This provides him opportunity to check blood pressure, weight, and urine.

The first sign of impending trouble is a slow rise in blood pressure or a sudden and excessive weight gain. When weight gain reaches two pounds a week or six pounds a month, incipient preeclampsia is suspected. Appearance of albumen in the urine comes next and, later yet, such symptoms as puffiness of hands and face, severe and continuous headache, and blurring of vision. Ambulatory treatment may be sufficient to cure or control mild toxemia. The patient rests at home lying in bed on her side much of the time and is forbidden to add salt to her food at the table or in the kitchen. She is presented a list of foods with a high salt content so that she can avoid them. Salt substitutes are available for those who object to unsalted food.

If ambulatory treatment is unsuccessful or if the toxemia is moderate or severe when first detected, hospitalization is necessary. Then the patient is placed at complete bed rest lying on her side. Lying on the back allows the large pregnant uterus to press heavily on the big abdominal blood vessels, the vena cava and aorta, increasing the likelihood of certain complications. She is given a low-sodium, high-protein diet. Small doses of a sedative, such as phenobarbital, are prescribed. If the pregnancy is thirty-seven weeks or more, after a day or two of hospitalization pregnancy is usually terminated by inducing labor or, when this is not feasible, by Cesarean section. If pregnancy is less than thirty-seven weeks temporization may be practiced to allow the baby to achieve greater maturity.

Both preeclampsia and eclampsia are about four times as common in twin than in single pregnancies, which strongly suggests that the elusive causative factor is in some way related to the fetus or placenta. In twins there are two babies and a larger mass of placental tissue.

Toxemia still ranks among the three chief causes of maternal mortality.

Fetal Death *in Utero*

In occasional pregnancies the fetus dies at some time between the twentieth week of pregnancy and its birth. Some of the more frequent causes of this mishap have been mentioned in this chapter: toxemia, premature separation of the placenta, and placenta praevia. Others, such as congenital malformations and erythroblastosis, are taken up in Chapter 20, and still others, such as maternal diabetes, in Chapter 11. Be assured it is not related to anything the mother did or failed to do. The death of a fetus within the uterus does not jeopardize the mother's health; in fact the maternal organism shows no reaction to it except for gradual loss of the weight gained in pregnancy and regression of the enlarged breasts of pregnancy to their prepregnant size, a sign pointed out by Hippocrates, the father of medicine, twenty-four hundred years ago.

Psychologically, it is very difficult both for the patient and her family. It all seems so useless and unrewarding. Then, too, there is a certain revulsion to carrying anything dead within the body. This is a complication of obstetrics which thoroughly tests the maturity and emotional stability of all concerned, even the doctor's.

Diagnosis of fetal death is frequently called to the doctor's attention by the patient's reporting that she has not felt the baby move for a day or two. This prolonged absence of fetal movements is significant only in the last few months of pregnancy; previous to this the patient's failure to note such fetal activity for a day or two is normal. Careful examination by the doctor fails to detect a heartbeat. These two pieces of evidence—the cessation of fetal movements in late pregnancy, and the doctor's inability to hear the fetal heartbeat—are not absolute, since the healthy fetus occasionally may be quiet for twenty-four or forty-eight hours, and in rare instances the sound of the fetal heart is temporarily impossible to detect. More absolute evidence can be obtained by a fetal electrocardiograph. Therefore when doubt exists a tracing is made through the mother's abdominal wall, frequently in the hospital where you are booked to deliver. A live fetus almost invariably gives a positive tracing (EKG).

Labor may begin spontaneously any time from a few hours to sixty days after the fetus's death, the average interval being two to three weeks. When labor occurs it is usually normal and relatively easy. A few days after fetal death the doctor will almost certainly attempt to initiate labor by the injection of Pitocin. If this fails he may use a technique called "salting out." Under local anesthesia a needle is introduced into the uterus through the abdominal wall at a point just below the navel. A half-pint or more of amniotic fluid is withdrawn, and a half-pint of 20 per cent sterile salt solution is injected into the amniotic cavity within the uterus through the same needle. Labor then commences in twelve to twenty-four hours. Few failures to initiate labor occur.

Approximately as many babies die before labor begins and during labor and delivery (1.5 per cent) as during the first month of life. The former is termed fetal death (stillbirth), the latter, neonatal death, and together, perinatal death (3 per cent).

Danger Signals—When to Notify the Doctor

The attainment of superior medical care is a bilateral undertaking between doctor and patient. If a doctor lacks competence or fails in diligence, ideal care cannot result, no matter how cooperative the patient. On the other hand, no doctor, no matter how expert and conscientious, can render even adequate care unless his patient cooperates. Part of patient cooperation in pregnancy requires that she inform him promptly of any deviation from normal health, unless it be of an obviously minimal variety such as a cold or a minor stomach upset. A list of the main danger signals follows:

1. *Vaginal bleeding* at any time during pregnancy. If it is just staining (less than normal menstrual flow) in the first half of pregnancy the news will keep till morning, but in the second half notify the doctor day or night, irrespective of the amount of bleeding. This does not include pink, mucoid discharge at term.

2. *Puffiness of the face, eyes, or fingers*, particularly significant if very sudden. Swelling of the legs and ankles when the face and hands are uninvolved is usually not significant, especially in hot weather.

3. *Severe, unremitting headache*, especially in the second half of pregnancy.

4. *Dimness or blurring of vision*, especially in the second half of pregnancy.

5. *Severe abdominal pain*, particularly if constant, no matter in what area of the abdomen or in what week of pregnancy.

6. *Vomiting* several times within a few hours.

7. *Fever over 100 degrees Fahrenheit*, particularly when associated with a chill.

8. *Painful urination* or burning on urination.

9. *Rupture of the membranes*, resulting in the escape of watery fluid from the vagina. The nearer you are to your term date, the less the significance.

10. *Absence of fetal movements* for twenty-four hours, from the thirtieth week on.

10

Miscarriage, Legal Abortion, and Premature Labor

The loss of a baby during pregnancy before it is far enough along in its development to survive outside the uterus (viable) is called "miscarriage" by most laymen. As in normal birth, the fetus is evacuated from its home in the uterus and expelled through the vagina. It was common medical practice to distinguish between abortion and miscarriage. "Abortion" was the term confined to the very early variety, before the embryo has actual form, and "miscarriage" the term for the later variety, after the embryo begins to resemble a baby. Medical usage now refers to both as "abortion."

Laymen often make another distinction, using the term "miscarriage" for involuntary abortion and "abortion" for those artificially induced. Again medical science makes no such distinction. Any pregnancy terminated before a fetus is developed to the point at which it can possibly live after its birth is an abortion, no matter when or how it occurs.

Spontaneous Abortion

According to three careful studies, between 14 and 18 per cent of all pregnancies—one in six—terminate spontaneously before the fetus is of sufficient size and development to survive. Two-thirds occur late enough so that fetal tissue can be identified. One-third are so early that the menstrual period is simply delayed and a positive pregnancy test, if taken, becomes negative. The very early conceptus is so small that it is not differentiated from the passage of menstrual material. The ordinary borderline between possible salvage of a baby and its likely demise after birth when born alive is 1000 grams—2 pounds, 3 ounces. This weight is normally attained between the twenty-seventh and twenty-eighth weeks of pregnancy. Of course, I do not mean to indicate that all babies above this intrauterine stage and weight survive, nor necessarily that all below succumb. The smallest infant on record to live was a 14-ounce baby, reported by Monro in the *Canadian Medical Journal* in 1939.

Most abortions or miscarriages occur long before the twenty-eighth week; actually three in four happen before the twelfth week, and only one in four during the sixteen weeks between the twelfth and twenty-eighth weeks. Most abortions occur shortly after the beginning of the tenth week, counting from the onset of the last menses.

Factors Influencing Incidence

While we still do not completely understand the causes of abortion, they are much better known than they were even a few decades ago.

In a study that my colleagues and I made, we found that three conditions are associated with a low frequency of abortion: youth, ability to conceive easily, and the absence of previous abortion. A woman under twenty-five who conceives within three months after she first tries to become pregnant and who has never aborted before is the most likely to leave a hospital nine months later with a baby. In this group the chances of abortion are only four in one hundred.

At the other extreme are the older women (more than thirty-five years of age) who require six months or longer to conceive and who have had an abortion. In this group the chances of miscarrying are forty in one hundred. Notice, this still leaves sixty who will bear their babies. And the forty who miscarry can try again and perhaps the next time be among the lucky sixty instead of the unlucky forty.

By finding out why a particular patient miscarries, the doctor may be able to prevent a recurrence. This is the reason that when you have symptoms of impending abortion your doctor will ask you to save any tissue expelled. If he cannot analyze it himself, he will send it to one of several special laboratories, where the material will be examined and a report sent him.

Some causes of abortion are related to the physical condition of the mother: fibroid tumors of the uterus, deep tears of the cervix (mouth of the womb) following a previous birth or abortion, extensive operations on the cervix, or congenital malformations of the reproductive organs (abnormal uterus or cervix from infancy). Acute infections associated with high fever, such as pneumonia, typhoid, pyelitis, and untreated malaria, may cause abortion. Profound anemia, rarely encountered in this country but sometimes seen in Africa and Asia, may be responsible. Herpes with genital lesions also carries increased risk of abortion in pregnancies less than four months. The acute conditions clear up and do not imperil subsequent pregnancies. Occasionally an abdominal operation, particularly if the site is near the pelvic organs, may produce abortion. Serious accidents are well tolerated by the fetus unless the mother suffers severe hemorrhage with shock. It is questionable whether psychic shock is ever the cause.

But many perfectly healthy and normal women miscarry, and some miscarry repeatedly. Our biggest problem as doctors is what causes such "normal" miscarriages and what we can do about them, because most abortions occur without discoverable cause.

In actuality the human fetus grows from a seed, and this human seed behaves generally like the seeds of all living things. The possibility of imperfect seeds is universal throughout the animal and plant kingdoms, and abortion is only another expression of the fact that the complicated processes of life and reproduction are often subject to possible misadventure.

Defective Germ Plasm

Many years ago I heard the late Dr. George Streeter, distinguished head of the Carnegie Institute of Embryology, discuss this topic before the learned members of the New York Obstetrical Society. He stood upon the rostrum, the eyes of the audience fixed upon him and, like a small boy with a pocket full of treasure, drew from his tuxedo vest two unopened pods of ordinary garden peas. "Gentlemen," he began, as he publicly shelled his peas, "I cannot be sure, but I'll hazard the guess that these pods will contain one or two bad, runted peas—defective germ plasm conceptions." They did.

Try it yourself. I think you may then be inclined to regard abortion less a freak abnormality and more as a common occurrence among all live things which develop from minute beginnings.

Actually, three out of four abortions are caused by faulty seeds, defective germ plasm. This means simply that things are not proceeding properly, and the conception ceases to develop; after days or weeks it is expelled normally. Medically speaking, such an abortion is a fortunate occurrence, although the woman who does not understand this is upset by her supposed misfortune.

If the conception is expelled because it is not progressing normally, either the embryo is nonexistent or defective, or else the placenta is deficient and so cannot supply adequate nutrition for the fetus. Often both embryo and placenta are abnormal.

Theoretical Causes of Defective Germ Plasm

We do not really know what causes a defective conception, except that nature is not always benevolent and kind. But we assume the cause to lie in one of four places: the sperm, the egg, the process of fertilization, or the implantation of the fertilized egg.

1. The fertilizing sperm may have been a dud and may have transmitted, instead of the father's apparent health and vigor, some hidden lethal factor. In this case the baby, if it had developed, would not have been normal anyway, and nature has provided abortion as a means of avoiding this consequence. Women who have been terribly disturbed by an involuntary abortion may be comforted to know that by this they have perhaps been spared a more serious misfortune.

2. The same may be true of the egg. Not all eggs are good eggs, or are potentially capable of developing into healthy babies.

3. The sperm and the egg may both have been normal and healthy, but their union may have been faulty. Fertilization is a very complicated physical-chemical process, as I demonstrated in Chapter 2, and does not always occur successfully, even though the two bits of germ plasm involved are healthy.

4. The sperm and the egg may be healthy and the fertilization normal, but the conceptus (the fertilized egg) may not have found a suitable environment in which to grow. That is, the fertilized egg may somehow not be implanted properly in the uterus, where it has to live and grow for nine months. Sometimes if it is planted in the wrong place, especially in the lowermost portion of the uterus, frequent bleeding will occur during early pregnancy and abortion will follow. A bulb or seed will not flourish if planted too deep or too superficially, or in improper soil. The human egg behaves similarly.

It is remarkable that implantation of an ovum succeeds as often as it does. Immediately after burrowing into the uterine lining the cells on the outside of the small spherical egg must take up food from adjacent maternal cells and later tap blood vessels to create little stagnant pools of blood to feed from. Then treelike branches of fetal cells sprout forth, the thousands of villi that begin forming the placenta. The complexity of all this is staggering to contemplate. If at any point one of these mechanisms fails growth ceases and abortion follows.

Genetic Basis for Spontaneous Abortion

During the past few years anatomical confirmation of the highly theoretic concept of defective germ plasm has been obtained by the microscope. Through improved techniques of tissue culture and exciting advances of cytogenetics, the science which permits determination of the normality or abnormality of the chromosomes in each cell, it has been determined that in about 36 per cent of spontaneous abortions the cells of the abortus show chromosomal aberrations. The chromosomal errors found in the cells involved the lack of one or more chromosomes, or an extra one or two, or broken-off parts of one chromosome attached to another. These errors of nature are incompatible with continuation of life, and early fetal death occurs. Chromosomal abnormalities are found more frequently in abortions occurring to women over forty years old and under age eighteen. The incidence of chromosomal abnormalities is relatively high in fetuses aborted before the end of the third month and relatively rare after the fourth month. The earlier an abortion takes place, the greater the likelihood of chromosomal aberrations. From the studies thus far reported, it appears that an abortion associated with defective chromosomes is a happenstance and shows no tendency to repeat. Women who abort a succession of pregnancies ordinarily abort fetal tissue with normal chromosomes.

The Reaction of the Uterus to Defective Germ Plasm

A fetus that is not developing properly will die, and then it is like foreign material in the uterus. The normal reaction of the body is to expel foreign matter. We try to cough up a small bone in the throat, or blink a cinder from the eye. Similarly, the muscular contractions of the uterus force out the dead conceptus, which, through its death, has become foreign to living tissue, the uterus.

The defective germ-plasm conceptus usually stops developing and dies six or seven weeks after pregnancy begins, that is, after the last period, but four or five weeks after actual fertilization. It remains in the uterus for another three or four weeks before being expelled. Thus the actual process of abortion, as I have stated, most often occurs between the tenth and eleventh weeks.

Late Abortions

Ordinarily abortions caused by maternal disease or some abnormality of the uterus or cervix occur between the thirteenth and twenty-eighth weeks. Abortions occurring during this period are very likely to result in a well-formed fetus which is either living or has very recently died.

Superstitions about Abortion

There is a firmly ingrained belief that abortion is likely to occur at the precise time a missed menstrual period is due and, therefore, many women take unusual precautions during the eighth week and again during the twelfth week. Since statistically most abortions take place during the tenth and eleventh weeks, it is easy to upset this superstition and to assure the reader that such time-oriented restrictions are quite unnecessary.

Undoubtedly many physicians of yesteryear, as mystified about the cause of a miscarriage as the patient, eagerly accepted her pat explanations. A woman of ancient Greece was frightened by a clap of thunder (to be sure it was not the first time Attic thunder had frightened her during the pregnancy), and she miscarried two days later. A Roman matron was riding in her chariot when it hit a rut in the street which the Roman city fathers had neglected to repair. And three days thereafter she aborted. The circumstances were reported to the respective physicians, who duly noted them in their clinical records. When later these doctors became authors of medical treatises, they constructed their theories for the cause of abortion from the cases they had noted down earlier. When later authors also wrote books, they added to their own guesses those copied from the authorities who preceded them. And the "causes" of miscarriage multiplied almost as rapidly as the human race. Even today one of the most difficult tasks in medicine is the separation of happenstance from cause.

How to Prevent Spontaneous Abortion

As stated on previous pages, I forbid neither travel, horseback riding, nor any activity to the normal woman in early or late pregnancy. My leniency is based on the premise that you cannot shake a good human egg loose any more than you can shake a good unripe apple from the apple tree. If you could, there would be no work for abortionists, nor would the strong wind out of the north leave any fruit to ripen in the orchard. Nature sometimes makes mistakes, but she fanatically preserves her seed and the fruits therefrom which are normal and which are not mistakes.

What a particular doctor prescribes when a woman bleeds vaginally in early pregnancy depends on two highly variable and equally important factors—the doctor and the patient. And since by no stretch of the imagination am I either your, the reader's, physician, or a paper substitute for him, the first thing to do is to report the bleeding to your doctor and ask him for instructions.

The usual treatment is bed rest combined with the administration of various hormone preparations. When I adopt this form of therapy—and occasionally I do—it is because the patient expects it and would consider herself neglected if I did not prescribe it.

Since early miscarriages are usually caused by defective germ plasm, by the time bleeding occurs the conceptus has already been dead a week or two, and no medication can restore life to dead matter. On the other hand, if the bleeding is very light and passing, then it is probably caused by some small complication that will not result in abortion. If so, the bleeding is harmless and will disappear by itself or perhaps after simple local treatment applied to the cervix.

If my patient is calm and understanding, I explain these matters to her when the bleeding starts. If after the explanation and my confession that miscarriage is a field of relative uncertainty and ignorance, she elects the usual orthodox hormone treatment, I prescribe it—no miracles promised. Many patients choose to continue their activities and are happier and less anxious when they do.

If the bleeding occurs after the twelfth week, when it is more likely that the conceptus is normal and some unknown, perhaps medical or mechanical, factor is responsible, bedrest and perhaps medicines make more sense. I may at this period occasionally use them if examination first shows the uterus to be developing normally in size and not far smaller than it should be, which would indicate the retention of a dead conceptus.

Interval between Abortion and Another Pregnancy

How long should a woman wait after aborting before she tries to become pregnant again? If defective germ plasm is proved responsible, then attempts to start another pregnancy should be begun immediately after the first menstrual period, which usually comes about four weeks to the day after the abortion. It is only a question of combining a good sperm with a good egg; the more often you try, the better your chance of hitting the right combination.

If the abortion was definitely not caused by defective germ plasm, i.e., fetus and placenta were normal, and a complete physical and laboratory examination does not reveal what caused it, then I usually advise a waiting period of about six months. Something caused pregnancy to terminate very prematurely and, since I cannot find out what it was and correct it, I propose to wait and hope that it will correct itself.

The Repetition of Abortion

What are your chances of a successful pregnancy if you have aborted once before, or twice, or three times? If it was only once, you have practically as good a chance as any woman who has never aborted—even without any treatment. If you have aborted twice in succession, your chances without treatment are somewhat reduced, perhaps to three in five. And if you have had three successive abortions, then the chances of your bearing a child without medical aid are perhaps less than fifty-fifty.

In other words, if you have aborted once, you do not have too much to worry about when you try the second time. If you have aborted two or more successive times, then you had better go to an especially well-qualified doctor and follow his advice carefully.

Your chances of producing a living child if you are a chronic aborter—that is, have had three or more successive miscarriages—have been considerably improved by modern medicine. One obstetrician reports that dietary instructions plus thyroid treatment have helped 80 per cent of his chronic aborters to carry their pregnancies successfully. Other authorities use other hormones. Yet others have achieved miracles with psychotherapy plus liberal amounts of vitamins B and C. This multiplicity of successful therapeutic agents is confusing. It seems to boil down to the fact that there is a strong psychic component in repetitive abortion, and if the patient is sufficiently reassured by the authoritative attitude of her specially qualified physician, the psychic component is largely eliminated. This, plus meticulous care by the specialist who makes the problem of repetitive abortion a primary interest, probably explains the good results from so many different methods of treatment.

The Story of a Typical Spontaneous Abortion

It is somewhat hazardous to enumerate medical signs and symptoms for the benefit of lay readers. They immediately search for them in their own cases, and if the signs are present or absent they are prone to misinterpret their observations. Therefore, I should like to caution against self-diagnosis in this situation.

In a typical abortion the couple has required a few months more than the usual two or three months to conceive. The woman is free of all pregnancy symptoms except the missed menses. The absence of any nausea is striking. She goes to her doctor's office when two months "pregnant," and says to him, "I feel great; if it were not that I missed, I wouldn't know I was pregnant." On pelvic examination the doctor makes a mental note that the uterus feels slightly firmer and smaller than it should for nine weeks' duration, but since many normal pregnancies at first give the same impression, he holds his peace. Ten weeks after the onset of the last menses the girl notices a brownish stain on the toilet tissue after voiding. On more careful inspection, the stain is found to come from the vagina, but there is no pain. Her breasts either never enlarged, or if they did, have gone down in size. The stain appears and disappears; it is a kind of dirty smudge mixed with mucus. Sometimes it is brown-red in color. During the night the staining stops, but on first getting up it is particularly noticeable. This simply means that the small amount of blood lost during the night is retained as a pool in the vagina and, when she assumes an upright position, it drains out. In a few days there is a dull ache in the lower abdomen, and the brown bleeding is now bright red. Some hours later cramps like exaggerated menstrual cramps appear. She begins to bleed more freely, the blood is a brighter red in color, and there is the passage of a few egg-sized clots. When the cramps have reached a crescendo she passes a peach-sized clot which is firmer and shaggier than the others. The cramps suddenly cease; the bleeding slows to a trickle and soon becomes just a stain. This is the story of a complete abortion.

On examination of the peach-sized mass, the doctor discovers that it is the whole egg sac, which may contain a badly degenerated fetus or no fetus at all. In either instance the process is all over and no curettage is necessary.

An Incomplete Abortion

In perhaps half the cases there is continuation of bleeding with clot formation, despite the passage of some firmer tissue. This indicates that some placental tissue still remains. Under such circumstances the abortion is usually completed after hospitalization by either hypodermic injections of the drug Pitocin, causing the uterus to contract, which may squeeze out the placental fragments, or by one of two simple operations. The first, in the jargon of the medical profession, is termed a "D and C," the letters standing for dilatation and curettage. The patient is first anesthetized; then, through the vaginal route, the cervix is dilated or stretched with a series of graduated cigar-shaped metal dilators until sufficiently open to admit a small rakelike instrument, a curette. The cavity of the uterus is then raked clean of remnants of afterbirth. The second operation is completion by aspiration. If the cervix is open a small metal or plastic tube, a cannula, is inserted into the uterine cavity and, using about 40 mm of Hg negative pressure, the remaining placental tissue is sucked out, usually in two or three minutes. It is much like employing a tiny vacuum cleaner. In many institutions this is handled as an outpatient procedure in the hospital's emergency unit. If the cervix is closed either general or local anesthesia has to be given first to permit cervical dilatation before aspiration is feasible.

The Danger from Abortion

Today women do not die from spontaneous abortion. Danger from severe blood loss, a rare occurrence, is neutralized by adequate transfusions, and possible, though infrequent, infection is readily controlled by available antibiotics.

The danger of despair, the feeling of frustration, is less easy to control. But remember, abortion is an unfortunate failing on nature's part, not yours. And if you are philosophical and courageous enough to try again, it is more than likely that with your doctor's help you will be successful.

Induced Abortion

The term "induced abortion" includes all previable terminations of pregnancy initiated by artificial means, in contrast to spontaneous abortions, which initiate themselves. One might differentiate them by saying that the former is manmade; the latter, God-made.

There are two kinds of induced abortions, legal and illegal. A legal abortion is an abortion carried out by a licensed physician within the statutory grounds spelled out by the law of the political jurisdiction where the procedure is to be performed. An illegal abortion is an abortion performed by a woman upon herself, or by a person other than a licensed physician, or by a licensed physician on indications or premises other than those permitted by laws of the state.

Early History

Induced abortion is an ancient procedure and its first performance long antedates recorded history. It was practiced by primitive peoples on every continent; ubiquity adding proof of age. The earliest medical manuscript extant, a Chinese herbal 5000 years old, recommends mercury as an abortifacient. The priest-physicians of the pharaohs in papyri written 4000 years ago evidenced knowledge of induced abortion. Plato advocated abortion on eugenic grounds for women less than twenty years of age and over forty, believing that they created inferior infants. He advocated the same fate for pregnancies implanted by men over fifty-five. Aristotle recommended abortion for women who already had many children to help control the population of the overcrowded city-state Athens. Soranus, the greatest gynecologist of antiquity, in a famous book written about 130 A.D., discusses which is preferable, abortion or contraception. With a modern tone to his words he argues for the latter, since it is safer, he wrote, to prevent conception than to eliminate it.

Religious Attitudes

The history of religious and ethical attitudes toward abortion is interesting. The ancient Babylonian Code of Hammurabi vigorously penalized induced abortion, specifying crucifixion for the perpetrators. As abortion is only mentioned once in the Bible, it can be assumed that it was little practiced by Jews (Numbers xxii) in the Biblical period and that it presented no problem to Christ's disciples. Judaism through the centuries has prohibited abortion unless a recognized rabbinical authority agrees in the individual instance that there is medical or social need. One of the most interesting cases arose during the era of Hitler terror, when any Jew who became pregnant was summarily killed with special indignities. The chief rabbi of Kovno, Poland, ruled that under such conditions abortion was permissible, since if it was not done two lives would be lost, and if done, only one life. Orthodox Judaism is still extraordinarily restrictive about abortion, but the Conservative and Reform wings of the Jewish faith have become as liberal about abortion as most of the Protestant groups.

Christianity took early cognizance of abortion and the first teachings of the Church forbade it under all conditions from the moment of conception. This decision was strongly reinforced by the fourth-century writings of Saint Augustine. Later the Church became concerned with the exact time of ensoulment, theorizing that before ensoulment there was no life and hence abortion would be no sin. The great thirteenth-century Church Father, Thomas Aquinas, promulgated the view that there was neither life nor ensoulment until the fetus moved and therefore abortion was not sinful in the first sixteen weeks of pregnancy. This view lasted for three centuries, and then the Church fixed ensoulment at forty days after conception. Abortion during the first forty days of pregnancy was considered no sin until 1869, when the Church ruled that life begins at the moment of conception and therefore abortion at any time is a grave sin. This is the position which the Catholic Church holds today; it never sanctions abortion per se, even to save the life of the pregnant woman. For well over one hundred years the major Protestant sects have sanctioned abortion, at first only for saving the mother's life, and later for health and eugenic purposes. This permissive attitude toward abortion has now evolved even further, resulting in support by several of the major Protestant denominations of abortion on demand, the decision being a personal one between doctor and patient.

Modern Abortion Laws

Before 1803 England had no specific abortion law, and the English Common Law had jurisdiction over abortion, holding that abortion was legal until the fetus moved. The 1803 English statute made all abortions a crime, but abortion before fetal movements was a lesser crime than abortion after fetal movements. The American Colonies, and subsequently the United States early in its history, were bound in many areas by English Common Law. Connecticut, the first state to pass an abortion statute, in 1820 made all abortions illegal, the penalty not being affected by duration of pregnancy. New York, in 1828, was the first political jurisdiction in the world to introduce an exception, abortion being permitted "to preserve the life of the mother."

Professor Cyril Means, a legal scholar, has researched the genesis of the New York law. The statute was passed by a Protestant legislature, not on ethical grounds but specifically to promote maternal health. This was in the days before anesthesia, asepsis, antibiotics, or transfusion, and death was common from the operative procedure of abortion, even within a first-class hospital. At the New York Hospital, between 1803 and 1830, eight legal abortions had been performed with five women surviving, a death rate of 37.5 per cent. During the same period childbirth at the New York Hospital was associated with a 2.8 per cent mortality. Therefore, to protect women against the inherent dangers of the operation, in 1828 the legislators insisted that its risk be permitted only when the physician involved believed there was no other means to preserve the life of the pregnant woman. Within several years all of the states either copied the exact verbiage of the New York statute or approximated it. In some it was phrased to promote "the safety of the mother," and a few stated that an illegal abortion was a criminal offense but did not define "legal abortion."

Modern Incidence in the United States

Until 1967 legal or "therapeutic" abortion was rarely performed, there being two legal abortions in the United States for every 1000 births, a total of about 8000 per year. The primary medical condition meriting abortion until about 1940 was organic disease involving heart, lungs, or kidneys. However, with the great improvement in general medical care, especially the discovery of specific drugs for infections, the need for abortion as a health safeguard in cases of organic disease acutely receded. At about this time the vague concept of abortion for protection against aggravation or initiation of emotional illness, so-called psychiatric grounds for abortion, rapidly became the chief indication. In reality psychiatric grounds soon became the subterfuge through which sophisticated and affluent women could acquire legal abortion for personal reasons. This resulted in a relatively high abortion rate for the private patient and a much lower rate for a clinic or ward patient, especially if cared for in a municipal hospital. In New York City in 1962 the legal abortion rate for private patients was 3.0 per 1000 births, 0.5 for clinic patients in voluntary hospitals, and 0.1 for patients in municipal hospitals.

During the period that 8000 legal abortions were performed in the United States, it is estimated there were one million illegal abortions, 20 per cent of the total pregnancies. I emphasize the word "estimated," because there could have been half as many or twice as many. Illegal abortion was even more discriminatory than legal abortion, the safety of the operation being correlated to the fee paid. Five hundred or one thousand dollars would buy the services of a clandestine physician-abortionist and twenty-five dollars those of a wholly unqualified granny-midwife or an operating-room orderly. And those without any money aborted themselves with hat pins, coat hangers, or slippery elm sticks. As a result deaths from illegal abortion were concentrated among the poor.

Liberalized Abortion Laws in Other Countries

In the meantime liberal laws concerning the performance of abortion had been introduced into other countries. Russia was the first, allowing abortion virtually on request shortly after the conclusion of World War I, a policy which has been maintained except for the interval from 1935 to 1955. Abortion statistics are still not available from Russia. Beginning in 1935 the four Scandinavian countries introduced partial liberalization resulting in 50 to 70 abortions per 1000 births. In the past year Denmark has further liberalized its statute and Sweden is likely to do so, and undoubtedly the proportion of abortions to births will increase. In 1948 Japan introduced abortion on demand, perhaps as a method of population control, though it was publicized as a health and eugenic measure to combat illegal abortion. In the early sixties Japan recorded over a million legal abortions annually; today with wider use of contraceptives the annual number has been reduced to 800,000. Japan, largely through abortion, rapidly brought its birth rate down from 34.5 births per 1000 population to 18, where it is today. The Eastern European socialist countries except for Albania followed Russia's lead in 1955 and 1956, permitting abortion virtually on request. In contrast to Russia several have published annual abortion figures. Hungary shows 30 per cent more legal abortions each year than births (1350 to 1000) and Poland half as many abortions as births. In Eastern Europe and Japan 95 per cent of the abortions are done early, at twelve weeks or before, resulting in splendidly low mortality figures, 2.5 and 4 deaths per 100,000 legal abortions, respectively.

The Movement for Legal Abortion in the United States

Because of the patent hypocrisy and subterfuge in legal abortion and of the socioeconomic discrimination in both legal and illegal abortion a strong movement in the United States arose to liberalize the fifty archaic, unenforceable state statutes. Then too, cognizance of the fact that, unlike other felonies, the crime of being aborted is committed, not by hardened criminals but by good citizens persuaded many that change in our abortion laws was required. A law which good citizens contrive to fracture, and usually without penalty, is a bad law.

In 1962 a group of eminent legal scholars, after much study, proposed a revised penal code for this country which included a model abortion statute. As the group was called the American Law Institute (A.L.I.), it is known as the A.L.I. law. In it the Institute spelled out three indications for the performance of legal abortion:

1. Health—if continuation of the pregnancy "would gravely impair the physical or mental health of the mother."

2. Eugenic—if the doctor believes that there is substantial risk that "the child would be born with grave physical or mental defects."

3. Humanitarian—if the pregnancy resulted from rape or incest. This included impregnation, with or without consent, of a child of fifteen years of age or less.

Shortly thereafter the World Health Organization, the eminent medical division of the United Nations, broadened attitudes toward health by redefining it. Health, it said, is "a state of complete physical and social well-being and not merely the absence of disease and infirmity."

In 1967 five states adopted statutes modeled on the A.L.I. bill. The first was Colorado. California, one of the five, was forced to omit eugenic conditions, since Governor Reagan stated he would veto any bill including such a provision. Subsequently eight other states similarly liberalized their laws. Scrutiny of results achieved in those states with A.L.I. bills left areas of dissatisfaction. In the main the new legislation did not reduce sufficiently ethnic and economic discrimination and the prevalence of illegal abortion. Therefore, in 1970 the four states Hawaii, Alaska, New York, and Washington, in the order named, removed abortion from the criminal code and made it an ordinary medical decision between doctor and patient. Three of the four states instituted such administrative restrictions as a residency requirement and permission of spouse. On July 1, 1970, New York State implemented the most liberal abortion law in the world. It contains no requirement of residency, age, marital status, or permission of spouse. Any woman less than twenty-four weeks pregnant is allowed abortion if she wishes it. The procedure must be performed by a physician licensed to practice in New York State, in a facility approved by the State Board of Health when done outside of New York City and by the City Board of Health within the City. The new law specifies that a physician is not required to perform an abortion and no hospital must make its facilities available for abortion. Fifteen of the sixteen states that have liberalized abortion have done so through legislative action. The sixteenth, Washington, accomplished it by popular ballot on November 3, 1970, when abortion was removed from the criminal code by 56 per cent of the electorate.

By 1972 the United States Supreme Court is likely to have rendered a decision on the legality of two state abortion statutes. Texas and Georgia cases had been placed on the fall docket of 1971. Texas still had the old statute, permitting abortion only to save life, while Georgia was one of twelve states with an A.L.I. type of partially liberalized statute.

What Has Been Accomplished by Liberalizing Abortion Laws?

In the first place, in most jurisdictions where the law remains unchanged there is a more liberal interpretation of statutes previously believed utterly restrictive. And in such states as California, with a partially liberalized law, each year the interpretation by the medical and legal professions is broadened to permit more legal abortions. The California figures were 6000 in 1968, 16,000 in 1969, 70,000 in 1970, and 110,000 estimated for 1971. I estimate that the annual 8000 legal abortions in the United States before 1967 increased to at least 400,000 in 1971.

Accurate figures are available from the Health Services Administration of the City of New York for abortions performed within the City for the first twelve months under the new state statute: 165,000 legal abortions were performed in hospitals and free-standing abortion clinics certified by the City. Abortion in a physician's office is not permitted. Sixteen per cent were performed in municipal hospitals, 16 per cent in special outpatient abortion clinics, and the remainder in private and community hospitals. Fifty-five per cent of the patients were from out of state. Fifty-four per cent were single, 16 per cent widowed, divorced, or separated, and 32 per cent married. The largest age group was twenty to twenty-four (37 per cent); the second largest was fifteen to nineteen (23 per cent). The ethnic composition was white, 74 per cent; non-white, 22 per cent; and Puerto Rican, 4 per cent, but for those who were residents of New York City, the proportion was white, 48 per cent; non-white, 42 per cent; and Puerto Rican, 10 per cent. Fifty-seven per cent of the total 165,000 were for a first pregnancy and 9 per cent for the fifth or greater. Three-quarters of the pregnancies were twelve weeks or less when aborted and 3 per cent were more than twenty weeks. There were eight deaths, six among the one quarter of the patients more than twelve weeks pregnant. The death rate was computed at 5.3 per 100,000 abortions.

These are the basic facts. What interpretation can be placed upon them? First, socioeconomic, ethnic discrimination in abortion seems to have been virtually eliminated. When 42 per cent of the abortions done for New York City residents were performed on nonwhites who comprise 18 per cent of the population, and 10 per cent on Puerto Ricans, who are 8 per cent of the population, it is clear that the poverty-ethnic ban on legal abortion has been lifted. Another way of expressing this is to point out that among New York City residents there are six legal abortions for every ten black births, four for every ten white births and three for every ten Puerto Rican births. Abortions in the municipal hospitals and on the wards of community hospitals are largely paid for by Medicaid. Fees in the free-standing outpatient abortion clinics are $150 to $200. They only abort women pregnant twelve weeks or less.

Private-patient hospital abortions are likely to cost $500 to $600, the expense about equally divided between physician and hospital. There is every prospect that competition will reduce this cost substantially.

There are several nonprofit referral agencies which potential patients may contact. If they reside in a state where the laws are still restrictive and enforced they can be referred to a liberal state in the area which has no residency requirement. A country-wide network of Clergyman Abortion Counseling units is available, as well as referring Planned Parenthood affiliates in over 190 cities.

Secondly, but of primary importance, lives are being saved. The estimated mortality rate from illegal abortion is 100 per 100,000 operations, in contrast to 5.3 for legal abortion in New York City. Dr. Milton Halpern, the Chief Medical Examiner, reports that there were seven deaths in New York City from illegal abortions during the first three months of the new law and none in the succeeding nine months, after the law was thoroughly implemented. A maternal mortality rate includes deaths from abortion, legal and illegal; abortions form a significant component of pregnancy deaths. This is illustrated by recent New York City statistics. The maternal mortality per 100,000 live births was 54 from October 1969 to March 1970, and was reduced to 26 since the new abortion law, from March 1970 to October 1971. There is further evidence that illegal abortions in New York are decreasing, since admissions to hospitals for incomplete abortions have decreased almost 50 per cent in the past year. It was common for abortion to be initiated by the patient herself or a paramedical person and for the process to be incomplete, the fetus being passed with all or part of the placenta remaining in the uterus. Such a patient would seek hospital admission for completion of the incomplete abortion. However, some incomplete abortions are an aftermath of spontaneous abortion.

Opposition to Abortion

Even though liberalized abortion appears to be functioning successfully as measured by several parameters, its success has not silenced the vocal opposition. There are many sincere individuals who equate abortion with murder and on these grounds never find it justifiable. Others feel that abortion is ethically immoral unless dictated by serious medical necessity and oppose it on socioeconomic grounds. There is the unsubstantiated claim that legal abortion is frequently followed by serious psychiatric complications. Perhaps this may be true in isolated cases in which the operation is accompanied by a patient's deep sense of guilt. Certainly no unprejudiced study has proved unfavorable psychic reactions to be common.

Those who favor a liberal abortion policy recognize that abortion is not to be accepted as the first line of defense against unwanted conception. The primary defense should and must be the consistent use of effective contraception. However, those who support liberal abortion feel that a back-up procedure to failed contraception, or failure to use contraception, is essential. Dangerous, discriminatory illegal abortion must be eliminated. Furthermore, in this era of overpopulation each child should be granted the birthright of being born gleefully wanted.

The argument continues. However, it appears to me that abortion will become partially or completely liberalized in all fifty states within the next decade either by legislative or court action. Both medical and public-health groups favor it as well as the major religious groups, except for the Catholics. When those who are still doubtful examine the good results they should become protagonists.

The Task Ahead

There are three medical issues which need to be stressed. First, contraception is psychically and physically to be much preferred to abortion for the prevention of an unwanted birth.

Second, the decision to have abortion should not be taken lightly, and if doubts are present in the individual about its wisdom consultation with an understanding counselor—physician, minister, social worker, or empathetic layman—is prudent.

Third, when once the decision is made, implement it at once. The earlier in pregnancy abortion is done the simpler and safer the procedure. Abortions at less than twelve weeks are far quicker, more free of risk, and less expensive than those beyond twelve weeks.

Abortion Techniques

When pregnancy is less than twelve weeks either D and C or uterine aspiration is performed vaginally. Both procedures are discussed under "incomplete abortion" on page 139.

Aspiration is rapidly replacing the previously standard technique of D and C. Among more than 137,000 abortions performed vaginally in New York City, July 1, 1970 to July 1, 1971, 63 per cent were by aspiration, the remainder by D and C. Uterine aspiration may be done without anesthesia in pregnancies less than eight or nine weeks. A small plastic cannula is inserted through the undilated cervical canal and suction applied. More usually, even in early pregnancies, a local anesthetic solution, a cocaine derivative, is injected on both sides of the cervix, which paralyzes and numbs its nerves. This permits cervical dilatation with little or no pain, and only slight discomfort from the aspiration procedure within the uterus itself. Aspiration without anesthesia or with local anesthesia permits the patient to leave the hospital or clinic in a half hour or at most two hours. A general anesthetic, usually an intravenous injection, postpones the patient's discharge for four to six hours. It requires nearly that long for the anesthetic to wear off completely.

A D and C is either done under a local or general anesthetic. The bleeding is usually more with D and C than with uterine aspiration. Discharge within one to several hours is also now rather generally permitted after a D and C.

No operation is free of potential complications, and D and C and aspiration evacuation are no exceptions. Among the complications there may be hemorrhage, perforation of the uterus by an instrument, or removal of only part of the placenta resulting in an incomplete abortion. The first two are likely to require emergency hospitalization for treatment. Incomplete emptying of the uterus would assert itself by bleeding and cramps one or several days after the abortion. Another possible complication may be the development of fever from infection.

Ordinarily convalescence from early abortion is rapid and complete. Perhaps the doctor will instruct you to laze about the house for two days. A douche is unnecessary, unwise, and usually forbidden. A shower is preferable to a bath for the first forty-eight hours. If there is bleeding, not just staining, particularly with cramps or passage of clots, or the appearance of fever over 100° F., notify your doctor promptly.

After twelve weeks of pregnancy, the conceptus is usually too large to permit emptying the uterus with ease and safety by aspiration or by a D and C. The technique now used in 90 per cent of such cases is salting out. However, salting out is technically difficult before the sixteenth week. Therefore if the patient is first seen at thirteen or fourteen weeks it is likely the operation will be postponed two or three weeks. We briefly discussed salting out on page 129 while discussing a dead fetus, but here I should like to go into more detail. A long injection type of needle is introduced under local anesthesia through the abdominal wall just below the navel into the uterine cavity. Frequently a narrow stiff tube of plastic, a catheter, is threaded through the needle and the needle withdrawn, leaving the catheter in place in the amniotic sac within the uterus. About a half-pint of amniotic fluid is withdrawn and an equal amount of a strong salt (20 per cent) or glucose (50 per cent) solution is injected through the needle or catheter, which is then also withdrawn. The fetus dies promptly and contractions of the uterus commence within twenty-four hours, and in six hours or less the patient miscarries spontaneously.

Less frequently hysterotomy is done to terminate second trimester pregnancies. A small abdominal incision is made under anesthesia, the uterus incised and evacuated; the operation is virtually a miniature

Cesarean section. As long as the abdomen is open, if the condition which necessitated interruption of pregnancy is destined never to improve sufficiently to render pregnancy safe and the couple consents, or the couple has determined they will never want another child, sterilization is carried out at the same time. The sterilization part of the procedure is simple and quick; each Fallopian tube, or oviduct, is tied and severed. By interrupting the pathway, a permanent roadblock is created, so that the egg can no longer descend to meet the sperm, nor can the sperm ascend to meet the egg. Such a sterilization technique removes no tissue; neither ovulation, menstruation, nor the production of hormones is altered. Therefore there is no possible effect on body weight or sexual functions, except that coitus can be practiced without chance of pregnancy.

Use of Rhogam

Any patient who is Rh negative and who was impregnated by an Rh positive male should receive Rhogam to prevent possible Rh sensitization after induced abortion or completion of an incomplete abortion. The necessity is less absolute after uncomplicated spontaneous abortion, though nevertheless a worthwhile precaution. Use of Rhogam will be discussed in detail when considering erythroblastosis on page 330.

After Abortion

Unless sterilization is carried out at the time of abortion, effective contraception should be employed as soon as intercourse is resumed. Menses are likely to reappear four to six weeks after abortion. Abstinence should be practiced for at least one week or until all staining disappears.

Research on a New Method of Abortion

The ideal method of abortion would be to produce uterine contractions at any stage of pregnancy by administering a drug and stimulating the uterus to evacuate itself. This would be medical abortion in contrast to the surgical methods described above. The idea of medical abortion is ancient, and the pharmacology of every century is replete with methods that do not work unless they make the woman so ill that her life is endangered at the same time. Women plagued with an unwanted pregnancy in the days of Imperial Rome, according to Soranus, were prescribed a series of oral medications, debilitating enemas, hot baths, rides in an ox-cart over rutted streets, and venesection, bleeding until they fainted. Soranus neglects to state how often the vigorous therapy worked and how many Roman matrons survived it. Modern pharmacopias list ergot and quinine as abortifacients. However, neither terminates a normal, developing pregnancy; they may cause evacuation of a defective pregnancy a day or two before nature would have done it.

When injected, a drug extracted from the pituitary gland, pituitrin, and more recently synthesized as oxytocin, will initiate labor near term. But it is useless in producing abortion unless administered in dangerously high dosage.

In the early 1930s Dr. Raphael Kurzrok noted that whenever he was doing an artificial insemination and semen gained entrance into the uterine cavity, the uterus reacted with violent contractions and virtually spewed the fluid out of the cervix. Next he removed a small strip of uterine muscle at Cesarean section, suspended it in a water bath and added semen. The semen stimulated the uterus to contract vigorously. A few years later the Swedish Nobel laureate in biochemistry Ulf von Euler took up the problem where Kurzrok had left off. He thought the yet-to-be-identified substance was formed by the male prostate gland and was found only in its fluid and therefore named it "prostaglandin." Subsequent research by von Euler and several Americans has shown that there are at least fourteen different prostaglandins with various pharmacologic actions found in several organs including the uterus. These remarkable chemicals are long-chain fatty acids. Three, E_1, E_2, and F_2 alpha, act upon uterine muscle causing contractions. Currently the prostaglandins are given, as is intravenous glucose, by the constant-drip method into a vein, and the abortion results are extremely promising. Dr. Sultan Karim of Makerere University in Uganda aborted fourteen out of fifteen pregnancies ranging for nine to twenty-two weeks. The whole procedure took from four to twenty-seven hours. D. M. P. Embrey of Oxford succeeded in twenty-eight out of thirty cases with pregnancies from nine to twenty-eight weeks, with infusions running six to sixty hours. There is reason to believe that the prostaglandins may be effective when given by mouth or by instillation as a suppository in the vagina, where they are readily absorbed. Either of these avenues of administration would be simpler than the intravenous route. It is perfectly possible that abortion may become an at-home do-it-yourself procedure in several years. What a boon that would be.

Premature Labor

When the newborn infant weighs less than 5½ pounds (2500 grams) or more than 2 pounds, 3 ounces (1000 grams), it is considered to be a premature infant. When the baby weighs between 2 pounds, 3 ounces and 1 pound, 1½ ounces (500 grams) it is classified as immature. All fetuses with birth weights less than 1 pound, 1½ ounces are designated as abortions. In these definitions no reference is made to the duration of pregnancy. This is because duration of pregnancy is so difficult to determine with exactitude, since menstrual periods are so variable and menstrual and coital data are frequently so unreliable. Ordinarily a 5½-pound baby is about four weeks from its expected delivery date and a 1-pound infant is delivered around the twentieth week of pregnancy.

Of all babies born in the United States 7.7 per cent weigh between 2 pounds, 3 ounces and 5½ pounds. The incidence varies with the socio-economic conditions and the race. As stated earlier in this book, in the Scottish study the most privileged tenth of the population had a 4 per cent prematurity rate and the less privileged, 8 per cent. In the United States the white incidence of prematurity is 6.8 per cent and the nonwhite, 12.9 per cent. Forty-nine per cent of twins weigh less than 5½ pounds at birth; this high rate of prematurity arises from two causes: the usual earlier termination of twin pregnancies over single pregnancies (258 versus 280 days) and the fact that two infants in the uterus are less well nourished than one.

Other causes of prematurity are toxemia of pregnancy, placenta praevia, premature separation of the placenta, maternal illness with a severe infection, such as pneumonia or untreated syphilis, but in 60 per cent of cases no obvious reason exists.

In these cases an apparently normal patient, most frequently a primipara (a woman who is bearing her first child), either begins labor or, in about a third of the cases, ruptures her membranes when approximately more than twenty weeks pregnant, but less than thirty-six. Many years ago I studied the fetal membranes in such cases to determine if they had an abnormally low bursting point. I found the strength of the membranes the same as in term births. Occasionally postpartum examination will reveal some congenital abnormality of the uterus or cervix as the cause, such as a bicornuate, or double, uterus (a uterus with a septum or a tissue partition down its middle), or a cervical tumor, such as a low fibroid.

When labor starts there is nothing that will stop it with certainty. Occasionally it stops of its own accord. Some interesting reports have appeared with the successful use of intravenous alcohol given by a continuous-drip technique over many hours. The good results are said to be due to action on the pituitary gland, the high blood level of alcohol preventing it from elaborating and discharging pituitrin, the chemical hormone which stimulates uterine contractions. Apparently in some instances, when the alcohol is stopped, the trigger mechanism which initiated labor is no longer sprung. The drug Diazoxide, a smooth-muscle relaxant, is also being studied for its ability to halt premature labor. If the patient ruptures membranes prematurely, and labor has not yet begun, the physician keeps her flat in bed, perhaps on antibiotics, hoping that the onset of labor will postpone itself. Occasionally it does for several essential weeks.

There is a tendency in some patients for premature labor to recur; in others it is an isolated phenomenon in their reproductive careers. The labors themselves are not unusual, except for the fact that they are likely to be more rapid. The management of labor differs from term labors, as will be discussed in the chapter on labor. In some cases of repetitive premature labor or late abortion the patient may be found to suffer from a weakness of the uterine muscle where it encircles the uppermost part of the cervix. In medical terminology, the condition is termed "incompetent os syndrome." Diagnosis is made mainly on the basis of the patient's history. A typical history is repetitive abortions in mid-pregnancy or very premature labors in which the membranes rupture before labor commences. In the proper case, an operation can be performed to strengthen and support the weakened ring of muscle by a circular, constricting, broad, nonabsorbable suture. The operation is usually performed between the fourteenth and sixteenth weeks of pregnancy. Some obstetricians prefer to do the "circlage" procedure before the patient starts another pregnancy. A second type of operation is to cut out a wedge of cervix involving the lower uterine muscle. The wedge is like a slice of cake. The two cut edges are sewn together, constricting the opening where uterus and cervix join. This is always done in the nonpregnant state. These operations truly work miracles in cases correctly selected. Delivery may be by Cesarean section or vaginally, depending on the type of operation or the variety of suture material. The handling of such a complication requires the services of an experienced obstetrical-gynecological specialist. A recent study shows thirty-five living children in thirty-nine cases (90 per cent), while previous to the operation only 22 per cent of the patients' infants survived.

The unfortunate thing about a premature labor, whether its onset be spontaneous or the result of necessary termination of pregnancy prematurely is the poor fetal survival rate in the very low-weight categories.

At Kings County Hospital in Brooklyn 10 per cent of white babies weighing 2 pounds survived; 20 per cent of those weighing 2 pounds, 3 ounces; 40 per cent weighing 3 pounds; and two-thirds with a birth weight of 3 pounds, 5 ounces. When the birth weight reached 2500 grams (5½ pounds), 97 per cent survived, nearly the same survival rate for babies born with greater birthweights.

Nonwhite babies in the lower-weight categories have consistently better survival rates than white babies in the same weight groups. Newborn survival depends significantly upon two factors, birthweight and gestational age (by this is meant the length of the pregnancy). Nonwhite babies weigh about three-quarters of a pound less at term, at forty weeks, than white babies, and are proportionately smaller throughout pregnancy. White babies weighing between 2 pounds, 3 ounces and 3 pounds, 5 ounces have a gestational age of twenty-eight to thirty-one weeks, while nonwhite babies of the same weight have a gestational age of thirty to thirty-three weeks. The more advanced the gestational age, the more mature are the infant's vital organs—lungs, kidneys, liver. This explains why in the Kings County study, at a birth weight of 3 pounds, 5 ounces, two-thirds of the white babies survived, in contrast to four-fifths of the nonwhite infants.

About 80 per cent of early deaths in infants with premature weights occur within the first twenty-four hours and well over 90 per cent take place during the first week of life. Therefore survival of a "premie" beyond the first day carries a favorable prognosis and beyond the first week, an excellent one.

11

Diseases and Operations during Pregnancy

There is no illness to which the pregnant woman is immune, unless it be some menstrual disorder. It is not within the scope or intent of this book to consider each major deviation from normal health and discuss its effects on the course of the pregnancy, or, in turn, pregnancy's influence on the ordinary life cycle of every disease. Let us content ourselves with discussing some of the commoner major medical and surgical problems as they occur in a pregnant woman.

Heart Disease

In the course of the last three or four decades there has been a radical change in the physician's attitude toward heart disease and childbearing, as well as in his treatment of this complication. Today motherhood is denied only to women with the most severe degree of heart impairment. Previously it was not uncommon to perform therapeutic abortion in cases of only moderate severity. If therapeutic abortion is required it is done early, never after the sixteenth week. The strain then of abortion is as great as the strain of labor.

This change in attitude arises from the magnificent results obtained through modern advances in the management of pregnancy and labor in the cardiac patient. Today such cases are carried on calorie-restricted, low-salt diets so that weight gain is kept below that permitted normal pregnant women. Whenever there is evidence of retention of tissue fluid, kidney-stimulating drugs are administered to promote urinary excretion. Rest and freedom from physical effort are demanded. If more than minimal heart disease exists it is generally advised that the pregnant woman rest in bed ten hours each night and, in addition, that she lie down for a half hour after each meal. Light housework and walking on level ground is permitted, but climbing is restricted. No heavy housework or shopping is allowed. A live-in mother's helper is a great asset. Colds and other infections of the upper respiratory tract are treated with great respect in pregnant women with heart disease, and confinement to bed and antibiotics are promptly prescribed. Heart drugs of the digitalis series are given whenever indicated. Physicians have learned that cardiac patients do infinitely better if they are allowed to go into labor spontaneously at term and deliver vaginally, than if their pregnancies are terminated four or five weeks prematurely by Cesarean section, as used to be done. Today antibiotic drugs are given routinely to such patients during labor and the first few days thereafter, since infection and fever may penalize the damaged heart. If the heart shows the slightest evidence of losing its ability to carry on its intended function, labor, and at times delivery, is conducted in an oxygen tent. Pain-relief agents and anesthetics are carefully chosen and carefully given. It is also important to relieve the pregnant cardiac woman of fear and anxiety, which tend to make the pulse beat rapidly, which is bad for such a patient, particularly during labor. The best way to dissipate fear and anxiety is reassurance by frank discussion between the patient and doctor. Airing fears, in itself, helps dispel them. With such meticulous attention women with heart disease, except those with an advanced form of the malady, may be allowed several children. The extent of the heart lesion and the socioeconomic situation, whether or not the burden of housekeeping can be temporarily lifted, are potent factors influencing safe family size in the individual case. Tubal ligation (sterilization) is frequently performed on the cardiac patient after she has produced a small family. Usually it is carried out on the fourth or fifth day, rather than on the first day, as for a normal woman.

Sometimes, in the exceptional instance, heart surgery is carried out in indicated cases during pregnancy. Ordinarily such procedures are performed before conception and in the intervals between pregnancies.

Tuberculosis

If I were asked to name one of the most exciting advances in obstetrics, I would nominate the diagnosis and treatment of tuberculosis. If there is anything in the patient's history or physical examination to suggest arrested or active tuberculosis, the doctor will want a chest X-ray. The fetus can be well protected. If an old healed lesion is found on X-ray, the "wonder drug" isoniazid is prescribed as a prophylactic measure during the last few months of gestation to prevent the tuberculosis from being made active by delivery and the early postdelivery period. On the other hand, if physical examination, sputum tests, or X-ray reveals an active tuberculous infection, pregnancy is allowed to continue, and in most cases the woman can be treated successfully at home by a combination of three drugs: isoniazid, streptomycin, and para-aminosalicylic acid. This is a far cry from the situation a few years ago, when a large proportion of the active cases of tuberculosis discovered in early pregnancy had a therapeutic abortion and then went to a sanatorium for months or years.

Modern medicine has demonstrated that pregnancy offers no obstruction to the therapy and cure of tuberculosis. The patients are treated as though they were not pregnant; even lung surgery is performed if necessary.

Diabetes

Before the introduction of insulin in 1921 few diabetic women became pregnant, and when they did catastrophe often resulted. The death rate for both mother and infant was alarmingly high. With the use of insulin, diabetics have become normally fertile, and when the disease is kept under intelligent medical control pregnancy no longer threatens the mother's health or life. Dr. Priscilla White of Boston, a great authority on diabetes, reports 99.8 per cent maternal survival in a very large series of pregnant women with diabetes.

However, diabetes, even when properly controlled, still gives relatively unsatisfactory fetal results. The miscarriage ratio is only slightly elevated over that of nondiabetic women, but for not completely understood reasons the fetus of the diabetic woman has a tendency to die before labor during the late weeks of pregnancy. Since such a risk is greatest during the last two or three weeks, most physicians terminate the pregnancy of the diabetic three, four, or sometimes six weeks before the calculated term by either inducing labor or performing a Cesarean section. The best results are obtained if during pregnancy and delivery the patient is under the joint care of an expert in diabetes and an expert in obstetrics. To achieve optimum fetal results the mother is admitted to the hospital one or several weeks before the date chosen for delivery, depending upon the severity of her disease, in order to have the diabetes under exact control before the birth.

The baby of a diabetic mother, particularly the one born to a mother who has recently acquired diabetes, tends to be excessively large. Babies of diabetic mothers often have a difficult first forty-eight hours, primarily from respiratory problems, but when this period has passed they do as well as any other newborns. At first they require vigilant care by expert nurses and physicians. The congenital malformation rate is slightly increased by maternal diabetes.

Venereal Disease

The performance of a routine blood test for the diagnosis of syphilis, usually termed a "Wassermann," is made obligatory during pregnancy by the laws of most states. A positive test is assumed to be caused by a syphilitic infection—unless, in the rare case, it is proved due to some other medical condition. The test becomes positive four to six weeks after one contracts syphilis. Today's treatment of syphilis with penicillin is wonderfully rapid and effective compared to previous therapy with arsenic, mercury, and bismuth.

Six to nine million units of long-acting penicillin are given in divided doses by intramuscular injection. If the patient is allergic to penicillin two grams of erythromycin or tetracycline are given daily for fifteen days. Since cured syphilis bestows no immunity, reinfection is always possible. Treating the mother treats the baby in the uterus as well, since penicillin readily crosses the placental barrier, and the child is born totally free of any evidence of the disease. On the other hand, when syphilis in the mother remains undetected and untreated the child may die in the uterus, or, if born alive, will be gravely ill, showing the stigmata of congenital syphilis.

Gonorrhea may complicate pregnancy. However, in untreated cases its main effect on reproduction is to render some husbands or wives irreparably sterile. If the mother harbors the gonococcus, the causative organism, in the vagina or cervix it may cause pelvic infection after delivery or infect the eyes of the newborn during passage through the lower birth canal. As will be detailed in the chapter on the newborn, preventive measures frequently are carried out as a routine within a few minutes of birth on every baby, whether it be born to a bishop's wife or a prostitute. The presence of the gonococcus in pregnancy is sometimes established by stained smears examined microscopically, but more often by bacterial cultures from the cervix, urethra, vagina, and rectum. Treatment is ordinarily a daily intramuscular injection of 2.4 million units of procaine penicillin for two to four days. Other antibiotics are also effective if penicillin sensitivity precludes its use. Cured gonorrhea also establishes no immunity. Obstetrical clinics report a 5- to 6-per cent incidence of positive gonococcus cultures.

During the past few years there has been a disturbing increase in syphilis and gonorrhea. Very likely this bespeaks greater premarital and perhaps extramarital sexual activity, as well as less reliance on the condom, which is not only an excellent prophylactic against unwanted pregnancy, but an excellent prophylactic against the dissemination and acquisition of venereal infection. Two statistics highlight the gravity of the problem during the past decade. The Los Angeles County Hospital has observed a sixfold increase in the incidence of congenital syphilis, wholly preventable if the mothers had presented themselves for adequate prenatal diagnostic care. It is estimated that the number of cases of gonorrhea contracted each year in the United States totals one and a half million.

German Measles (Rubella)

It was neither known nor suspected until 1941 that the very mild and common infectious disease, German measles, or rubella, was capable of causing serious congenital abnormalities in the unborn fetus if its mother contracted the disease during early pregnancy. An Australian ophthalmologist named Gregg was suddenly presented with a remarkable number of infants with congenital cataracts of the eye, born to the wives of soldiers living in the vicinity of neighboring army camps. By diligent sleuthing he discovered that all of the mothers had had German measles in very early pregnancy. Studies of other rubella epidemics all over the world showed that many other fetal defects could result from German measles during pregnancy, such as other eye lesions besides cataracts, heart malformations, deafness, microcephaly (pin-head), mental retardation, slowing of intrauterine growth, and chromosomal changes. In addition, German measles caused an increased incidence of miscarriages and stillbirths. The type of abnormality had relationship to the week of pregnancy when rubella occurred. The earliest weeks lead most frequently to eye difficulties, the sixth or seventh week to malformation of the heart and later infections to deafness. Infection after the thirteenth week, the end of the third month, left little likelihood of any major malformation, but resulted in impaired health in some children.

There has been much division of opinion concerning the incidence of fetal damage. All agree that some women with German measles even in very early pregnancy have completely normal babies and that the severity of the mother's illness bears no relationship to either the occurrence of fetal abnormalities or their severity. The general consensus is that infection during the first four weeks of pregnancy (until the conclusion of the sixth week after the last period) causes at least 50 per cent of damaged infants or fetal deaths; during the next two weeks the incidence drops to about 25 per cent, and during the third month to perhaps 15 per cent.

What is German measles, or rubella? A virus infection with an incubation period of one to three weeks, the disease begins with slight fever, catarrhal symptoms, sore throat, pains in the legs. A day or two later a general pinkish body rash appears. Swollen glands soon become palpable. Within a few days to a week the rash disappears without scaling of the skin. The disease is often so mild that the victim does not know she has had it, and furthermore, other medical ailments are so similar that they may be misdiagnosed as German measles. Misdiagnosis is less likely during an epidemic. German measles most frequently occurs in children since about 85 per cent of the adult population is already immunized by previous infection. There is geographic variation in susceptibility. Ten to 20 per cent of adult women in the United States are susceptible to rubella, but in the Far Western states the figure is 50 to 75 per cent. Having had the disease bestows permanent immunity. However, since several minor diseases mimic rubella, some who think they have had it did not and vice versa. Very severe epidemics occur about every twenty-five to thirty years and mild epidemics every eight to ten years. The United States had a very severe epidemic in 1964–1965. In Connecticut alone there were 200,000 cases of rubella during the winter and spring of 1964–1965 in a total population of 2,500,000. It is estimated that throughout the country the 1964–1965 epidemic caused 8000 stillbirths and at least 20,000 children born with birth defects.

How does such a mild disease do so much fetal damage? The causative agent is a specific virus which causes a viremia, that is, causes the mother's blood to swarm with these ultramicroscopic organisms. The virus of rubella, like other viruses, passes from the mother's blood via the placenta to the fetus. If this occurs very early in pregnancy, it overwhelms the fetus since it has not yet developed general immune mechanisms to defend itself adequately. The organ system most damaged is probably the one which at that time is making its greatest growth spurt in the blueprint of fetal development.

There are two new developments which will have an important impact on the management of rubella and pregnancy.

In 1967 the National Institutes of Health in Washington developed the hemagglutination inhibition (HI) test, which determines whether one has previously acquired immunity to rubella through having had German measles. Addition of a special preparation of rubella virus to a suspension of newly hatched chicks' red blood cells causes the cells to clump together. However, if the virus is first combined with the blood serum to be tested and then added to the chick blood-cell suspension, and if no clumping occurs, it proves antibodies were present in the blood specimen and immunity exists. The patient's antibodies neutralized the virus and prevented red-blood-cell clumping. If clumping occurs it demonstrates the absence of antibodies in the test specimen and the lack of immunity.

The HI test has two practical applications. Ideally the absence or presence of immunity to rubella should be determined for every woman before contemplating pregnancy. If positive the test will give her a feeling of reassurance, but if she is not immune she is forewarned and, as will be discussed later in this section, measles vaccine is probably advisable. If there is the possibility that she may be pregnant and the test is negative, precautions should be taken against acquiring rubella. For example, if you are less than three months pregnant and some relative or friend gets German measles, be tough and isolate yourself from him and his recent contacts, particularly children. In the presence of an epidemic of rubella a nonimmune teacher with the possibility of pregnancy should temporarily abandon the classroom.

A second and important use of the new test is its ability to establish a positive diagnosis of rubella if there is doubt. Blood taken within four to five days of the appearance of the rash (the earlier the better) is still negative or weakly positive for antibodies. Then if the test is repeated in one week or longer, it will have become strongly positive if the diagnosis is German measles. In other words, the test goes from negative to positive, or if by the time blood is taken there is already a weakly positive test, in the week's interval, it will have become strongly positive. The blood level, or titer, of antibodies will have risen substantially.

The second important development in the field is a protective vaccine. Three of the commercial vaccines are made from a strain of virus developed by the Division of Biologic Standards of the National Institutes of Health at Bethesda and a fourth from a case of German measles at "Cendehill," France, properly named Cendevax. All are attenuated live-virus vaccines. The live virus is grown in a cell culture of monkey or dog kidney or of duck embryo, and transplanted to new uninfected cell cultures thirty to sixty times, until the repeated passages have sufficiently weakened its virulence. Then when injected into a person who is not already immune it either causes no disease or at the most a minimal attack which is not contagious to others. The vaccine creates an effective titer of antibodies, the individual developing immunity to rubella. There is uncertainty how long vaccine-induced immunity to rubella lasts. It appears that it is not permanent like the immunity acquired by infection. For if a vaccinated person after a few years is exposed to a case of German measles the antibody titer may go up, suggesting a new viremia, or circulating virus in the blood, even though the exposed individual shows no clinical signs of the infection. It is not known whether the viremia under these circumstances may affect the fetus.

There are two schools of thought in regard to mass vaccination programs. The American plan is to vaccinate all boys and girls between the ages of four and seven years, and when this has been accomplished, it is believed, the disease will be virtually eliminated. If it is not eliminated, adolescent girls may have to be given a booster shot to increase the antibody titer in preparation for potential motherhood. England seems to favor no vaccination in childhood, allowing a large proportion of the population to be infected and to acquire natural immunity, and then testing all adolescent girls and vaccinating those who are negative. Young matrons whose tests are negative should be vaccinated and strictly warned against pregnancy for a minimum of ninety days after vaccination.

What practical conclusions can be drawn for the present?

1. If there is a local vaccination program against German measles, have your children participate.

2. In the meantime do not isolate your children from individuals with German measles and be happy if they catch it. If there is doubt as to whether it is German measles get an accurate diagnosis by antibody titers.

3. If you are contemplating a family, have yourself tested. If the test is negative, be vaccinated. Do it immediately postpartum, when you are undoubtedly taking precautions to avoid pregnancy. At other times, postpone pregnancy by using effective contraception for three months after vaccination.

At one time it was thought advisable to give an injection of gamma globulin to a pregnant woman who had been exposed to German measles. The consensus of experts is opposed to its use. It rarely, if ever, prevents the disease but may lessen its severity sufficiently to confuse the diagnosis —which is no solution to the problem.

What ought you to do if you are unfortunate enough to have contracted German measles during the first three months of pregnancy, the diagnosis having been verified either by the new antibody test or by a physician knowledgeable in exanthemata (infection diseases associated with a rash)? The choice lies between taking your chances and continuing pregnancy or having an abortion. As I have stated, abortion done in a hospital by a well-trained physician carries virtually no operative risk. Which course to pursue will depend on such factors as your religious beliefs, your age, the fertility of your marriage, and the size of your family. You and your husband should consult your obstetrician at once and on the basis of these multiple factors explore what is the proper decision for you.

In nearly every state, even in states with highly restrictive statutes, abortion is done legally for rubella. If you live in one of the benighted states where this is not the case, make arrangements in a neighboring state. No doubt you will have to go to a non-Catholic hospital, for I know of none which permits abortion for any cause. If your own physician is resistant to performing abortion for proved rubella, you have every ethical reason to consult another physician who does not share his opinion.

As for my own feelings, I believe that in almost every instance abortion should certainly be done if verified German measles occurs in the first two months of pregnancy; if between two and three months it is prudent to have an abortion, but the necessity is less urgent. After three months abortion is probably unnecessary.

Poliomyelitis

With the widespread use of vaccines, infantile paralysis is becoming a rarity in the United States. Previous to the vaccine era, it had been noted that pregnant women were not only more susceptible to a polio infection, but the death rate from the infection was higher among them. Also, fetal loss was about 33 per cent. If a pregnant woman has not previously been immunized against polio she should be immunized at once. Both the Salk and the Sabin vaccines are safe for immunization during pregnancy.

Influenza

There is no evidence that influenza causes congenital malformations. However, a pregnant woman is more susceptible to the infection, especially during epidemics. Furthermore, the disease victim is more likely to develop lung complications during pregnancy. Therefore, a pregnant woman should isolate herself if possible from other influenza sufferers. Vaccination against influenza is probably of value during pregnancy, especially during an epidemic or when one is anticipated.

Other Viral Infections

True measles, chicken pox, mumps, scarlet fever, glandular fever (acute infectious mononucleosis), and whooping cough apparently do not affect the normality of the fetus, regardless of the week in pregnancy when the illness occurs. As a matter of fact, the only viruses implicated in this respect are German measles virus, the coxsackie virus which causes cytomegalic disease, and certain strains of herpes virus. The latter two viral infections are quite uncommon.

Toxoplasmosis

A parasitic disease acquired from eating raw or uncooked meat and occasionally from household pets. It is normally very mild in its manifestations in the adult, frequently mimicking flu but associated with swollen glands. In its acute stage the parasite can be transmitted to the fetus by transplacental migration and causes serious damage often resulting in abortion, prematurity, or death. Surviving children show some disability, largely damage to the eyes or brain. A study in West Berlin found evidence of toxoplasmosis in 13 per cent of the pregnant women tested for the parasite and serious damage to 4.6 per cent of the pregnancies in the women with positive tests. In other studies positive tests have been reported in 13 to 59 per cent of the populations surveyed. In most instances the symptoms are so mild that a person does not know when he is infected. In the active phase of toxoplasmosis the parasite can be stained in centrifuged body fluids. There is evidence that one baby in every 1000 in the United States is born with congenital toxoplasmosis.

Once a woman has acquired toxoplasmosis and developed antibodies against it she cannot transmit the parasite to her fetus. Similarly, if a mother has given birth to a toxoplasmic child she can be assured that all subsequent children will be free of the disease. Only acute infection, just before or during pregnancy, makes the fetus vulnerable, and some recent studies indicate that the disease may be transmitted only in the last six months of pregnancy. To prevent acquiring the disease during the period when the fetus is vulnerable, a pregnant woman who has never had toxoplasmosis should avoid eating raw or rare meat.

Immunization of the Fetus

Antibodies resulting from childhood diseases which the mother contracted previous to conception remain circulating in her blood for an indefinite period, and are transferred via the placenta to the fetus in each pregnancy. As a result, the infant is born with immunity to a disease to which the mother has become immune. The duration of this type of acquired immunity in the child is brief, lasting from three to six months. An exception to this general rule is whooping cough, for even though the mother has had the illness, most newborns are highly susceptible.

Surgical Emergencies

Surgical emergencies arising during pregnancy are usually treated as though the patient were not pregnant. If a surgeon feels that he would be compelled to operate if the woman were not pregnant, he will usually operate when she is pregnant. This generalization is particularly true for appendicitis, acute gall-bladder conditions, which are particularly frequent during pregnancy, strangulated hernia, thrombosed hemorrhoid, kidney stone, etc. On the other hand, if the surgical problem presents no emergency, such as removal of tonsils, cure of hemorrhoids, repair of a simple, unstrangulated hernia, plastic operations on the vagina for loss of urinary control or descent of the pelvic structures, surgery is better postponed until three months or more after delivery.

Abdominal operations on the reproductive organs are sometimes necessary during pregnancy; the commonest is removal of a cyst of the ovary, or a fibroid tumor attached to the uterus by a slim stalk about which the tumor may twist. If possible, one postpones removing an ovarian cyst until after the eighth to twelfth week since the corpus luteum of pregnancy may be in the cystic ovary, and its removal very early in pregnancy causes abortion in many cases. Removal of the ovary containing the corpus luteum (the gland formed at the site of the ruptured Graafian follicle) after the twelfth week is completely safe.

Otherwise operations during pregnancy are unlikely to cause abortion or premature labor, or affect the fetus in any way. The fetus tolerates amazingly well anesthetics which do not seriously reduce the oxygen level in the maternal blood.

Dental extractions or fillings may be performed whenever indicated. Local anesthesia is preferred to general anesthesia. If the latter is necessary during pregnancy, most physicians prefer sodium pentothal, cyclopropane, or ether to plain nitrous oxide, the dentist's "laughing gas."

Psychiatric Illness

Emotional difficulties of varying intensity may first assert themselves during pregnancy, or existing emotional illness may be aggravated by pregnancy. Treatment is not affected by the fact that the woman is pregnant. A psychiatrist or a psychiatric clinic should be consulted and therapy followed as advised. Tranquilizers, shock, or even hospitalization may be recommended just as though the patient were not pregnant.

It is not uncommon for a woman to become quite depressed, tearful, and irritable in early pregnancy, particularly if she is ambivalent or hostile to the pregnancy. Her mood swing may be aggravated by queasiness or nausea. As she feels better physically and adjusts herself to the thought of having a baby, the mood clears and she becomes herself again.

Fear and apprehension of the unknown certainty apply to having a baby. To lessen such concerns by providing reliable information on what lies ahead is the function of a book like this one. However, there is no substitute for a frank discussion with your doctor. Fear of illness and death is little justified on the basis of recent statistics. Never in history has there been a safer time to give birth. If one removes from the figures illegal abortion deaths and preventable deaths charged to failure to seek or obtain adequate prenatal care, it becomes apparent that one faces only a minuscule mortality risk from pregnancy and delivery, little higher than from auto accidents. Pain in labor can be minimized by psychoprophylactic childbirth or by drugs, or by a combination of both. Fear of something happening to the baby is justified, but the brighter side of the picture is that after you reach the twenty-eighth week of pregnancy you have better than 97 chances in 100 of producing a living, surviving baby and more than a 99 per cent chance that the infant will be born with no serious abnormality. The odds, especially with good care, are vastly in your favor. Nevertheless, if you have apprehensions do not incubate them by keeping them to yourself. Ventilate them to an expert—your doctor. It is only fair to him, as well as yourself.

12

The Mechanics of Labor

A Labor Pain

The neophyte always wonders how she will know when labor actually begins. Can she distinguish the pains of childbirth from intestinal cramps or an ordinary backache? The throes of labor are unique for several reasons. In the first place, unlike other pains, they rise in *slow crescendo*, remain *fortissimo* for a brief period, and close in moderate *diminuendo*; or they are like a scale* that makes a leisurely ascent to its high tone and is held aloft for a few beats before the several descending notes are sung. The transcription of a labor pain into music would be:

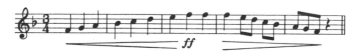

while ordinary pain would be scored

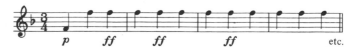

* It has been suggested by Mrs. Susan Peterson, a reader of a previous edition of this book, that a major scale does not convey the "grinding and twisting" sensation of a labor pain. For musically literate readers she offers this transcription as "a probably more accurate and certainly more contemporary idiom":

Labor Pain for Two Oboes

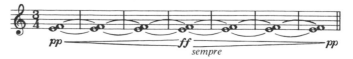

Another distinctive feature is that a labor pain is always associated with a contraction of the uterus. If a woman feels her abdomen during the acme of such a pain, she notices a large, board-firm mass, which becomes a softish, indentable mass once again when the pain is over. The chief characteristic of these pains is their rhythmic nature, their recurrence at fixed intervals. As labor progresses, the interval from the beginning of one pain to the beginning of the next is gradually shortened from fifteen or twenty minutes at the onset to three or four minutes when labor is well under way. In addition, the total length of an individual pain increases from less than half a minute at the start to more than a minute toward the end. Unlike most pains, labor pains have a complete remission between them, a happy respite in which the patient is comfortable. Usually labor pains occur first in the small of the back and after a few hours migrate down the flanks to center in the whole lower abdomen. Many compare them to exaggerated menstrual cramps, which are grinding and twisting in type. The pinkish vaginal discharge which ordinarily accompanies the pains of true labor is termed "show." It is blood-tinged mucus dislodged from the cervix as the latter begins to dilate. Sometimes this normal show, which is to be distinguished from abnormal bleeding (frank, undiluted blood), anticipates the onset of labor by a day or more.

False Labor

As I have already mentioned in Chapter 9, true labor may be preceded by one or several discouraging bouts of false labor, especially in women who have already borne children.

Cause Not Known

What causes labor to begin? Why does it start approximately 280 days after the first day of the last menstrual period? These are simple and definite questions which no one as yet can answer. From the appearance and disappearance of the hard abdominal mass, we know that contractions of the uterus occur irregularly throughout pregnancy (Braxton-Hicks contractions), but suddenly, for no explicable reason, these painless contractions become regular and painful; then labor has begun. Quite commonly, particularly in early labor, the entrance of the obstetrician is followed by a temporary lull in the intensity and frequency of pains.

Time of Day

Almost everyone will attest that the stork is a creature with perverse habits, preferring nocturnal to diurnal flights. Actually, this is not true; it just seems true. Being up at three in the morning to receive a "bundle from heaven" is an event, but missing lunch just an occurrence.

Furthermore, since many labors last for ten to twelve hours, they are likely either to begin or to end at night. John forgets that John, Jr., was born at 10 a.m., but he will not forget the snowy drive to the hospital at 3 a.m.

A biometrician placed this problem under scientific scrutiny and analyzed the birth hour for 134,335 deliveries which occurred in Nürnberg. The distribution in six-hour periods was approximately the same in each:

Time Period	Per Cent	Time Period	Per Cent
6:00 a.m. to 12 noon	25.85	6:00 p.m. to 12 midnight	24.25
12 noon to 6:00 p.m.	22.39	12 midnight to 6:00 a.m.	27.51
Total—(6:00 a.m. to 6:00 p.m.)	48.24	Total—(6:00 p.m. to 6:00 a.m.)	51.76

Time of Year

The United States Public Health Service publishes the birth and death statistics for this country annually, data most accurately prepared by the National Center for Health Statistics.

The material is so carefully checked and counterchecked that the latest volume is always at least eighteen months behind the current date.

The live births in a recent year were distributed monthly as follows, the number for the average months being placed at 100, making the year's total 1200, each month's birth figure being adjusted for the length of the month.

January	97.4
February	99.6
March	99.6
April	95.3
May	93.3
June	98.0
July	103.6
August	105.1
September	107.8
October	102.5
November	99.3
December	99.8

The four late summer and early fall months (July-October) have the greatest number of births (34.9 per cent), which means that the greatest number of conceptions occur in late fall and early winter.

Rupture of the Membranes

In half the deliveries the bag of waters formed by the fetal membranes ruptures during the last hours of labor. Sometimes it remains intact to the very end, and the obstetrician has to speed the labor by rupturing it. The membranes are insensitive and can be punctured without anesthesia. A pointed instrument is introduced into the vagina and, guided by the doctor's fingers, tears a snag in them.

At the rupture of the membranes varying amounts of fluid immediately gush forth, and minor spurts may accompany each labor contraction thereafter. In one-eighth of the cases the membranes rupture before labor has begun (premature rupture of membranes), and such labors are termed dry labors. This is about twice as common in first pregnancies as in subsequent ones.

Dry labors have an undeservedly bad reputation; they are the same as labors which occur with membranes intact except they may be shorter. Actually there is no such phenomenon as a dry labor, since the cells lining the inside of the amniotic sac are constantly secreting fluid at the rate of a quart in two hours. If membranes are unruptured, as much fluid is absorbed as is secreted, but when membranes are ruptured a large portion of the water flows from the vagina.

If the membranes rupture before the onset of labor and the patient is within a few days of term, in nine instances out of ten labor will commence within twenty-four hours—more than likely in less than six hours. Most obstetricians will attempt to start labor by a dilute intravenous Oxytocin drip in patients at or near term, if labor has not commenced within twelve or twenty-four hours. On the other hand, if membranes rupture prematurely and the patient is many weeks or even months from term, there may be a very long latent period before labor's onset—sometimes thirty or forty days, or longer. It is routine to place these patients at complete bed rest at home or in the hospital. Allowing pregnancy to progress several vital weeks may mean the difference between no baby and a baby. A recent patient ruptured her membranes at twenty-seven weeks and did not go into labor until six weeks later. As a result of the fortunate long latent period she now has a splendid son. However, unless the pregnancy is of twenty-six weeks or longer duration, the chance for a successful outcome is probably less than 2 or 3 per cent.

Doubt often exists as to whether the membranes have ruptured. Toward the end of pregnancy, pressure on the bladder by the fetal head sometimes causes the involuntary passage of urine, which may be confused with the loss of amniotic fluid. The submission of the fluid to a chemical color test (nitrazine paper) usually gives the answer. A yellow to olive-green color of the nitrazine paper moistened with the fluid is negative, while a blue-green to deep-blue color usually means amniotic fluid and ruptured membranes.

Normal Length of Labor

There have been a number of careful studies on the normal length of labor, and, as in most such studies of large groups, there are many cases which do not approximate the average. In my own experience I can recall two dramatic dissenters, women who actually had their babies with the first pain. I shall recite the case history of one.

During my residency one of the senior staff members sent a patient into the hospital a few days before her expected date of confinement. He told me that she was a most unusual lady, like the Hebrew women in Exodus—"Lively, and are delivered ere the midwives come." He had been engaged as accoucheur on the three previous occasions, but had never once even caught up with the stork. This time, however, he was obstinately determined to win from his feathered colleague, and he asked me to call him early in her labor. At 2:20 a.m. the nurse telephoned. She said the patient had awakened, had had no pains, but felt queer. With firemanlike haste I leapt into a pair of pants and dashed. As I arrived on the delivery floor, I collided with the stork, who was zooming down in a daredevil landing. After encasing my unwashed hands in sterile rubber gloves, I received the child, born after a single pain. It was all over by 2:31. There was no point in notifying the senior doctor until the next morning, but I immediately went to the telephone and called the husband. His only response was, "Why in the hell can't you fools ever call me in time?" With commendable restraint, I slammed down the receiver.

This extreme example should fill the reader with neither apprehension nor false expectancy, since no first babies and very few subsequent babies are born after the first few pains. One of the staff of the Johns Hopkins Hospital published an analysis of the total length of labor in 10,000 deliveries—that is, from the onset of the first pain until the whole process is over, including the extrusion of the afterbirth. He reported three values: mean, median, and mode. Mean is average. Median is the central value; that is, exactly as many women had labors longer as had labors shorter than the median figure listed below. The modal value is the commonest value observed, the precise duration of labor most frequent in the total series. The researcher divided his patients into primipara (first labors) and multipara (all labors subsequent to the first):

	Mean (Hours)	Median (Hours)	Mode (Hours)
Primipara	13.04	10.59	7.0
Multipara	8.15	6.21	4.0

It is generally agreed that median and modal values in a study of this type are more significant than mean values.

A recent study demonstrates that if a ten-year period or longer intervenes between births, the length and character of the labor is likely to be more like that of the primipara than of the multipara.

Several investigators have reported on the incidence of very rapid labors—labors lasting less than three hours—and relatively long labors—those requiring more than twenty-four hours. One woman in a hundred may anticipate that her first child will be born in less than three hours, and seven in a hundred may expect such good fortune in subsequent births. Approximately every ninth woman requires more than twenty-four hours to deliver a first child, and every thirty-third, children subsequent to the first.

Effect of Age on the Length of the First Labor

The effect of age on childbirth is an important problem, particularly important at this time when marriage is often postponed until the woman is toward the end of her reproductive span. At this period many women avoid maternity because of the insurmountable hazard which they believe their age adds to labor. This erroneous supposition is the result of uninformed lay opinion, aided by quasi-scientific medical observations.

In an analysis of the effect of age on childbirth, we can rule out of consideration the multiparous woman, for if a woman has once borne a child her age at a subsequent birth little affects the speed and progress of labor unless the previous birth was many, many years before. We shall focus our attention on the effect of age upon the first childbirth. How much is labor lengthened, and how much increased risk is there to mother and child?

Almost all observers agree that a first pregnancy after the age of thirty-five, when women are classed as elderly primiparas, is attended by an increase in length of labor. Today we believe that the difficulty is due to the replacement of some of the easily stretched elastic tissue cells and muscle cells of the uterus and birth canal by less easily stretched connective tissue cells. Even though women are still young at thirty-five, from the standpoint of childbearing their span is more than two-thirds over.

When one compares a large group of women thirty-five or over giving birth to first children with a group of women of assorted ages in their first labor, he finds that the more elderly women are penalized an average of one and one-half hours; when they are compared to women twenty years old or younger, the difference is approximately four hours.

In all the studies on elderly primiparas, the maternal and fetal risks were slightly higher than in an average age group, but the increase was so insignificant that no woman is justified in being deterred from motherhood by it. Women thirty-five or over when undertaking their first pregnancy can confidently anticipate a very happy outcome if they receive the proper type of obstetrical care.

Youth and Childbearing

Despite the fact that the relatively elderly woman does satisfactorily, there is no way of gainsaying the fact that the best ally of successful childbirth is youth. It is a message which the medical profession must constantly reiterate to the women of America. This in no sense should be interpreted as a clarion call for teen-age motherhood. It is my firm conviction that young couples should postpone parenthood until the schooling of both husband and wife is complete and they are economically and emotionally prepared to start a family. When this time arrives, they should plan the size of the family and the spacing of births and begin to initiate that plan. In this critical period of overpopulation no couple need feel that they have a debt to mankind to replace themselves. All children should be born with the invaluable heritage of being keenly wanted by parents who are capable and anxious to care for them.

I learned the value of not postponing childbearing from a patient several years ago. When I first saw her she was thirty-four and had been twelve years married. She was a department-store buyer and so engrossed in her career that she could never afford the time to start a family. When she suddenly realized age was catching up, she got pregnant very efficiently, and excitedly came to see me. On examination, I found that she had a fibroid tubor of the uterus many times the size of her early pregnancy, and when, because of complications, the whole uterus had to be removed, leaving her forever childless, she kept sobbing to me in a kind of chant, "Why didn't someone tell me you should have children while young?"

Apart from all socioeconomic considerations (of course in actual practice they can never be ignored), the ideal age for a woman to start a family, from the purely obstetrical viewpoint, is between the ages of eighteen to twenty.

According to a 1968 report of the National Center for Health Statistics the age group of twenty through twenty-four had the greatest number of first births in the United States; the fifteen-through-nineteen five-year sample ran a close second. The figure given under each five-year age span is the number of women within that age bracket who gave birth to their first living child per 1000 estimated female population. We shall list the groups in order of frequency:

Age Group (Years)	No. of Women Per 1000 Having Liveborn First Children
20–24	76.5
15–19	50.9
25–29	29.7
30–34	7.3
35–39	2.5
40–44	0.5

The number of women in every 1000 for the specific age group who gave birth to a baby, irrespective of whether it was their first or tenth, was as follows:

20–24 years	167.4 babies per 1000 women
25–29 years	140.3 babies per 1000 women
30–34 years	74.9 babies per 1000 women
15–19 years	66.1 babies per 1000 women
35–39 years	35.6 babies per 1000 women
40–44 years	9.6 babies per 1000 women

The figures above are not current and are cited from a period when the United States birth rate was higher than now. It is likely that the rate per 1000 women is lower in each category but the proportions remain similar.

How Many Labor Pains Are Required?

"How many pains make a baby?" is the facetious form in which the layman phrases a serious scientific query. As can be surmised, there is extraordinary variation, just like the number of pitches in a nine-inning ball game. According to one Swiss study, first labors required an average of 135 contractions and multiparous labors, 68.

The Forces Involved in Birth

Before discussing delivery, we must first consider the forces involved in birth.

It is necessary to imagine the baby confined in a large, gourd-shaped, elastic bottle, the muscular uterus. This lies within the mother's abdomen, the bottom of the bottle under her ribs, and the mouth deep in her pelvis. The cervix is about a half-inch long when labor begins, and it is almost tightly closed. Before a full-term baby can be expelled from the uterus, the round neck must be stretched to a diameter of four inches (ten centimeters), the minimum necessary to allow the baby to pass from the uterus into the narrow, stiff-walled, five-inch corridor (pelvis and birth canal) which leads to the outside world.

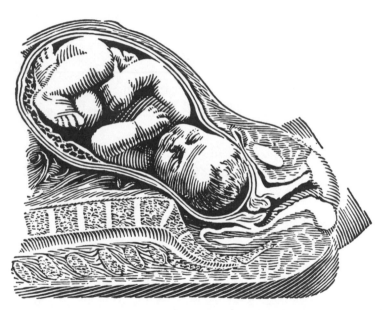

Fetus at full term, before the onset of labor. The pelvic floor is thick, the cervix closed, the uterus relaxed

The motive power that dilates the mouth of the uterus and propels the child through the resistant birth corridor is mainly the force generated by the contractions of this large muscular organ. This largest muscle of the body, far heavier and greater than the powerful biceps of a heavyweight champion prizefighter, forms a complete elastic casing about the child except for the small opening at its neck—the relatively weak point in the wall. When the muscle fibers contract, the pressure within the uterus is greatly increased—the process is like compressing a water-filled rubber bulb—and this increased pressure is transmitted to the constraining walls.

Many computations have been made of the force of a single labor pain, and figures varying from four to one hundred pounds have been obtained by separate investigators. From their data, an average of between twenty-five and thirty pounds seems likely. This force is directed against the cervix in two ways. The uterus has a completely separate inner lining, the membranes which contain the child and the amniotic fluid. During a pain both the baby and the fluid surrounding it are put under thirty pounds of pressure in all directions. When the membranes are intact, this force drives the fluid against the cervix; when they are ruptured, the baby is driven against it. Through pressure exerted by either the fluid or the baby, the cervix is forced open, stretched open from within. In addition to this pressure from within (dilatation), the neck of the bottle is shortened and pulled open by the contraction of the muscle fibers of the lower portion of the uterus, to which the muscle fibers of the cervix are attached (retraction). About nine of the ten and one-half hours of a primiparous labor and five and three-quarters of the six and one-half hours of a multiparous labor are occupied in stretching the opening in the cervix to its maximum four-inch diameter. This phase of labor is called the first stage, the stage of cervical dilatation. When the cervix is fully dilated, the baby no longer meets resistance in the upper birth canal, and the whole force of the uterine contractions is spent in driving it through the lower birth canal. In this stage of labor (the second stage) the force of the uterine contractions is greatly augmented by involuntary contractions of the woman's abdominal muscles, to which are added her own bearing down efforts. Instinctively she fills her lungs with air, fixes her diaphragm by closing her epiglottis, and increases her intra-abdominal pressure by straining as though at stool. These activities increase the uterine pressure to about sixty pounds. The primiparous woman expels her infant after an hour and a half of the second stage; the multipara requires a second stage only half as long. The second stage of labor, the expulsive stage, is the period between complete cervical dilatation and birth. The third stage, or placental stage, the time elapsing from the birth of the baby to the delivery of the placenta, lasts but a few minutes.

13

A Spontaneous Birth

When to Notify the Doctor

Most doctors want to be called as soon as rhythmic pains are established or the membranes rupture, no matter what the hour. If it is your first baby there is less rush than if it is your fourth. If at night you are in doubt, try to go back to sleep. Real labor will keep you awake. A considerate patient who hesitates to call at two in the morning may be solaced by the knowledge that disturbing an obstetrician is not the same as disturbing any other of mortal breed; for he is a rare species of night prowler who through years of specialized training is able to turn sleep off and on at will, has indeed learned to be almost independent of the god Morpheus, thus acquiring the worn look that distinguishes him from such diurnal healers as psychiatrists and dermatologists.

Do Not Eat if in Labor

At the request of one of my medical colleagues, an anesthesiologist, I insert a timely note of warning. After labor begins eat nothing until you consult your doctor; it is safe to drink clear liquids such as broth or tea. If you are very hungry he may let you eat jello, crackers, or similar foods. Do not drink milk, as the gastric acid forms a solid from it. Many anesthetic accidents have occurred when the patient entered the delivery room with a full stomach, then vomited and aspirated stomach contents into the lungs while going under or coming out of a general anesthetic. Even if you are scheduled to have psychoprophylactic, or natural, childbirth an emergency could arise requiring general anesthesia.

Recently one of our patients delivered a few hours after a dinner of corn. She vomited and sucked some of the kernels into her lungs. Prompt bronchoscopy (inserting a periscope-like instrument down the windpipe) and the removal of several kernels averted serious consequences.

Why the Hospital?

Until the second decade of the twentieth century it was mainly streetwalkers and the very destitute who sought hospital deliveries; available accommodations were in keeping with the standards of such clientele. Since 1910 there has been a complete revolution. Magnificent obstetrical institutions have been built for poor and rich alike, who use them in increasing numbers—regardless of class or financial station. By 1942, two out of three births in the United States were conducted by doctors in hospitals and by 1959, 96 out of every 100. The United States has become an urban nation and all but the most remote rural areas have a hospital, and wherever there is a hospital women from miles about converge on it for delivery. Virtually 100 per cent of the babies born each year in New York City are delivered in the hospital by physicians or nurse-midwives under medical supervision. This latter form of obstetric care is still sufficiently infrequent to be statistically unimportant.

Why have hospitals become the vogue? There are two reasons: the patient and the doctor. The patient prefers the hospital because it is more comfortable when she is in labor and assures her days of rest after delivery, entirely isolated from domestic cares. Delivery at home, moreover, requires complicated preparations. Most important of all, the patient has faith in hospitals. She is confident that the modern hospital is equipped to meet any sudden complication, and she knows that in a hospital when her own doctor is out of the building a competent staff member is available to substitute.

The doctor prefers the hospital for several reasons. In case of emergency—in obstetrics emergencies occur with lightning suddenness—the hospital can save the patient's life with a transfusion, a Cesarean section, the use of an oxygen tent, etc. Any complication of pregnancy, labor, and the puerperium (the six-weeks period following childbirth) can be better diagnosed and treated there because of laboratory facilities and consultation staffs. Obstetrical analgesia—pain-relieving drugs in large doses—can be given with safety only in a hospital. To have his cases centralized rather than scattered over a large metropolis is essential to the busy obstetrician.

Much has been written about the relative safety of the home and the hospital for childbirth. I know of no evidence to prove that the home is safer. The ideal hospital is one considered Class A according to the standards of the American College of Surgeons, and one with a separate maternity unit directed by a qualified staff of obstetricians. Such a hospital is superior to any home, unless the home is so elaborate that a complete private hospital can be set up. Hospitals are constantly improving in this country, and almost everywhere there is a community-supported institution which is safe for obstetric care.

Preparations for the Hospital

The labor of a woman who has borne a child before may be so sudden and unpredictable in its termination that she is usually sent to the hospital as soon as the doctor is reasonably certain the call is no false alarm. In his management of the primiparous woman he takes advantage of the psychological fact that most patients calculate the length of labor from the time they enter the hospital and not from the actual onset of pains. Labor is shortened in the mind of the primipara by keeping her at home during the first several hours and sending her to the hospital only when pains become regular and five or six minutes apart. In the early phase of a first labor keep yourself occupied. Perhaps you should summon your husband from work to keep you company. A movie or a visit to the art museum might be just what you both need.

Departure for the hospital to have a baby is an event surcharged with drama, some inherent, some engrafted. You can lessen the latter by accepting two pieces of advice. Above all, be calm. Then the next most important admonition is, be prepared! Either pack your suitcase two weeks in advance or prepare a list of things to bring along; otherwise, in the excitement of the moment, necessities may be left at home. Do not take baby clothes, since most hospitals will not allow you to use your own articles in the nurseries. As far as your own things are concerned, bring the minimum; most patients bring too much. Toilet articles and accessories, a robe, bed jacket, slippers, and two or three pajama tops or shorty nightgowns are the primary requisites. You will also need two nursing brassières, not the ones that come with a protective pad. Pack two sanitary belts to hold napkins in place; the hospital provides napkins. Entertaining literature, stationery for thank-you notes, your address book, and perhaps a small portable radio complete the cargo. At most hospitals television is available for rental.

Be sufficiently farsighted also to have a little bag packed with baby clothes and diapers and perhaps your own going-home frock, so your husband won't have to scatter things about in searching for them with masculine ineptitude.

If you already have children at home, make arrangements with a neighbor or relative for emergency baby-sitting coverage. See to it that the sitter can get there under her own chaperonage; fetching her first may use up strategic time at the last minute.

If you have no car, make preliminary arrangements about transportation in advance. If you are at term and live a distance from town, and paralyzing sleet or snow threatens, it might be safer to spend the night in the environs of the hospital. If you are snowbound, the State Police are magnificent in such an emergency.

It is well to rehearse with your doctor which door to use in entering the hospital at any hour. Ringing the wrong bell at two in the morning and getting no response is, to say the least, frustrating.

Be sure to bring with you any necessary insurance cards and perhaps your checkbook. Some hospitals ask for a deposit when you arrive if you have not already given one at early registration.

Arriving at the Hospital

After you arrive at the hospital the routine varies from institution to institution, in some measure depending on its size. In many, the pregnant woman is met at the front door by an attendant with a wheel chair who trundles her to the admitting office. There her registration card is removed from the file of undelivered cases, and notations are made on it, including the number of the room assigned. The patient, with the husband bringing up the rear, bag in hand, is then either wheeled to the delivery floor, where the labor rooms are situated, or taken directly to her own room.

Admission to Delivery Floor

At the Mount Sinai Hospital a woman in labor goes directly to the delivery floor, where the nurse in charge greets her with a cheerful, "How are *you*, Mrs. Jones? It's nice to see you here; we have been expecting you. We hope you will have a pleasant stay. Do not hesitate to call upon me or my staff for anything which will add to your comfort." If these are not her exact words, at least the content is similar. The husband is relieved of the bag and told to go to the waiting room and return in three-quarters of an hour.

The woman and nurse enter one of several labor rooms, which are light and cheerful with pastel-colored walls, curtains at the windows, and modern French prints on the walls. The regular adjustable hospital bed has a comfortable foam-rubber mattress; in addition there are attractive chairs, a bedside table-cabinet combination, and an Executone two-way conversation connection with the nursing station. Each labor room has its own lavatory.

Process of Admission

The head nurse is relieved by a student nurse or an aide, who divests the patient of her clothes, which are then listed on a form to be signed by the patient. The clothes are put into a paper bag, properly tagged, and sent to a locker area. The laboring woman has been given a plain, abbreviated heavy cotton gown, which partially fastens in back; when she is standing, it comes about halfway down the thigh. Temperature, pulse, respiration, and, in some institutions, weight are taken. A specimen of urine is obtained and venipuncture done. The hemoglobin (the amount of iron pigment in the blood) or hemotocrit (proportion of red blood cell mass to blood fluid) determined. Some of the blood is sent to the lab to be on hand for possible cross-matching, if transfusion should be necessary, and for Rh and perhaps VDRL (Wassermann test) determination. If labor is not far advanced, pertinent historical data are recorded.

Admission Examination

The woman's doctor or, in one of the large teaching institutions, the resident on duty performs the admission examination. Heart and lungs are examined, blood pressure taken, and abdomen palpated to determine accurately how the baby lies. The fetal heart is located and its rate counted. As the final act of this first examination, either a vaginal or rectal examination is performed to discover how far labor has progressed. The progress of labor is gauged by two criteria: the amount the cervix has dilated, and the depth to which the presenting part has descended in the birth canal. The opening in the cervix is round, and the amount of dilatation is expressed in terms of the diameter of this circular opening. When labor begins the opening is less than 2 centimeters ($\frac{4}{5}$ of an inch, or a single finger-breadth); a completely dilated cervix is 10 centimeters (4 inches, or five finger-breadths) in diameter. The depth of descent is measured by the relation of the presenting head or breech to a little bony prominence on either side of the pelvis, the ischial spine, situated midway down the birth corridor. The corridor is about six finger-breadths in length from the inlet where the baby enters to the outlet from which it emerges, and progress is expressed in the number of finger-breadths that the presenting part of the baby is above or below the midpoint milestones, the ischial spines. The presenting part advances from a minus-three station through zero to plus three, when it becomes visible as the doctor spreads apart the lips of the vagina.

If the admission examination proves that labor has begun, the genital area is washed and the hair shaved or clipped by a nurse. Clipping has the advantage of allowing one to escape the uncomfortable itching which usually happens when shaved hair regrows. Unless labor is too far advanced, an enema of warm soapy water is given. In many hospitals, you will be allowed to expel the enema on a toilet. In others you will be given a bedpan. In the latter case ask the nurse to place the bedpan on the edge of the bed and to put a chair beside the bed. Then you can rest your feet on the chair and can sit upright. Don't be in a hurry to get off the toilet or bedpan; otherwise you may expel liquid stool with subsequent contractions.

Conduct of First Stage

During early labor, if facilities permit, the husband is welcomed as a visitor in the labor room. The laboring woman is encouraged to walk about or to occupy herself with reading, knitting, etc. Most women feel more comfortable during labor in an upright position. The only time it is necessary to lie down is during the doctor's examination. When tired, you should rest. One of the unique occupations of labor is for husband and wife to time and record the occurrence and length of the contractions. Clear fluids such as water, broths, and tea are permitted in the beginning phase of labor.

Pain Relief in Labor

When the contractions of the uterus become frequent and moderately severe, in the primipara at approximately four-centimeters' or two-fingers' dilation, and in the multipara as soon as labor is well established, analgesic and amnesic drugs are administered unless you have elected to have one of the psychologic methods of pain relief. Perhaps one can call the former method medicated and the latter nonmedicated child-birth, although this is not entirely accurate since all of the psychological methods favor the use of drug relief if the laboring woman finds it necessary.

It is important at this point to differentiate clearly between an analgesic, an amnesic, and anesthetic. An analgesic simply diminishes the sense of pain; aspirin, for example, is a mild analgesic. An amnesic is a drug with the specific property of creating forgetfulness; it erases the memory of current events. The recipient has no knowledge of what occurs between the time he is given the injection and several hours later when its effect wears off. An anesthetic obliterates all sensation, either through the production of transitory unconsciousness (general anesthetic) or by temporarily interrupting the pathway by which sensory nerves communicate pain and other sensations to the brain (conduction anesthetic).

The History of Pain Relief in Obstetrics

When did medical science first concern itself with the sufferings of the parturient woman? From time immemorial it had always been considered woman's sacred heritage to bring forth children "in sorrow." Had not God ordained it?

I have searched a dozen authoritative obstetrical texts of the sixteenth, seventeenth, eighteenth, and early nineteenth centuries, and there is not a single reference to the use of drugs for the relief of pain in travail, although many pain-relieving drugs were known and employed in general surgery and medicine. For a kinswoman who injured her back when six months pregnant, the greatest obstetrician of Renaissance France, Mauriceau, prescribed in 1668 "at two several times a small grain of Laudanum in the Yolk of an Egg, a little to ease her violent pains." However, his famous book contains not so much as an "I am sorry" for the pains of labor. Some of these early authors devoted pages to the instruction of medical personnel in the proper conduct of tedious, painful births, but not a word was included about mitigating drugs.

Not only were labor pains unrelieved, but nothing was done to relieve the horror of obstetrical operations. Without an anesthetic or any other drug, Chamberlen, the inventor of the forceps, worked unsuccessfully for three hours to deliver a rachitic dwarf by means of his then secret instrument.

After giving up my vain search for early examples of the relief of pain in childbirth, I chanced upon an essay by Sir James Young Simpson of Edinburgh, the intrepid innovator who conducted the very first delivery under anesthesia. Ninety-eight years before my search of early medical sources for a reference to pain relief in birth, his search had been equally fruitless.

Simpson administered the first obstetrical anesthetic during the delivery of a poor woman in the slums of Edinburgh. She was "etherized shortly after nine o'clock" on January 19, 1847. Simpson immediately realized the full import of the occasion. By chance, on the same day he was apprised of his appointment as one of Victoria's Scottish physicians. He considered this the lesser of the two events, for three days later, in reporting them to his brother, he wrote, "Flattery from the Queen is perhaps not common flattery, but I am far less interested in it than in having delivered a woman this week without any pain while inhaling sulphuric ether. I can think of naught else."

Gauss of Freiburg, Germany, was the first to institute and advocate pain relief during labor. In 1907 he introduced a combination of morphine and scopolamine for this purpose. The former diminished pain; the latter dimmed memory. He called his technique *Dämmerschlaf,* "twilight sleep"; while under its influence the patient remained in a kind of midstate between consciousness and unconsciousness.

No phase of modern childbirth is more in flux than the conquest of its pain.

To understand the question, one must distinguish between the pain of labor preceding birth and the pain of actual birth itself. We shall term the one labor pain, the other birth pain.

At the Johns Hopkins Hospital, more than four decades ago, when I cut my eyeteeth in the art of midwifery, obstetrical pain relief was simple. Labor pain was treated either by what we called vocal anesthesia—pep talks along the well-grooved line, "It can't hurt as much as you make out"—or by the injection of a small dose of heroin, an opium derivative. The medical use and prescription of heroin was legal then, but became illegal shortly thereafter, morphine being substituted. Just before the birth the heroin was supplemented by nitrous oxide gas given intermittently with the last ten or twenty labor pains. (Nitrous oxide is familiar to most because of its use in tooth extractions.) For birth pain the patient was inexpertly anesthetized into unconsciousness by nitrous oxide, nitrous oxide and ether, or chloroform.

The whole field has now become immeasurably improved and complicated.

Analgesics

Many drugs and combinations of drugs are available to the obstetrician for the relief of labor pains. They may be given by mouth, rectally, or by hypodermic injection directly in a vein or deep into a muscle. The intravenous avenue is most rapidly effective, as the drug placed into the circulating blood immediately affects the brain; when given by another route, it must first be absorbed into the circulation before it can act. Today the most popular drug is Demerol (meperidine, a synthetic morphinelike compound) given in combination with scopolamine. The latter, a member of the belladonna family, is the amnesic, the eraser of memory; the former deadens pain and creates an overpowering urge to sleep when given in sufficient quantity. Occasionally other analgesic drugs, such as Sparine or one of the barbiturates (Seconal) is added to the two standbys. One of the more recent tranquilizer drugs (Phenergan, Vistaril, Valium) may be given with Demerol, omitting scopolamine. This combination produces analgesia and sedation without much amnesia. However, the absence of restlessness, which is a common reaction to scopolamine, makes the patient easier to manage.

In successful cases, under the influence of one of the drug combinations, the patient soon falls into a deep, quiet sleep between pains, but groans and moves about in a restless manner with each pain, particularly if scopolamine is used. The somnolent state continues into the second stage of labor and for several hours after delivery. When the patient wakes, the obstetrician is rewarded by hearing her ask, "Doctor, when am I going to have my baby?" The quickest way I know to prove that the child is already born is to guide the patient's hand to her own abdomen. Puzzled, she seeks for the familiar mountainous lump; when she finds it gone and replaced by a sunken valley the silliest, happiest grin steals across her face.

The relief of labor pain is tricky business. Each time a drug is given the doctor must ask himself three questions: "Is this drug, in the dose prescribed, safe for the mother? Is it likely to lengthen labor by diminishing the force of the contractions? And may it be injurious to the baby?" As stated in an earlier chapter, most drugs given the mother, no matter by what route of administration, rapidly gain access to her blood and forthwith pass through the placenta into the fetus's blood. This is the case when analgesic drugs are used. As a group the analgesics are nervous depressants, depressing not only the sensation of pain but other nervous mechanisms, including respiration. The mother's breathing center, located in the brain, is relatively resistant to their depressing effects, but not so the respiratory center of the newborn, which is highly susceptible to such inhibitory influences. For this reason particularly, and to a lesser extent for the safety of the mother and the possible slowing effect on labor, the obstetrician must be chary of the amount of pain-relieving drugs he prescribes during labor. All too often he must reluctantly turn a deaf ear to the laboring woman's importunate pleadings for more and yet more drugs. Her goal is total eradication of pain; his goal is maximum relief within the bounds of safety for mother and child. Not only drug dosage but the timing of administration requires care. If given too early, before labor is well established, drugs may halt or lengthen the process. I am always puzzled by the woman who says, "My doctor knocked me out with the very first pain, and I didn't feel a thing." She either forgets because of the amnesic beneficence of scopolamine or dramatically distorts the truth.

Psychological Pain Relief

Twilight sleep was slowly accepted in this country and even more slowly in England, but by the late thirties it was deeply entrenched, particularly in the United States, and very widely practiced. However, not all obstetricians and not all women were equally enthusiastic. There were obvious advantages, but disadvantages as well. Among the latter was the fact that most twilight-sleep patients were unable to cooperate and push the baby out so that many deliveries became forceps births.

Then too, more babies were born depressed. Some women, though grateful for the pain relief, felt cheated by not being consciously present during their child's birth—happy termination of nine months inconvenience with no knowledge of it until hours later.

A counterreaction set in against extensive medication during childbirth. This leads to exciting and productive results, the development of several psychological methods of pain relief in labor.

Natural Childbirth

The first of these was "natural childbirth," developed by the late Dr. Grantly Dick-Read during the late thirties in England. He published his theories and the program applying them in his now famous books, *Childbirth Without Fear, Natural Childbirth Primer,* and *Introduction to Motherhood.*

Dick-Read felt that childbirth is essentially a "normal and physiologic process" and most of the pain stems from poor conditioning brought about by the influence of a Biblical emphasis on pain in labor, old wives' tales, and distorted reports in lay writings. His key concepts were that fear and a muscularly unrelaxed, tense state are the chief sources of pain and difficulty during labor. Read advocated the elimination of fear through knowledge, which dispels terrorizing mystery from the birth process. This is done by professional instruction through discussions and the use of visual aids, such as pictures and diagrams. He would also prevent the patient from being left alone during labor. Solitude at such a time breeds fright. In addition, patients are taught relaxation exercises during the prenatal period so that they may apply the techniques during labor and delivery. They are taught how to pant during a labor pain and how to relax skeletal as well as vaginal and perineal muscles. Read advised that the term "labor pain" be expunged and "contraction" substituted. He forcefully insisted that the contractions of the first stage are not minded at all by those who learn and employ his teachings, and that the expulsive phase of the actual birth is easily tolerated because of the physical satisfaction which results from giving in to the instinctive urge to expel the baby. Read claimed that anesthesia, even the deadening of sensation by local anesthesia, is unnecessary for most properly prepared subjects.

Read attested that the gratification which the mother feels in being awake and an active participant in the process of birth gives rise to a feeling of exultation and a sense of accomplishment which no other experience in life bestows. He stated explicitly that any patient employing natural childbirth who needs help from pain-relieving drugs or anesthesia should never be denied them.

Hypnosis for Labor and Delivery

Hypnosis for obstetrical pain relief has been employed experimentally since the middle of the nineteenth century, at first in France and later in Germany and England. Since 1950 several scientific studies and some popular books concerning hypnosis for labor and delivery have been published in the United States. The best known of the latter is William Kroger's *Childbirth with Hypnosis*. There is no doubt that in some instances hypnosis is spectacularly successful; the patient delivers in a trance, experiencing no pain. In fact I have witnessed a Cesarean section performed on a highly receptive subject with no other anesthetic than hypnosis. The drawbacks to this technique are its unpredictability —not all pregnant women are equally successful candidates for hypnosis —and the extravagant amount of time the physician-hypnotist must invest in the prenatal conditioning of his patient. Because of these deterrents, hypnosis is still viewed as a trick in its application to birth.

The LaMaze Psychoprophylactic Technique

Pain relief by conditioned reflex, an outgrowth of the work of the great Pavlov, the psychoprophylactic method, came to America from Russia via France. It was brought to France in 1951 by the late Dr. Fernand LaMaze. I met Dr. LaMaze at his leftist Metal Worker's Hospital in Paris a year later. Though a very large man, almost elephantine in appearance, he seemed gentle and kind. Despite the partial language barrier between us, he took much time and great pains to tell me about his program. In 1959 the American Society for Psychoprophylaxis in Obstetrics was founded. It now has many affiliated branches throughout the country.

Two of several excellent American books on psychoprophylactic pain relief are *Thank You, Dr. LaMaze*, published in 1959 by Marjorie Karmel, who tragically died far too young, and *Six Practical Lessons for an Easier Childbirth* by Elizabeth Bing, published in 1967. Mrs. Bing was the physiotherapist associated with our "education for childbirth" program at Mount Sinai, and this discussion of psychoprophylaxis will be largely based on her interpretation. In this country, psychoprophylaxis has virtually replaced Dick-Read's natural childbirth.

Let me try to explain the philosophy of the LaMaze method. When pain is perceived, there are other simultaneous sensations, resulting from visual, auditory, or tactile stimuli. By concentrating overpoweringly on one of the other stimuli, pain instead of occupying central importance assumes peripheral importance. A simple example follows. Suppose you have a bad headache and you go to see a first-rate film. You probably do not feel the headache while the picture engrosses you, but when it ends the headache reappears. Your concentration on the film was strong enough to eliminate temporarily perception of pain, but when you stopped concentrating on the film the headache once more became the focus of your attention. Also, an athlete in the midst of a contest may not feel a broken bone, but after the game the hurt is fully evident.

One way to increase one's perception of pain is to over-anticipate it. You go to the dentist and when he touches a tooth with an instrument the slight discomfort is magnified by apprehension into pain. Many women view childbirth with similar apprehension, and by anticipating and concentrating on the expected sensation of pain its effect is multiplied.

The basic tenets of psychoprophylaxis are: first, a thorough understanding of the processes of labor and childbirth alleviate unnecessary tension and apprehension, the pain multipliers; second, muscular relaxation helps the body's efficiency and increases comfort during labor and delivery; third, there is undeniable pain and discomfort during childbirth which by a conditioning process can be displaced from a central to a peripheral location in one's consciousness through the substitution of another center of concentration. The new center of concentration is the special body function, breathing. Active, difficult, and varying techniques of breathing are taught in psychoprophylaxis. To employ them properly requires strong central concentration.

In her book, Mrs. Bing writes as though she were addressing a class. "You will learn to change your breathing deliberately during labor, adjusting it to the changing characteristics of the uterine contractions. This will demand an enormous concentrated effort on your part. Not a concentration on pain, but a concentration on your own activity in synchronizing your respiration to the signals that you receive from the uterus. This strenuous activity will create a new center of concentration in the brain, thereby causing painful sensations during labor to become peripheral, to reduce their intensity."

The husband's role is crucial in the psychoprophylaxis program. He attends the classes and becomes an assistant teacher, for he must help his wife learn and practice the respiratory exercises and muscle-relaxing techniques in daily homework. In these practice sessions he is timekeeper and ticks off the passing seconds in a feigned series of uterine contractions. At all times and particularly during labor and delivery he must offer his wife moral and physical support. The delivery team consists of the laboring woman, the husband, the physician, and the nurses. To work effectively each must know his or her role thoroughly and do it well. The couple is told that more than 60 per cent of women feel relatively little pain using psychoprophylaxis, but many will require relief through drug medication in varying amounts. If this becomes necessary there should be no sense of failure or shame, since physical factors, such as the size of the baby, its position, the size of the pelvis, and many other things vary from individual to individual and from labor to labor.

Psychoprophylaxis is usually taught to a half dozen couples as a group in six weekly sessions beginning toward the end of the seventh month. In the first session pregnancy, the three stages of labor, uterine contractions, and delivery of the baby and placenta are presented through discussion and visual aids. Session 2 is largely concerned with muscle-relaxing techniques. Sessions 3 and 4 discuss the three phases of uterine contractions during labor, "latent, accelerated, and transitional," and the tempo and depth of breathing to be carried out during each phase. The wife and husband are taught how to massage the abdomen and back during strong contractions. Session 5 concentrates on birth, the second stage of labor, what happens during actual delivery and how to prepare for it, the husband's role during delivery, and how the woman stops pushing down on medical command. The content of the sixth session is how to recognize real labor, what articles to take to the hospital, an account of hospital labor routines, a review of breathing patterns during labor's three phases, the use of medication, the great moment, and what follows.

To make psychoprophylaxis successful the hospital and its staff must permit the husband to be present in both the labor and delivery rooms. An anesthetist should be constantly available in case a situation develops that dictates a sudden operative delivery. Ordinarily the only anesthesia used is a small amount of local injected into the fourchette (the skin area at the rear of the vagina) or perineum (the bridge of tissue between vagina and anus), as the physician may elect to enlarge the vaginal birth ring by making a clean cut in this area with a scissors (episiotomy) to prevent a ragged birth tear.

Couples who choose psychoprophylaxis under ideal auspices—competent preparation, an enthusiastic thoroughly indoctrinated physician, and a hospital skilled in the technique—report a sense of rapture or near mystical bliss. A birth so conducted creates a feeling of togetherness and mutual accomplishment for wife and husband. The father being able to witness and help with his own child's birth and the mother being able to view the whole procedure through a focused mirror on the opposite wall creates a unique, positive life experience.

"Which Is for Me: Psychological or Medicated Pain Relief?"

I am sure that many readers ask themselves the above question. I am equally certain that I cannot answer it for them. Nevertheless, through extensive experience, I can make some observations which may prove helpful.

Do not make the decision on the basis as to which is safe for you and your baby. Both are safe. Your baby has a greater likelihood of being awake and alert with a psychological method of pain relief.

Do not make the choice because some relative, and this includes your husband, prefers one or the other method for you. In this, you have no one to please except yourself.

Psychological pain relief is well suited to the woman who feels that having a baby is the greatest of life's many experiences and does not want to miss a minute of it. She wants to be wide awake when contractions become strong to sample what they are like. She wants to feel the pressure of the baby on her pelvic muscles and wants the thrill of helping push her baby out. She wants to know when she is taken to the delivery room and, above all, to hear her baby's first cry; while still on the delivery table, perhaps before the cord is cut, she wants to cradle the baby in her arms before it is even cleaned up.

In contrast is the woman who has a low threshold for pain, who hates to be in pain. She looks forward to several children and fears that if labor and birth are too uncomfortable she will lack the spunk to stage a repeat performance. She is very likely to spend a half century with her child, and missing the first few hours of their association seems a very brief fragment of the whole. To her, temporary separation from reality at such a time, through the boon of safe analgesia and anesthesia, is a welcome goal.

Then there is the woman who falls in neither group. She is uncertain. In this case, I advise giving psychological childbirth a trial. Read the books, take the classes, if they are available in your community. Be perpared! Fortunately, a decision in favor of unmedicated or lightly medicated childbirth is not irrevocable. Try labor without drugs. It may be much easier than you anticipated. If the going gets rough, ask for a little medication, perhaps half of the standard dose. Then, if you still find it too rugged, ask for full drug relief and retreat into the bliss of temporary severance from reality.

Above all, do not feel defeated if you find you want full medication. No one else but you is really concerned; therefore have the type of labor which best suits your needs. Certainly if you tell your teen-age daughter fifteen years hence that you had her by medicated or psychological techniques, she could not care less.

Choosing the Doctor and Hospital for Psychoprophylaxis

Explore your doctor's attitude if you want to give psychological pain relief a sincere try. If he is out of sympathy with your choice, forget it. Or if you are certain you want psychoprophylaxis, be wise enough to choose a doctor who favors it. Do not be embarrassed when you make your first appointment to ask whether the doctor is experienced in psychoprophylactic childbirth and practices it. If not, ask to be referred to a colleague who does. Then you and the doctor must choose a hospital which welcomes husbands in the labor and delivery rooms.

Under any form of pain relief, psychological or medicated, the presence of your own physician during labor is an important ingredient in successful pain relief. Confidence in him and the elimination of apprehension, uncertainty, and fear are in themselves powerful pain relief medicines.

Abdominal Decompression

A plastic shield that produced negative pressure when applied to the abdomen of the laboring woman was introduced in 1959. It was stated by the innovator that negative abdominal pressure reduces both the pain and the length of labor. Studies by several observers fail to corroborate either claim.

Anesthetics

Obstetrical anesthesia, rendering a patient completely insensible to pain during actual delivery, has come of age. Until the last decade or two it had been the stepchild of the science of anesthesiology. In contrast to the attitude toward anesthesia in general surgery, it was felt that literally anybody could put a woman to sleep to have a baby. When deliveries were conducted at home, it was common practice to convert the husband or some other relative into temporary anesthetist. And in hospitals novice anesthetists, senior medical students, or inexperienced interns were frequently used for delivery anesthesia. As a matter of fact obstetrical anesthesia is difficult anesthesia—first, because you have the interests of two patients, mother and baby, to consider, and these interests are sometimes antithetic. In the second place, the obstetrical patient is often poorly prepared for anesthesia. The surgical patient is admitted to the hospital for rest and preoperative starvation at least eighteen hours prior to a scheduled operation. On the other hand, the woman in labor may enter the hospital just after a hectic day of domesticity, climaxed by a big, indigestible dinner. The importance and difficulties of obstetrical anesthesia are constantly gaining recognition, so that more and more births are being attended by two medical experts, the obstetrician and the anesthesiologist.

Several anesthetics are available to eliminate birth pain. They can be divided into two main categories, general and conduction—the latter also termed local or regional. A general anesthetic affects the whole body, creating anesthesia by temporary but complete unconsciousness. A conduction anesthetic functions differently. It simply interrupts the pathway from a specific area where the pain stimulus is received to the brain cells, where it is appreciated as pain. An electric light offers a homely analogy. The stimulus is the wall switch, the conduction pathway the wires in the wall, and the electric bulb on the ceiling the brain which receives the stimulus. If the conducting wires are cut, the bulb will not light, no matter how many times you flip the switch.

General anesthetics until relatively recently were almost wholly inhalation anesthetics, gases inhaled into the lungs and absorbed immediately into the bloodstream. In obstetrics it is common practice to intubate when administering an inhalation anesthetic, since so often the woman may come to deliver shortly after a meal. When the patient is asleep a metal tube is passed from the tooth area through the larnyx into the upper trachea (wind pipe). Hence, since the larynx is blocked by the tube, if vomiting should occur the gastric contents cannot be sucked into the lungs and is harmlessly aspirated from the mouth through a tube. If intubation is used a sore throat may follow anesthesia for several hours.

Since the blood bathes the whole body, the anesthetic gases in the blood soon reach the brain, and when in sufficient concentration unconsciousness results. Another method is to bypass lung absorption by injecting the anesthetic agent, a water solution of a chemical powder, directly into the bloodstream. The general anesthetics, no matter whether inhalation (nitrous oxide, cyclopropane ether, fluothane, etc.) or intravenous sodium pentothal soon pass across the placenta into the baby's circulation and may narcotize it (make it sleepy). When general anesthetics are superimposed on heavy doses of analgesics, a fair proportion of sleepy, sometimes very sleepy, babies results. And they do not announce their entrance into the world with loud trumpeting, but come around quickly with conservative, careful handling. They later become indistinguishable from babies of mothers who did not receive general anesthesia plus heavy analgesia.

Conduction anesthesia acts locally, relatively little is absorbed into the mother's bloodstream, and only small amounts find their way across the placenta to the baby's circulation. Therefore babies born to mothers given conduction anesthetics are likely to howl lustily the minute they are born.

There are three ways in which conduction, or regional, anesthesia may be used in obstetrics. One is by local infiltration. When the baby is ready to be delivered, the doctor eliminates birth pain by injections of one of the cocaine drugs into the lower birth passage, thus numbing the perineum, the area between the rectum and the vagina, as well as the lower vagina itself. The obstetrician may accomplish this by injecting the whole area widely with the drug, or by injecting a single spot on either side, blocking the nerve fibers as they fan out from the main nerve trunk, a procedure termed pudendal block.

In the second method, called spinal, the conduction anesthetic is injected into the spinal fluid surrounding the lower spinal cord. The needle is introduced into the spinal canal by inserting it in the midline of the lower back between two vertebrae, and a single dose of drug administered. The needle is then withdrawn. One may use either an ordinary water solution of the drug or a dextrose or sugar solution. The former diffuses rapidly, bathing the lower portion of the spinal cord, and produces complete anesthesia to the navel or above. The latter mixture is hyperbaric—that is, heavier than the spinal fluid—and if the patient is kept sitting upright for thirty seconds after the injection and then lies down immediately, the dextrose anesthetic solution sinks to the bottom of the spinal canal, numbing only the lowermost nerve trunks. This produces anesthesia in a restricted area, an area which ordinarily contacts a saddle when one is riding horseback; therefore, this form of spinal is termed saddle-block. Since a spinal stops labor it cannot be given for labor pain, but only for birth pain. Spinal anesthesia is ideal for delivery except for two drawbacks. First, about 6 per cent of spinal anesthetics are followed by severe and sometimes protracted headache which eventually disappears without any aftermath. This is caused by leakage of spinal fluid into the back muscles through the puncture hole made in the dura (a tough membrane that covers the spinal cord and the brain), the leakage in turn reducing spinal-fluid pressure. Within one to several days the hole seals itself, the spinal-fluid pressure rises, and the headache disappears. By using a very fine needle headache was reduced to 0.3 per cent in one series of cases. The second drawback is that they not infrequently induce a temporary drop in blood pressure; therefore, the patient must be carefully observed, with blood-pressure readings every five or ten minutes during the first hour after injection.

The third type of conduction anesthesia is extradural; the anesthetic is not injected into the spinal canal and placed in direct contact with the spinal cord itself, but into a space lined by ligaments and bone which is external to the dura. A cocaine derivative placed within the space bathes the spinal nerves in the area as they make their exit through apertures in the dura, and thus exert their anesthetic effect directly on the nerve trunks themselves.

One form of extradural is caudal (Latin: *cauda*, meaning "tail"), so named because if human beings retained their embryonic tails the point of injection would be just at the base of the tail, into the so-called caudal space. This extradural space is below the level of the spinal cord itself; the drug simply bathes the descending nerve trunks. A caudal anesthetic is usually given continuously—that is, additional amounts are injected into the caudal space as soon as it is evident that the numbing effect is beginning to wear off. This requires that a needle be left in place. An interesting modification is the substitution of a plastic catheter (tube) for the needle. The tiny catheter is threaded into place through the large needle, the needle withdrawn, and the protruding end of the catheter fixed securely in position by adhesive tape. Additional doses are administered through the indwelling catheter.

A second form of extradural is lumbar epidural. A spinal puncture is made between two of the lumbar vertebrae (lowest five vertebrae) just as one does in an ordinary spinal puncture. The big difference is that the needle is not inserted as deeply: instead of lodging in the spinal canal inside the dura it remains outside of it in the extradural space. Just as in caudal anesthesia a catheter can be inserted through the needle, the needle withdrawn, and the catheter left in place. This permits continuous analgesia-anesthesia through the last half hour of labor and for delivery as well.

Extradural caudal and epidural are unique since they may be used in the same patient as combined analgesic and anesthetic techniques to eliminate labor pain as well as birth pain. Injections are begun when labor is well established and the cervix has become partially dilated, and are continued until after delivery. Extradural sounds like the answer to a matron's prayer, and when it works well it truly is. It never causes the unpleasant headache aftermath which may curse spinal and saddle-block anesthesia.

Why isn't extradural anesthesia the perfect obstetrical pain-relief method that modern obstetrics has sought so earnestly? First, it is technically difficult; great skill and experience are required to lodge the needle in the caudal or lumbar epidural space. Second, the patient must have a vigilant nurse or physician constantly at her bedside to check when more drug is needed and observed for fluctuations in blood pressure. In many hospitals such available technical personnel is an unobtainable luxury. If given too early, or if the labor is not of the rapidly progressive type, it may prolong labor. In the past few years lumbar epidural has been used more frequently than caudal, primarily because the accurate insertion of the needle is technically simpler.

Other methods of conduction pain relief are being tried. One of the most promising is paracervical block. This technique places the anesthetic agent on either side of the cervix and the lower lateral borders of the uterus where the pain nerve fibers run. It is used primarily for labor pain. An additional anesthetic is necessary for birth pain, like pudendal or saddle-block.

In summary, then, modern obstetrics has made tremendous progress in the relief and even elimination of the pain of childbirth. Today no woman need suffer as her grandmother did. The obstetrician has a bag full of techniques, from psychoprophylaxis to paracervical block. He will choose the technique with which he is experienced, one he considers eminently safe for the mother and baby, and one that is best suited to the particular patient. Two authorities in this field, Doctors Robert Hingson and Louis Hellman, summarizing a study of over 10,000 deliveries by various anesthetic techniques, show quite clearly that as far as the baby is concerned any type of birth anesthetic given the mother is equally safe. The only important variable as far as fetal results are concerned is the competence of the anesthetist in administering the particular method he uses.

Delivery

Having discussed pain relief at length, we can rejoin the parturient in the labor room. By this time she has probably received Demerol and scopolamine, unless she has chosen psychoprophylaxis, and her husband has been dismissed and sent to the waiting room to join other expectant husbands and their retinues of expectant grandparents and aunts and uncles. The laboring woman is oblivious to all this; she is sleeping soundly between uterine contractions, perhaps snoring. When a contraction comes she wakes, tosses about, moans, and, as soon as it subsides, returns to sleep. Her own doctor, the nurses, and resident physicians are constantly going in and out of the room. It is likely that the sides of her bed are equipped with movable metal guard rails, which are kept raised except during an examination. Analgesia makes one behave as if drunk, and the guard rails protect the patient, restrain her from jumping or falling out of bed if she is momentarily left alone. At frequent intervals a doctor or nurse checks the fetal heart with a stethoscope, noting its rate and regularity. At less frequent intervals a physician determines the extent of labor's progress by rectal or vaginal examination. Now the pains become longer in duration and more frequent, occurring every three or four minutes, and the "show" becomes bloody. When examination reveals the cervix fully dilated and the baby descended to the vaginal floor, the patient is transferred to the delivery room.

The Delivery Room

A delivery room looks like a small operating room. It contains a complicated-looking anesthesia machine full of knobs and different-colored cylinders of various anesthetic gases. There is also an instrument table draped with sterile throws. An infant-resuscitation machine is off in one corner. The personnel are capped, masked, and sterilely gowned and gloved. Until recently few patients ever saw all this, but now, in the era of psychological pain relief and conduction anesthesia, many laboring women see not only the room itself but the whole process of birth by means of an adjustable mirror attached either to the wall or to the large, special, shadowless light in the ceiling overhead.

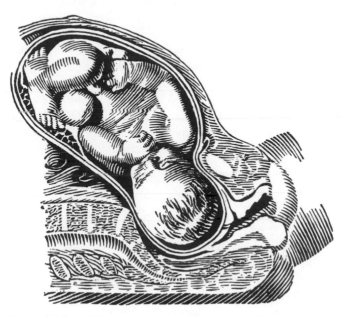

Early stage of labor. Uterus is contracting, cervix dilating; bag of waters is below head

The woman is transferred to the delivery table, a very broad type of operating table equipped with leg holders which, when she lies on her back, hold her legs wide apart. Her wrists are strapped to the sides of the table to prevent her from fingering the sterile drapes when they are applied. If the membranes are intact, the doctor ruptures them with a clamp or hook. Since the membranes are the fetal sac and not connected with the mother, their rupture or puncture is painless. At this stage, unless the patient has received epidural or spinal anesthesia, the baby's head pressing on the tissues of the lower vagina and bowel makes her bear down involuntarily, with a reflex desire to expel the offending mass. With each labor pain, because of the powerful force generated by the contraction of the large, muscular uterus, aided by the mother's vigorous straining, the baby descends lower and lower, and soon its scalp appears at the entrance to the vagina.

Simultaneous with descent the baby's head rotates until the middle of the back of its head, the occiput, is in the twelve o'clock position

(O.A., occiput anterior), directly under the middle of the mother's symphysis. If you look at your wrist watch with twelve o'clock on top, I can explain it more clearly. Ordinarily when labor begins the occiput is at the half-past one position (L.O.A., left occiput anterior) or at half-past ten (R.O.A., right occiput anterior). For birth to be possible the force of the uterine contractions must spin an L.O.A. head to the right or an R.O.A. head to the left to permit birth through the birth passage. With the back of the baby's head squarely beneath the symphysis and his chin directly over the mother's rectum he presents the narrowest diameter of his head to the narrowest diameter of the pelvis. Some babies' heads have to rotate through greater arcs from nine or half-past seven or three or half-past five to twelve before birth is possible. Birth occasionally occurs with the occiput at six o'clock and the face at twelve, since this also presents a narrow transverse diameter of the head to the transverse diameter of the pelvis.

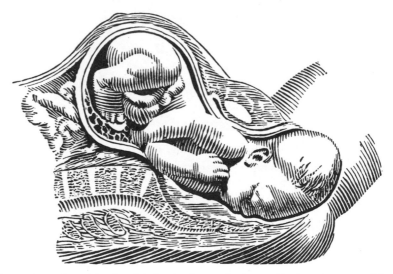

The end of labor. The head is beginning to be born. Occiput is at 12 o'clock, anterior

With each labor pain, the elastic vaginal orifice is further distended, and more and more of the baby's scalp appears, at first an amount which could be covered by a dime, then by a quarter, and finally fifty cents' worth.

At this point, unless the patient is experiencing psychological pain relief or is under the full effects of a continuous conduction anesthetic, general anesthesia is induced. The anesthetized patient is now brought into position at the edge of the table, with knees bent and thighs spread

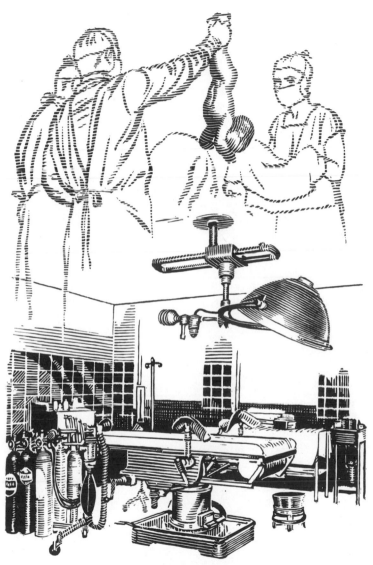

A modern delivery room

wide asunder by the metal leg rests. The vaginal region, the lower abdomen, and inner parts of the thighs are cleansed. The doctor surrounds the opening of the birth passage so completely with sterile towels, over which he places a large sheet with a perforated eighteen-inch square, that it appears as though birth is occurring through a window.

The Birth

As labor progresses, the baby's head protrudes farther and farther, and the perineum (the tissue lying between the vagina and the rectum) is stretched to an unbelievable degree. Now the head no longer recedes between pains but continues to bulge through the vaginal opening. Since, because of overdistention, vaginal tears are almost certain to occur in the perineum, most doctors anticipate them at this point (with the patient completely anesthetized if she is having general anesthesia; if not the area has been anesthetized by some type of conduction or local anesthetic) by making an incision in the perineum before the head emerges. The simple operation is called an episiotomy. The episiotomy cut is made with scissors. The arguments favoring episiotomy are: an incision is straighter, less jagged, and simpler to repair than a tear; and an incision made before a tear occurs prevents the vaginal tissues from being overstretched and makes vaginal relaxation less likely following childbirth.

Now the child's head is pushed out by an assistant who applies pressure on the mother's abdomen, or the obstetrician makes upward and outward pressure on the chin through the thinned perineum and virtually lifts the head out. The head when fully born spontaneously turns to the left or right, depending toward which side of the mother the baby's shoulders are, and is grasped by the doctor, who places one hand beneath each side of the jaw. As the head is guided downward, the front shoulder slips out; then a pull upward brings forth the rear shoulder. With continued gentle traction, the chest, trunk, and lower limbs follow easily.

When delivery is completed, the child is held by its heels, head down. Using a rubber bulb or tube, the obstetrician sucks accumulated blood or mucus from the mouth and nose. By now the child begins to breathe regularly and cry. The navel cord is clamped three inches from the abdomen and cut. The child is then handed to a nurse, who blankets and deposits it in a warm crib.

Evaluation of the Infant's Condition at Birth

The face and scalp of a baby in good condition usually looks slightly blue as the head is being born, but becomes ruddy immediately with its first breath. Pallor is a poor sign. Immediate urination and, if the infant is a boy, erection of the penis are good signs. A useful and precise way of cataloguing the newborn's condition at birth was developed by Dr. Virginia Apgar when she was anestheologist at New York's Columbia-Presbyterian Hospital and is known as the Apgar Score.

Apgar Scoring System

Score	0	1	2
Heart Rate	Absent	Rate below 100 per min.	Over 100
Respiratory Rate	Absent	Slow, irregular	Good
Muscle Tone	Flaccid	Some movement	Active Motion
Cry	Absent	Cry, poor	Vigorous Cry
Color	Deep blue or pale	Body pink, extremities, blue	Pink all over

The baby is observed and the score recorded by a trained person at one minute and five minutes of age. A one-minute score of 3 or less indicates the baby is in poor condition, its life in jeopardy, and immediate resuscitative efforts indicated. A score of 7 to 10, ten being the maximum, demonstrates that the baby is in excellent shape. The five-minute score has been shown to be correlated with the baby's future, both survival and normalcy.

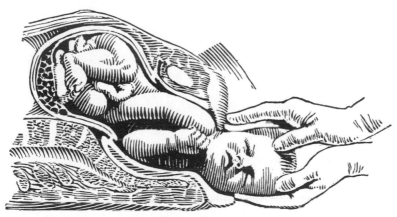

Head has been born; shoulder is being delivered

If the child requires resuscitation, it is given to a trained assistant to resuscitate. Here, too, there are many methods. Modern delivery rooms are equipped with one of several excellent machines which combine three features: suction to clear mucus and other secretions from the upper air passages, positive pressure to inflate the lungs in order to establish respirations, and a mask with constant oxygen to be put over the baby's face when its own respirations have taken over.

Less satisfactory methods of infant resuscitation are blowing one's breath into the infant's mouth, manually compressing and expanding the chest, or putting a tube past the larynx into the trachea and inflating the lungs. Injections of various drugs are advocated by some; others momentarily immerse the baby in ice water; and still others slap it vigorously. Patience, imperturbability, and exquisite gentleness will resuscitate more babies than all radical methods combined.

Tending to the Baby

A gadget resembling a bobby pin is substituted for the clamp on the three-inch stump of umbilical cord, where it remains until the cord dries and drops off. Usually no dressing is applied to the cord; it dries and desiccates better if exposed to the air. A drop of 1 per cent silver-nitrate solution or a little penicillin or tetracycline ointment is put in each eye to eliminate any chance of gonorrheal ophthalmia, eye infection due to the gonococcus bacterium.

The infant is immediately marked with the mother's name to prevent even the remotest chance of a mixup. There are several different methods of identification. At the Mount Sinai Hospital, when the mother is admitted to the labor suite, a bracelet of plastic with a cardboard insert marked with indelible ink is made in triplicate with her name and admission number spelled out. One bracelet is attached around the mother's wrist, and she wears it during the complete hospital stay. The other two completed bracelets are kept in reserve. As soon as the baby is born, one is placed around its left wrist and the other around the right ankle.

Delivery of the Placenta

The obstetrician next turns his attention to the delivery of the placenta. It is attached firmly to the uterus over an area about eight inches in diameter. After the child's birth the elastic uterus retracts and becomes much smaller, since it is no longer ballooned out by the fetus. Soft, its muscle fibers uncontracted, the uterus rests, following the strenuous work. In a variable number of minutes—usually just a few—it begins to contract again. The placenta is spongy, noncontractile tissue; the uterus, pure contracting muscle. With the further contractions of the undistended uterus, the area to which the placenta is attached diminishes marvelously. Since the placenta cannot contract and remains the same size, the flimsy attachment between the two is torn through, leaving the placenta free in the cavity of the uterus. With additional contractions of ever-increasing magnitude, the uterus obliterates its cavity by squeezing the free placenta downward into the capacious vagina. This occurs without the aid of man.

The uterus, after separating the placenta and expelling it into the vagina, assumes a different shape and position. When this occurs the uterus is grasped through the abdominal wall by a doctor or nurse and pushed downward toward the pelvis. The firm mass of muscle acts as a piston and thrusts the placenta halfway out; then the obstetrician gently pulls and twists the partially extruded afterbirth from the vagina. The membranes, being joined to the placenta, come away with it.

As soon as the placenta is delivered, the obstetrician examines it carefully to be certain it is complete. A placenta is formed by the fusion of twenty or so little placentae (cotyledons) which are more or less separate, but crowded compactly together. It resembles a mosaic of many smooth, even tiles, each tile representing a cotyledon; if the mosaic is complete, the placenta has been delivered intact. If there is a defect, one of the tiles missing, the accoucheur must put his hand in the uterus and remove the retained cotyledon, because otherwise it might cause immediate or late hemorrhage. I have oversimplified the problem; sometimes even the most experienced and meticulous obstetrician remains uncertain whether the placenta is complete, and if so he usually awaits developments.

Occasionally the normal mechanism of placental separation and extrusion does not function, and the placenta has to be peeled away from the wall of the uterus. With the patient anesthetized, the operator follows the navel cord high up into the uterus until he reaches the placenta. He then scratches it loose with his gloved fingers and removes it as he withdraws his hand. Most doctors perform a manual removal if the placenta is not delivered several minutes after the baby; they may do so sooner if hemorrhage occurs with the placenta undelivered.

At the site where the placenta was attached, pencil-thick blood vessels are torn across. The reason women do not ordinarily bleed from this wound is that the uterus is specifically constructed to meet the situation. Its muscle fibers run crisscross, that is, they interdigitate, and the blood vessels run in the interstices. It is like fitting the fingers of one hand between the fingers of the other. When the fingers are loosely fitted and held before the window, light comes through the web; but if they are tightly fitted, not even the tiniest beam filters past. In the same way as the light, the blood vessels of the placental site are shut off, the walls of the vessels squeezed together by the tightly contracted, interdigitating muscle bundles surrounding them on all sides. It is therefore essential that the uterus remain firmly contracted after the delivery of the placenta. Ordinarily this is accomplished by massaging the uterus off and on for an hour through the abdominal wall in a bread-kneading fashion. The modern obstetrician is greatly aided by two drugs, Oxytocin (obtained from the pituitary glands of cattle) and Ergonovine (obtained from a vegetable parasite which grows on rye). Both are now manufactured (synthesized) from chemicals in the laboratory. These drugs have a specific action on uterine muscle, causing it to contract firmly, and, when given in sufficient quantity, cause it to remain contracted. Each is given by injection, either intramuscularly or directly into a vein. The blood lost at delivery averages eight ounces, or half a pint. Since the woman's blood volume temporarily increases about a quart during pregnancy, she usually tolerates the loss of half a pint, or even several times this amount, with impunity.

Repair of the Episiotomy

The episiotomy—or if perchance one was not done, the perineal tear sustained—is repaired with absorbable catgut sutures, and since they are absorbable they need not be removed. The methods of repair, the length of the sutures, and the type of stitch vary so much from operator to operator that the usual lay question, "How many stitches did I have?" has no meaning. The answer, "Just a few," is truthful.

The Immediate Postdelivery Care of the Mother

The patient is either transferred to a recovery room adjacent to the delivery room or kept on the delivery table in the delivery room for one hour or longer, so that she can be carefully observed by doctors and nurses. The consistency of the uterus is constantly checked; if it is firm nothing has to be done, but if it is soft and toneless it must be massaged through the abdominal wall. When this does not harden it, a bottle of a dilute solution of Oxytocin in glucose water is fed into a vein over the period of an hour or two. The patient's blood pressure, pulse, and respirations are observed, as well as any evidence of abnormal vaginal bleeding. If the patient is being cared for in a recovery room, as soon as she is awake and conscious of her surroundings the husband is invited up so they may congratulate each other, and perhaps be introduced to the "little bundle from heaven."

The Postdelivery Care of the Baby

As soon as he has finished with the mother, the doctor while in the delivery room turns his attention to the infant, which has spent the first few minutes of its earthly existence snuggled in a warm crib. From this it is taken and laid on a table. The doctor examines the child for congenital defects. First he notes whether it has a harelip. Then he sweeps his fingers over the roof of the mouth to determine if the hard palate is normally formed; if the child has a cleft palate, its nose and mouth form a single cavity. The doctor looks to see if movement of the child's tongue is restricted by an excessive length and thickness of the fraenum (Latin: "bridle"), a small web of tissue that, when well developed, tends to bind the normally free front portion of the tongue to the floor of the mouth. The doctor may clip the fraenum with a pair of scissors; no bleeding follows, since the web has no blood vessels or more likely he lets it alone anticipating it will stretch later on. The doctor examines the skull to determine the distance between the bones. The bones on either side and the bones in front and in back are separated from each other by a narrow furrow (suture) covered only by skin. If the separation is abnormally great, it indicates unusual pressure within the skull, commonly caused by hydrocephalus, known to the layman as water on the brain. The doctor inspects the ears, for frequently a small accessory lobe grows like a mushroom from the true lobe. If this is present, a piece of silk thread is tied tightly about its stalk, and in a few days the accessory lobe drops off. He listens to the child's heart and lungs with a stethoscope. He determines whether the heart sounds are normal, for certain abnormal sounds (murmurs) denote abnormalities of structure. He also determines whether the lungs are expanding properly. He feels the abdomen for tumors. He then puts the child on its belly and examines the lower bony spinal column for defects. The presence of such a defect (*spina bifida*—"spine divided in two") can be determined without X-rays only if a small fluid sac overlies it. He next examines the genitals of the child, in the male paying special attention as to whether or not there is hypospadias, a defect in the underside of the penis which discharges the urine at the base of the penis instead of its tip. The scrotum, the pouch-shaped sac below the penis, is felt to see if both testicles have descended. Often, particularly in premature infants, one or both are still retained within the abdomen. The anus, the external end of the rectum, is observed to see if it is normally patent or if it is imperforate; if the latter, an opening must be made within the next several hours by a surgeon experienced in the procedure. Then the doctor examines the arms and legs. He observes whether the toes or fingers are webbed and if there are any accessory ones. Very often the extra digit is purely rudimentary, hanging by a thin strand of skin. Sometimes, however, it is well developed and as well attached as the other five fingers or toes. If it is of the former type, the doctor ties a silk thread about it and allows it to drop off a few days later. He examines the feet to see if they are clubbed, for remarkable results may be obtained if a club foot is put in a cast during the first few days of life. Then he rapidly passes his fingers over the whole bony framework to ferret out unsuspected fractures.

Mother Meets Baby

The baby is wrapped in its receiving blanket and, if the mother is awake, taken to her to be loved and held. This is a touching scene, and only a stony heart would not be moved by it. Most mothers, particularly first mothers, are awed, a little strange and frightened. One has to place the baby next to her and guide the mother's arm to encircle the infant. Opening the blanket and demonstrating the presence of ten toes and ten fingers, and the genitals to corroborate the sex, breaks the ice, and then mother and baby really start getting acquainted. If there is a recovery room and the mother is promptly transferred to it, the baby's introduction may be postponed until the father can join them.

The baby is soon transferred to the nursery, frequently in an electrically heated boxlike structure on wheels, where it is weighed, bathed, and diapered. Its temperature is taken rectally or under the armpit (the axilla). If it is below a certain level the infant is placed in a specially heated crib; otherwise, in a regular bassinet. If the infant has a birth weight of less than five pounds, it will no doubt be placed in a special nursery for prematures, and perhaps in an incubator with oxygen available.

The Moment of Triumph

After one or two hours, depending on hospital routine, the mother is wheeled in her bed to one of the postpartum floors. Hers is a victorious march; if a woman is ever a queen it is at this *triumphant moment* of her life.

14

Difficult Labor

Difficult labor is uncommon today. Its lessened frequency in modern childbirth stems from prevention, sorting out probable cases and delivering them by Cesarean section before labor's onset, and from the fact that there are many therapeutic measures which can be employed to prevent a labor from becoming difficult. Such measures are the stimulation of weak contractions by drugs, the inducement of rest during labor through sedation, the administration of glucose solution into an arm vein to eliminate dehydration, and the prevention of infection by antibiotics. But even granting the premise that the chance of having a difficult labor is slim, no discussion of birth would be complete without its inclusion.

Dystocia (Greek, meaning "difficult birth") has many causes. These can be classified under three headings: abnormalities of the expulsive forces, of the passenger, or of the passage.

Poor Contractions

The first of these, abnormality of the expulsive forces, is termed inertia of the uterus—that is, poor contractions. They may be too short, too feeble, too infrequent, or, as is usual, a combination of all three. The labor contractions may be subnormal throughout the travail (primary inertia) or normal at first and then become desultory (secondary inertia). Drugs to stimulate labor, such as Oxytocin, are used in exceedingly small amounts to treat inertia. Usually it is given as a constant infusion in an arm vein, a little of the drug being diluted 500 or 1000 times with glucose water. When an Oxytocin drip is started, it is likely to be continued until after the delivery. Another drug, sparteine, has been used in the place of Oxytocin. Its advantages over the latter remain unproved. Strong contractions often follow these aids to labor.

Contrary to expectation, the patient's physical condition at the onset of labor seems to have no influence on the character of the labor. Patients debilitated by wasting disease to the point of complete invalidism have as strong contractions as the most robust.

It seems wise at this point to continue to lay the ghost of dry labors. For some reason laymen have the idea that dry labors per se are longer, more painful, and more dangerous than labors with intact membranes. This is not true, according to several investigations. All agree that, if everything else is normal, not only is there no injurious effect from the premature rupture of membranes, but it actually exerts a beneficial influence on the length of labor.

Abnormalities of the Passenger

The second source of dystocia is abnormality of the passenger, the fetus. The most common complications in this respect are abnormalities of position and size. The normal position of the fetus during labor is with the head down, the breech up, the spinal column parallel to the long axis of the mother, and the back of the baby toward the mother's abdominal wall. The head is flexed so that the baby's chin practically rests on its breastbone. Labor in the average case is lengthened somewhat by the two most common variations from normal fetal position—posterior presentations and breech presentations. In the former, the baby presents head first, but its back faces the back of the mother instead of her abdomen (O.P., occiput posterior) and the length of labor is often increased. In a breech presentation, where the child presents with the breech down and the head up, the average duration of the labor is increased about one hour. The less common abnormalities of position—transverse (the long diameter of the child and that of the mother being at right angles), face (the head, instead of being completely flexed or bowed as usual, is extended so that the face presents to the pelvic inlet instead of the crown of the head), and brow (the head flexed only partially so that the forehead presents)—lengthen labor more than one hour. Strange as it may seem, the weight of the baby appears to have no effect on multiparous labors but exerts an appreciable one on primiparous labors. A first labor with a nine-pound baby is usually two and one-half hours longer than a first labor with a five-and-one-half-pound baby.

Abnormalities of the Passage

The third source of dystocia lies in abnormalities of the passage, the birth corridor, which includes the bony pelvis as well as soft tissues, the cervix and vagina.

The bony pelvis is roughly funnel-shaped. The child enters the circular mouth of the funnel (pelvic inlet) and issues forth from the spout (pelvic outlet). If any diameter of the pelvis is diminished below the limit of ordinary normal variations we classify the pelvis as contracted. The type of contraction depends, first, on the particular diameter affected and, second, on the cause.

Our modern concept of the obstetrical pelvis and its measurement (pelvimetry) dates from the middle of the last century, when two professors in Kiel each carefully measured the pelves of a thousand German women, and in this way established what measurements cause a pelvis to be classified as normal, borderline, or contracted.

Contracted Pelvis

Indications of pelvic size can be gathered from the patient's obstetrical history, by her height (taller women have larger pelves than women of shorter stature), by manual measurements, by how far the baby has already descended when labor commences, and by the labor's course.

At the pelvic examination during the first prenatal visit the obstetrician takes a key measurement for the estimation of pelvic size. He measures the diagonal conjugate (C.D.), the distance from the under surface of the symphysis bone in front to the top of the sacrum (the posterior bony wall of the pelvis) where it joins the last vertebra. If the measurement is five inches or longer, one can almost be certain that the upper part of the pelvis, the pelvic inlet, is not contracted. He also feels the general shape and contour of the bony pelvis, particularly to determine whether its lowermost portion is ample in size.

In a first pregnancy, by the time labor commences at term, the part of the baby presenting, the head or breech, should be engaged—that is, it already should have descended well into the pelvic inlet, the mouth of the bony funnel. Lack of fetal engagement at the onset of labor in births subsequent to the first does not suggest a contracted pelvis.

If after several hours of adequately strong labor there is little evidence of progress in either the baby's descent or dilation of the cervix, the properly trained physician will reconsider his previous favorable estimate of pelvic size.

Whenever the physician is suspicious of the adequate size of the pelvis, he has available an excellent technique for confirming or refuting these suspicions, X-ray pelvimetry. This is one situation in which the value of X-ray strongly outweighs the theoretic risks of radiation effects on mother or fetus.

X-ray Pelvimetry

If, because of a previous bad obstetric history or subnormal manual measurements, the physician determines at the patient's first visit to obtain X-ray pelvimetry, he will undoubtedly postpone the procedure until about the last week or so of pregnancy or until early labor. The postponement is motivated by his desire to avoid the theoretical risk of exposing the early fetus to X-rays, but, more important, it permits a meaningful comparison between the pelvic diameters and those of the fetal skull. X-ray pelvimetry can be done with equal satisfaction during labor.

Only by X-ray pelvimetry can the internal diameters of the pelvis be measured with precision. Numerous techniques are in use, and roentgenologists have individual preferences. All of the standard methods are satisfactory with scrupulous attention paid to technical details such as the positioning of the patient and the distance of the X-ray tube from the film. Ordinarily two pictures are taken: a front view from which one can measure the transverse diameters of the pelvis, and a lateral view from which the longitudinal diameters are read.

The experienced physician is not only able to obtain precise measurements of crucial pelvic diameters from X-ray pelvimetry but he also gains an understanding of the pelvic architecture which offers him valuable guidance in a problem case. He can determine whether the inlet is round, heart-shaped, narrowed or elliptical; he can see whether the walls of the pelvis tend to converge or diverge; and he can study the form of the sacrum. It may be important to know whether it is straight or curved, and whether it flares back or forward.

Large, modern maternity hospitals, like the one at the Mount Sinai Hospital, have an X-ray unit as part of the delivery-floor equipment. It renders valuable assistance.

Disproportion

In reality there is no straightforward entity such as a contracted pelvis or a normal pelvis. The true issue is whether or not Mrs. Jones's pelvis is large enough to deliver successfully baby Jones, with whom she will labor or is laboring. A pelvis technically contracted may be functionally normal, or a technically normal pelvis may be functionally contracted, as in the case of a woman with small but normal pelvic measurements who labors with an eleven-pound infant. Therefore in each labor one attempts to judge the size of the baby in relation to the size of the pelvis. If the baby is big and the pelvis small, examination demonstrating true disproportion between the two, unsuccessful labor is obviated by Cesarean section a few days before the due date or early in the labor.

However, if there is uncertainty about the possibility of a vaginal delivery, a test of labor is called for, which harms neither mother nor baby. Today such test labors are rarely allowed to last more than eight or ten hours; if at the end of the test period little progress has been made, a Cesarean section is performed. On the other hand, if the presenting part has descended and the cervix is dilating satisfactorily, labor is permitted to continue with full anticipation of a normal birth.

The baby's head is extremely malleable, since the bones forming the skull are still separated, not having fused together as they will by the age of eighteen months. Molding of the head by the forces of labor is very gradual, the head acting as though made of very stiff clay. Molding may make a big difference—the head may gradually decrease a half-inch or more in its critical transverse diameter during several hours of labor. When a baby comes breech first, the aftercoming head is born without the opportunity to mold. Therefore larger pelvic diameters are required to accommodate a breech birth than when the baby exits head first. Because of this, many physicians make it routine to secure X-ray pelvimetry in all breech cases, particularly in a first labor.

Causes of Contracted Pelves

Contracted pelves are due to heredity or environment. The generally contracted variety usually occurs in undersized, small-boned, fragile-looking women. In them it is largely an inherited stigma. General malnutrition and poor hygiene during the years of growth may exaggerate this inherited pattern. A typical generally contracted pelvis is about four-fifths the size of the normal pelvis.

Individuals in whom the inherited reduction in body height is decidedly more marked than is seen in small normal people are classed as dwarfs.

Dwarfs

Dwarfs present an interesting obstetrical problem. Medically we distinguish two types of inherited dwarfism: the true ateliotic (Greek: "not" + "complete") dwarf, a properly proportioned individual who differs from the normal only in his miniature appearance; and the chondrodystrophic (Greek: "cartilage" + "ill" + "nutrition") dwarf, an individual with very short arms and legs and a normal-sized head and trunk. Circus troupes contain both types.

The ateliotic rarely have children, but the short-limbed chondrodystrophic, so faithfully depicted by Velázquez, presents a very real obstetrical problem, since both sexes are normally fertile. This type of dwarfism narrows the pelvic inlet and, since the children are of normal size, dystocia invariably results. Before the modern surgical era and its relatively safe Cesarean operation, chondrodystrophic women rarely survived pregnancy. Today, of course, the chances for a live mother and a live infant are excellent. A chondrodystrophic parent of either sex may have normal children; in fact, this is usually the case, although there is no doubt that the deformity is more common in certain stocks tainted by it.

Rickets and Osteomalacia

Rickets and osteomalacia (Greek: "bone" + "softness") are the two environmental conditions which cause the greatest distortion and contraction of the pelvis. Rickets, a disease of infancy, is due to dietary deficiencies of calcium, phosphorus, and vitamin D, and at the same time a subnormal quantity of the ultraviolet rays from sunlight. Therefore it is mainly an urban disease, for though rural children may have rickets-producing diets, they get enough sunlight to compensate. It is a disease for which people with dark skin have a special predisposition since their skin pigment makes it more difficult for the ultraviolet rays to penetrate.

In a severe case the whole skeleton of the infant becomes soft and puttylike. Arms and legs bow; the spinal column becomes bent and angulated; and the ribs become beaded where they join the breastbone (the rickety rosary). At the same time the forehead protrudes on either side (rachitic bossae) and the pelvis becomes narrowed. A rachitic infant delays its walking because of pain in standing on its softened limbs; as a result, it spends its waking hours sitting. The whole weight of the upper body, transmitted down the spinal column, constantly presses upon the puttylike sacrum (the large bone that forms the base of the spinal column and the rear of the pelvic girdle); this makes the sacrum buckle forward, reducing the most important diameter of the pelvic inlet. In severe cases this diameter is so diminished that it offers an insuperable barrier to vaginal delivery. The lower portion of the pelvis, the pelvic outlet, is not contracted in rickets; as a matter of fact it is often widened, since the constant sitting posture of the child tends to spread apart the softened bones.

Osteomalacia, adult rickets, is unknown in this country but existed in northern China and in certain parts of India, and perhaps still does. In the latter country, it was intimately associated with the folk custom that decreed permanent indoor seclusion for the women of certain classes, a custom called Purdah.

Unlike rickets, osteomalacia contracts the outlet as well as the inlet of the pelvis—the sprout of the funnel as well as the bowl.

Both rickets and osteomalacia are best treated by prevention. A well-balanced diet, including cod-liver oil or other substances rich in vitamin D, and abundant sunshine during childhood and pregnancy make their acquisition virtually impossible. I am happy to say that during my medical lifetime rickets has almost disappeared from the American scene, a tribute to our efficient public-health agencies. This makes a striking contrast to forty-five years ago, when I assisted at, or performed, many Cesarean sections because of rachitic pelvic deformities. Today there are few if any such cases in all New York.

Pelvic Fractures and Limps

Very occasionally a poorly aligned healed fracture of one of the pelvic bones causes difficult birth. Either a large bone callous or distortion of the bony architecture may create an obstacle to pelvic delivery. This is seen mainly after automobile accidents.

A unilateral limp during childhood, which was so commonly seen after polio, may cause a flattening on one side of the pelvic bowl. The side affected is the side of the good leg. The child bearing all its weight on one leg flattens the still, malleable pelvic brim on that side, while the pelvis on the side of the withered leg remains normally rounded.

Soft-Tissue Dystocia

In rare instances, despite strong pains, a normal pelvis, an average-sized infant, and a satisfactory position of the fetus, the cervix dilates at an abnormally slow rate. These cases are spoken of as instances of cervical dystocia. Some of them follow previous operations or treatments of the cervix, while others show no discoverable cause. Cervical dystocia may prolong labor many hours, and even then the very last stages of dilation may have to be completed by some operative means. Treatment consists of patience on the part of patient and physician, to say nothing of patience on the part of the family.

Resistant vaginal tissues may prolong the second stage, the time intervening from the full dilation of the cervix to the birth of the child. This is especially common in comparatively elderly primiparas, women aged thirty-five or more, in their first labor. Strenuous athletic pursuits, especially horseback riding, thicken vaginal muscles, and this occasionally produces a soft-tissue dystocia. From this point of view—and from only this one viewpoint—the thin, emaciated, sedentary type of woman has an obstetrical advantage over her robust, muscular, athletic sister. Dystocia from unusually resistant vaginal tissues can be easily overcome by an episiotomy—cutting of the tissues. Occasionally fibroid uterine tumors (localized overgrowth of smooth muscle and connective tissue) block the pelvis. Whether or not a fibroid causes labor difficulty is more a matter of its location in the uterus than its size. A fibroid high up virtually never causes difficulty in delivery, while one low down in the pelvic region may very well do so. Rarely, a sizable cyst of the ovary may lodge in the pelvis behind the uterus, leaving insufficient room for the baby to enter the pelvis. In the presence of an obstructing fibroid or cyst, a Cesarean section is necessary unless the obstruction can be pushed out of the pelvis vaginally to allow space for the baby to enter. At the time of the Cesarean section, an ovarian cyst is always removed but the fibroid may not be, depending on the anatomical findings at the time of operation.

In writing this chapter I was constantly aware that a lay reader may have a tendency to overemphasize and personalize anything which smacks of the abnormal in birth. Instead of taking the cheerful attitude that the abnormal is the infrequent—an attitude which would be fully justified by facts—she says to herself, "It would be just my luck to have a tough time."

More than ninety-five out of a hundred readers will not have a difficult labor. They will be pleasantly surprised to discover how easy and simple the whole process is. To the remaining five or less we can give comfort by assuring them honestly that modern obstetrics accepts the challenge of the abnormal with total confidence, since it finds no abnormality beyond the reach of the knowledge and tools now available to it.

15

Obstetrical Operations

A significant trend in modern childbirth is the increase in the incidence of operative deliveries, causing a sharp decrease in the number of babies arriving unassisted. In this section I shall attempt to unearth the factors responsible for the rise in operative births.

One reason is that the constantly greater use of hospitals, antiseptics, and anesthetics has created an aura of surgical confidence, making an obstetrical operation not nearly so momentous a matter as it was twenty years ago.

A second factor is a subtle shift of values in the importance of the infant's life when compared to the life and health of its mother. Until recently, except to one religious group, the life and health of each mother were inestimably more important than those of her child; today the pendulum has veered a long way toward dead center. I have tried to discover the explanation for this shift in values. It is in part due to three things: the smaller number of children that parents produce, the more careful planning of pregnancies, and the reduction of the infant mortality rate. For the smaller families of this generation, the product of each pregnancy gains in importance, whereas when a woman already had ten children her eleventh was not so exciting. Then, too, most of today's pregnancies are planned pregnancies; they usually don't just happen. When a couple carefully plans to have a child and the result is a fetal death, there is a sense of deep frustration which the loss of an unplanned baby perhaps may not elicit to the same degree. And with the decrease in infant deaths there is the feeling that if the child is born alive, it is certain to be reared. This was not true in Paris in 1668, when the famous obstetrician François Mauriceau wrote, "We see daily about half of the young children die, before they are two or three years old." With the change in attitude, operative interference is often resorted to in order to save the baby, and with today's improvement in surgical techniques, the mother's life is not endangered.

A third source of the increase in operative obstetrics is the modern woman's insistence on short, relatively painless labors. I am not castigating her, for I dare say if I were metamorphosed into a laboring woman, I should probably join the chorus of "Don't let me stay in labor too long, and be sure it doesn't hurt." As is obvious to the reader from earlier discussions, several of the current techniques of pain relief require a forceps delivery; for heavy analgesia, and caudal and epidural, as well as spinal, anesthesia deprive the patient of her usual urge to bear down and spontaneously expel the baby. This increase in forceps deliveries is an increase in only the simplest type, the low or outlet forceps, an operation which carries no additional risk to mother or baby.

Good obstetrics cannot condone more complex operative procedures done solely to shorten labor, for under these circumstances delivery is carried out before the patient is ready, substituting a needless and dangerous procedure for one which would be simple and safe minutes or hours later. The obstetrician whose inexperience or excessive sympathy prompts him to make undue haste because of the importunings of an overanxious family or patient has frequent cause for regret.

It is impossible to fix the optimum obstetrical operative rate, for it depends on many variables. The type of clientele a particular doctor or hospital draws affects it; the greater the reputation of either, the larger the proportion of problem cases. As previously stated, analgesia and anesthesia are also important factors, as is parity (the number of previous deliveries). More important than the gross operative rate are the types of operations and particularly the obstetrical end result. Are the mothers left healthy and well, with future childbearing unprejudiced? Are the babies vigorous and uninjured?

Forceps Delivery

The majority of obstetrical operations are done by means of a special instrument, the forceps. This consists of two separate thin steel blades with inner surfaces curved to fit the sides of the infant's head. The blades are inserted separately into the vagina, opposite each other, and when their handles are articulated, the child's head is securely grasped between the blades. With moderate traction on the handles, exerted in the axis of the vagina, the head is extracted.

The word *forceps* in Latin means "a pair of tongs." It is said to have been derived from the earlier Latin words *formus* ("hot") and *capere* ("to take"). The obstetric forceps in its modern form, an instrument capable of extracting a living child without injury to it or to the mother, is an invention of the early seventeenth century. Previous to this, single-bladed and even double-bladed instruments, called hooks, were in use, but probably only for the extraction of a dead child. The old double-bladed instruments had a permanent articulation so that each blade could not be inserted separately; they looked like the once-familiar ice tongs.

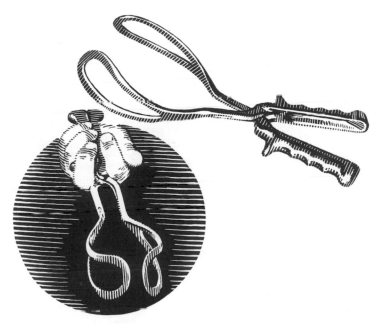

A common type of forceps

The inventors of the modern obstetrical forceps were a singular medical family—the Chamberlens. In 1569 the first of the English line, William, emigrated from France to London to escape Huguenot persecution. Most of the Chamberlens were Royal Surgeons or Physicians, and several English queens were delivered by them. This obstetrical dynasty of Chamberlen extended uninterruptedly from Peter the Elder's admission to the Guild of Barber-Surgeons in about 1596 to the death of Hugh, Junior, in 1728. They were no ordinary men; they lived hard and tempestuously, unwilling to confine their energies within the narrow scope of their professions.

History of the Forceps

The forceps were probably invented in about 1600 by Peter the Elder and kept as a hereditary family secret to be buried with Hugh, Junior, in

1728. According to modern medical standards, such conduct was wholly unethical, and any twentieth-century doctor who would dare a similar practice would find himself ostracized, read out of all medical societies, and anathema to decent people. However, it is obviously unfair to judge the behavior of one century by the standards of another.

How was the secret finally revealed? The existence of the forceps was hinted at as early as 1616 at a meeting of the Royal College when a slurring reference was made to the boast of Peter Chamberlen the Younger "that he and his brother, and none others, excelled in the management of difficult labors."

Hugh, Senior, emigrated to Holland in 1699 under suspicion of debt. While there he appears to have obtained some money, for he returned to England for two years before settling permanently in Amsterdam. While in Holland, probably at the time of his supposed flight, he sold the secret of the forceps to Hendrik Van Roonhuyze, the leader of Dutch obstetrics. During the succeeding years of the early eighteenth century the secret oozed out in England and on the Continent. William Giffard of London used the forceps openly on April 6, 1726, calling them extractors. He is generally considered "the altruistic and honorable physician who should receive full credit for introducing the forceps into general use in England." By 1733, when Edmund Chapman published the very first account of the forceps, there were already several models, and their use "was well known to all the principal men of the profession, both in town and country."

The retention of an important medical secret transmitted from generation to generation for a century and a quarter is unique in history. The Chamberlens were crafty enough to exclude all others from the room when they operated; they used the forceps unassisted.

Not because of its antiquity—for other obstetrical operative procedures antedated it—but because of its importance, delivery by forceps merits first place in the discussion of obstetrical operations.

Indications for a Forceps Delivery

A delivery by forceps can be done only under definite conditions: if the head of the child fits the pelvis without any disproportion, the membranes are ruptured, and the cervix is completely dilated. This means it cannot be done before the second stage of labor, except in the very rare case when the obstetrician stretches or cuts the last remaining undilated portion of the cervix to effect immediate delivery.

Indications for delivery by forceps are obviously divided into two broad classes—fetal and maternal. The sole fetal indication is acute distress of the unborn child, evidence of which is displayed by an irregular fetal heart with a rate below 100, particularly when coupled with the appearance of brown or dark green amniotic fluid in a head presentation. This change in the ordinarily colorless fluid is caused by contamination with fetal intestinal contents (meconium). If the fetus is in poor condition, the anal sphincter (rectal muscle) relaxes and allows meconium to be expelled. (The appearance of meconium in a breech presentation is normal and of no significance.) In the main there are two causes which account for these signs of fetal distress: a disturbance in the placental-fetal circulation, leading to deprivation of oxygen for the child; or pressure on the head of the child from the stress of labor. Any of a number of accidents may cause interference with the fetus's oxygen supply: the cord may prolapse (slip down) into the vagina, the abnormal situation permitting its compression between the child's body and the rigid walls of the pelvis; or the umbilical cord may become shortened from looping itself about the child's neck or body so that, as the child descends, the cord is made so taut that its blood vessels are constricted. Premature separation of the placenta may also interfere with the fetal-placental circulation by lifting up and putting out of function large areas of the placental bed. The second source of fetal distress, excessive pressure on the head, may result from a short, stormy labor or a very long one—either may cause cerebral concussion or even hemorrhage. When there is an acute slowing of the fetal pulse, particularly when associated with meconium-stained amniotic fluid, delivery is wise. If the head is sufficiently low in the pelvis and the cervix completely dilated, a prompt forceps delivery offers the best solution.

The maternal indications for forceps are many. The mother may be ill with heart disease, tuberculosis, a toxemia of pregnancy, or some other serious illness; if so, it is wise to terminate labor as soon as feasible and safe. Or perhaps the patient has been delivered in a previous pregnancy by Cesarean section and to protect the uterine scar from rupture one spares it some of the severe strain of the second stage of labor by a forceps delivery as early as possible. Then, too, mother and fetus may both be in excellent condition but a forceps may be indicated by lack of progress in labor. If the cervix is fully dilated, the head very low in the pelvis, and there is no progress for an hour, it is best to interfere for the sake of both mother and child. If the head is higher, usually a two-hour or longer period without progress after full dilatation of the cervix is permitted before a forceps is undertaken.

The indications I have described are agreed upon by all obstetricians, but this is not true of the so-called "prophylactic forceps," which may be done as a matter of routine as soon as the head impinges against the perineum, particularly in first births. Proponents of the prophylactic forceps, who include most obstetricians of this country, as well as the author, claim that it spares the fetal head from prolonged pressure against a rigid perineum, and that the mother is relieved of much of the strain of the terminal part of labor. Also, if one combines the prophy-lactic forceps with an episiotomy (anticipating a tear by cutting the perineum), the maternal tissues are left in better condition at the con-clusion of the delivery in some cases than if a spontaneous birth were allowed. Those opposed damn it with the catch phrase, "Meddlesome midwifery."

The Performance of a Forceps Delivery

Before a forceps operation the patient is anesthetized by general or conduction anesthesia, positioned on the table, cleansed, and draped. The operator performs a careful vaginal examination to determine the position of the head. This is done with the aid of familiar landmarks, the two soft spots (fontanelles) at the front and back of the child's head. The one in front is relatively large and diamond-shaped, while the one in back is small and triangular. The operator can corroborate his fontanelle findings by crowding his fingers alongside the head and sliding them above it to feel the baby's ear, since the front of the ear is fixed, while the back is loose and floppy.

After accurately diagnosing the exact position in which the baby's head lies, he picks up one blade of the forceps and inserts his other hand in the vagina. He then gently slides the blade along the palm of his vaginal hand so that it is insinuated between the vaginal wall and the fetal head. He then shifts the blade so that the child's ear underlies the center of the blade. Now properly placed, the first blade is held firmly in position while the operator introduces the second blade, manipulating it so that it comes to rest on a straight line opposite its fellow. For example, if we again imagine the pelvis as a clock with twelve in front at the top, and one blade is inserted at three o'clock, the other would be inserted at nine; or if the first blade is inserted at half-past five, the other would be placed at half-past eleven. The two handles are then locked. If the forceps are properly applied, the handles lock easily; if not, they must both be removed and reinserted. An experienced forceps operator knows that forceps injuries to the baby are the result of an imperfect application of the blades, and he will spend time and patience in getting just the application he desires. When he is satisfied that both blades are well applied to the sides of the head he begins his forceps extraction.

The head, as in a spontaneous birth, cannot be born by forceps unless a line drawn down the center of its long axis is parallel to the long axis of the pelvic outlet. Obstetrical forceps have two functions—to rotate and to extract. The operator first rotates the head so that these two axes are parallel, the blades at three and nine on our imaginary dial. He does this by turning the handles through the necessary arc. This accomplished, he begins the extraction, pulling steadily for fifteen or twenty seconds, then releasing traction momentarily before he pulls again. The cycle is repeated over and over. The head descends little by little with each tug; when it distends the perineum, an episiotomy is performed. Soon the head is almost completely born, the forceps blades slipped off, and delivery of the head completed by a lifting motion on the chin applied through the mother's tissues, the perineum. The delivery of the rest of the child is the same as in a spontaneous birth.

The amount of force necessary to perform a forceps operation depends on the point in the pelvis to which the head has already descended and on the size of the baby and the pelvis. An easy delivery requires relatively little force, but a difficult one requires brawn. Forceps operations are divided into high, mid, low, and outlet, depending on the point in the pelvis the head has reached when the operation is begun. The guide points which differentiate the various types are the same ischial spines I mentioned in describing a spontaneous birth. If the head has descended to the level of these spines, it is a mid-forceps; it is a high forceps when the head is above the spines, and a low forceps when the head is below them. When the scalp of the child is clearly visible on spreading open the lips of the vagina before the operation is begun, it is termed a perineal or outlet forceps.

High forceps has fallen into complete disuse because of the great damage which it so often causes to the maternal tissues and the child. Cesarean section, which is far safer for both patients, has been substituted. A high mid-forceps, one between high and mid, is also rarely done.

The incidence of forceps operations varies markedly in different clinics, depending on the parity (number of previous deliveries), race, and social status of their clientele. It is much higher among private patients, perhaps because their demands for speedy deliverance are more personalized by their own private accoucheurs. It also depends on whether or not the obstetric service practices routine prophylactic forceps.

There are as many models of forceps as there are kinds of baseball bats. In some instances a new forceps merely represents a slight modification of some pre-existing standard instrument—perhaps an inch longer or an inch shorter. In my opinion it makes relatively little difference which forceps is used as long as the operator is skilled in the use of that particular instrument to accomplish delivery under the circumstances presented by the case at hand. Obstetricians may sing paeans of praise for the Smith or the Jones instrument; but it is largely a matter of the instrument to which one has become accustomed by training and experience.

Vacuum Extraction

Many attempts have been made to replace the steel forceps with softer material to accomplish extraction, including a net to be insinuated over the child's head. The most successful is the vacuum extractor introduced in Sweden in 1954. It consists of a metal cup that is closely applied to the scalp. A controlled amount of negative pressure is created in the cup with a pump which sucks a segment of scalp into the cup, which seals it firmly in place. Direct traction on the head can be made by pulling on the rubber tube attached to the cup, or the head can be rotated by it. Vacuum extraction is very popular abroad but has never gained a firm hold in the United States. There are numerous reports of fetal damage—lacerations and hematomas of the scalp and infrequent brain hemorrhage. On the other hand European experience bespeaks its relative safety. When used it does not eliminate the need for episiotomy.

Breech Extractions

A breech extraction may be done without the aid of instruments. And as for its antiquity, I venture to guess that, if Mrs. Noah had two breech children, the second was delivered by extraction. Probably the first was allowed to deliver unaided; part of the child was born spontaneously, then further progress was temporarily arrested, and by the time birth completed itself the child was lost. For the second breech— if Mrs. Noah had two—Mr. Noah stood by and tugged on the child at the proper moment. In some such way the operation began. Since then science has evolved certain technical maneuvers which have increased the efficiency of breech extractions.

As stated in an earlier chapter, it is quite usual for the child to present as a breech (the buttocks over the pelvis, head toward the ribs) until the last four to six weeks of pregnancy, when most of them turn spontaneously to a head (vertex) presentation. However, 3.5 to 4 per cent persist as breeches, remaining so during labor. No cause is to be found for the majority of breech presentations. Even if there is no apparent cause for the breech, the likelihood for it to recur in subsequent pregnancies is increased; although even in these women the chances probably remain less than one in four.

A breech birth, except for a slight lengthening of labor in an average case, is no more difficult for the mother, nor has she increased likelihood to complications postpartum. On the other hand, a breech birth carries a somewhat greater risk for the baby than a cephalic (Greek: "head") delivery. However, the hazard today is materially less than it was years ago. The improvement is due to several causes. It has now become current practice to visualize and measure by X-ray the mother's pelvis when a breech presentation persists near term, unless the adequacy of her pelvis has already been proved by the previous vaginal delivery of a large baby. In the case of a breech presentation, a good-sized baby, and an unfavorable pelvis, risk to the baby is obviated by a Cesarean section before labor begins. Improved anesthesia has also paid its dividend in the reduction of breech mortality. Then, too, certain technical operative steps—notably the proper method of bringing down the baby's arms when they rest straight upward above the head, extended like a cheer-leader's, and the application of forceps to the after-coming head for its delivery—have contributed their part.

The labor of the patient delivering a breech is followed with unusual care, and the patient is taken to the delivery room as soon as the cervix is fully dilated. At this stage the fetal heart is listened to frequently, for one of the fatal accidents that may occur to the breech child is compression of the navel cord between the infant's body and the pelvis in the course of its descent. If at any time after the cervix becomes fully dilated the fetal heart becomes significantly slow or irregular, the operation of extraction is begun at once. If not, the patient is allowed to give birth to the breech, as far as its hipbones, through her own unaided expulsive efforts. The child descends through the vagina on its side, and when the hipbones come into view, the mother is anesthetized and prepared and draped as for a forceps delivery. If it is a frank breech (the legs completely bent at the hips straight at the knees so that the feet rest against the chest), the operator hooks a finger in each groin and pulls downward in the axis of the vagina. The legs soon drop out, and then he grasps and pulls on the child's thighs, trunk, and chest in turn, gently climbing up the body with his hands. Now the front axilla (armpit) comes into view, and the doctor inserts a finger in the upper vagina, with which he hooks the upper arm, and the whole extremity is flipped out. The rear arm is similarly delivered. When the baby is a footling breech—legs extended straight down, not flexed upward at the hips—delivery is simpler. As soon as the cervix is fully dilated and the feet appear outside of the vagina, extraction can be begun.

The head of the baby remains to be delivered. This can be done manually; the operator allows the chest and belly of the child to rest on his forearm and hand, two fingers of which he inserts in the vagina to make pressure on the upper lip and jaw of the infant. This keeps its head flexed, which aids in the delivery. The fingers of the other hand encircle the nape of the neck, which by this time is born and presents at the entrance to the vagina, and make downward and outward traction. By this maneuver the head is slowly born. The alternative operation is to apply forceps to the sides of the head after the shoulders are delivered and to do a forceps extraction of the after-coming head. We prefer the latter technique, particularly in a primipara.

Since cephalic (head first) deliveries are safer for the baby, during late pregnancy or even during the early hours of labor the doctor frequently attempts to convert a breech presentation to a head presentation. This is performed by grasping the fetus through its mother's abdominal wall, and turning it through 180 degrees by gradually pushing the breech to one side with one hand, and the head and shoulders to the opposite side with the other hand. When successful, this rotates the child to a cephalic presentation. Not infrequently the infant thumbs its embryonic nose *in utero* and reverts back to a breech presentation as soon as the doctor lets go.

Version

Just the reverse of cephalic version, podalic (Greek: "foot") version consists in turning the child from a vertex to a breech and extracting it at once as a breech. The procedure is technically termed an internal podalic version because the operator inserts his whole hand inside the uterus, reaches up and grasps the child by the feet, turning it completely upside down. The cumbersome name, internal podalic version, is usually referred to by the abbreviated term, version.

Version was the earliest obstetrical operation, except for breech extraction. It was used in antiquity, lost in the intervening centuries, and reintroduced in 1550. At this time the forceps had not been thought of, and Cesarean section, if used at all, was still a freak spectacle. Naturally, therefore, version became very popular in difficult cases. With the introduction of the forceps and the free and safe use of Cesarean section, version is used infrequently today.

Podalic version is indicated in two groups of cases: in transverse presentations, when the long axis of the child lies across the mother's pelvis; and in all head presentations in which it is believed that delivery can be more safely and rapidly accomplished by means of it. Of course it can never be done unless the cervix is completely out of the way by being fully dilated. The necessity for version in transverse presentations is obvious, since birth is mechanically impossible until the fetus is converted into a longitudinal presentation. In head presentations version may rarely be indicated if the head is very high or if the head is engaged and attempts at forceps fail. Today the more usual solution for such problems is Cesarean section. In cases of prolapse of the cord (slipping down of the navel cord into the vagina ahead of the child), with the cervix fully dilated, version may offer the ideal method of delivery, for it can usually be accomplished more rapidly than any other method.

Version is not attempted if there is disproportion between the size of the fetus and the pelvis, or when the membranes have ruptured sometime before and much of the amniotic fluid has drained away. For then the uterus fits so snugly about the child that there is danger of rupturing it in the process of turning the child.

The technique of version calls for the same anesthetization, draping, and preparation of the patient as are demanded by forceps and breech deliveries. In addition, some operators pour sterile liquid soap into the lower birth canal to make it slippery. The operator wears a special long rubber gauntlet, which encases his arm to the elbow. When the patient is deeply anesthetized, the whole hand is inserted into the vagina and the fetal head gently displaced. The obstetrician ruptures the membranes, passes his hand beyond the head, up into the uterus. He folds the baby's arms over its chest in a sort of Napoleonic stance. This aids in preventing the arms from passing through the pelvis at the same time as the head; for the excessive diameter of both arms plus the head blocks the pelvic inlet. The operator then grasps both feet of the child and pulls gently on them, while at the same time he manipulates the head with his external hand through the thickness of the sterile coverings and the abdominal wall. He pushes the head up as he pulls the feet down. This rotates the child so that its feet are over the pelvis and its head high up in the uterus under the ribs. The obstetrician then pulls the feet through the vagina, and the rest of the delivery becomes an ordinary breech extraction.

It is not uncommon to deliver the second of a pair of twins by version. This is usually simpler and safer than doing a version on a singleton, for the twin fetus is usually considerably smaller and the uterus is roomier, having been overdistended by its double tenancy.

The outlook for the mother is good if the contraindications to the operation are borne in mind; the main accident to be feared is rupture of the uterus. This is uncommon; it can be largely avoided by having the patient completely relaxed by deep anesthesia and by gentleness in the process of the actual turning. The outlook for the child is approximately the same as in the breech extraction.

Induction of Labor

By induction of labor is meant the bringing on of labor before it has begun of its own accord. If labor is induced between the twenty-eighth and thirty-sixth weeks, when the child still weighs less than five and one-half pounds, it is known as the induction of premature labor. Induction of labor with a baby weighing five and one-half pounds or more is induction of term labor.

Years ago the most common and almost sole reason for inducing labor was contracted pelvis, for if the child was born when quite small it could still pass through the woman's diminished pelvic diameters. Today, because of the increased safety of Cesarean section and the great fetal mortality caused by the birth of a premature child through the cramped confines of a contracted pelvis, this indication has virtually been abandoned.

We divide the reasons for inducing labor into those associated with the mother's safety, those related to the fetus, and reasons of convenience. The commonest maternal reason is the presence of one of the high-blood-pressure toxemias; the commonest fetal reasons are maternal diabetes and immunization of the mother to the Rh factor. The latter indication will become increasingly less frequent with the wider use of Rhogam, as will be explained in Chapter 20. In both conditions the baby may die undelivered in the last few weeks of pregnancy. If the baby dies for any reason during pregnancy and labor does not start spontaneously within a few days it is usually induced. In this unusual situation the salting-out technique described in the induction of late abortion is employed. Reasons of convenience may be divided into two categories: the patient's convenience and the convenience of the physician. The patient may have a pressing social obligation which she is very anxious to honor, such as being a bridesmaid at a wedding; or she may live thirty or forty miles from the hospital and be frightened at the thought of delivering en route. The latter fear is groundless unless she is a multipara. Convenience of the physician may include anticipated absence to attend a medical meeting or a long-planned vacation. Before a doctor will consent to induce labor for either the patient's convenience or his own, everything must be ideal for its performance. The baby must be at term and term size. It must be a cephalic presentation and the presenting head must be engaged with a soft, short partially dilated cervix. When such conditions are rigidly met, no difficulties are likely to be encountered by inducing labor.

The induction of labor without a strict medical indication is a highly controversial topic. Be guided by your own doctor's opinion and practices; do not try to persuade him one way or the other. Your safety and that of your baby are of paramount importance to him, as important to him as they are to you. You may be assured that he will do what he thinks is right and safe for you.

History of Induced Labor

Methods for inducing labor depend on understanding the physiology of labor. It is not surprising, therefore, that current methods are relatively recent. Until the beginning of the seventeenth century it was generally believed that the fetus made its exit from the uterus much as the chick pecks its way out of the egg, by its own efforts, pushing against the fundus with its feet and cleaving the portals of the womb asunder with the cone-shaped wedge of its hands joined as if in prayer.

It was not until the end of the eighteenth century that the first scientific method for inducing labor, the artificial rupture of the membranes (bag of waters) was originated. (From time immemorial it had been the practice artificially to rupture the membranes during the course of childbirth in order to accelerate it; to induce labor it is done before labor has begun, in the hope of starting the process.) The efficacy of this method depends upon the fact that the simple rupture of the membranes with the drainage of a small amount of amniotic fluid alters the pressure relations within the uterus, so that labor is initiated.

A second method is based on the fact that certain drugs will stimulate the uterine muscle to go into labor. Of the several drugs experimented with, the only one to withstand the scrutiny of time is pituitrin. In 1909 Blair Bell of Liverpool found that pituitrin, an extract of the tiny pituitary gland which lies between the brain and the roof of the mouth, was very efficient in producing contractions of the uterus immediately after delivery, and two years later it was first used to induce labor. Since then pituitrin has been broken down into its two active components, Pitocin and Pitressin; the former is used as Oxytocin in obstetrics. A new pituitrin-like drug, sparteine, is occasionally given by injection every hour or less to induce labor. It appears to be slightly less effective.

With this choice of methods, which does the doctor use today? He is likely to start the procedure with a hot soapsuds enema, which has the tendency to make the uterus more irritable, more sensitive to stimuli. Then he will either puncture the membranes by guiding a pointed instrument through the vagina into the cervical opening and up to the bag of waters, which he spears, or he will administer Oxytocin. Sometimes he combines the two techniques, first rupturing the membranes and starting Oxytocin forthwith, or he may reverse the order, initiating contractions by Oxytocin to be followed soon thereafter by puncture of the membranes. Oxytocin for this purpose is usually given intravenously in a continuous, slow, dilute drip, five to seven drops having been added to one pint of glucose water. However, some doctors prefer to give Oxytocin by intramuscular injection, injecting one or two drops every half hour. Linguets of Oxytocin placed beneath the tongue and cotton nasal pledgets saturated with Oxytocin have also been used as routes for its administration. Induced labors are normal in all respects, except they are likely to be somewhat shorter, particularly when Oxytocin is employed.

When the patient is several weeks from term and there is urgent medical need for initiating labor, conditions are usually unfavorable for rupture of the membranes. In these cases Oxytocin also may not work. But if one precedes Oxytocin by a thorough stripping of the membranes from their attachments near the cervical opening by a finger introduced through the cervix, without rupturing them, Oxytocin will have a greater likelihood of starting labor.

A new chapter in the induction of labor is being written by the prostaglandins, referred to in the earlier discussion of induced abortion. These as yet experimental compounds appear to be effective in starting uterine contractions at all stages of pregnancy. In a few years when toxicity, dosage, and methods of administration have been thoroughly studied and evaluated they may well supplant Oxytocin.

Cesarean Section

In terms of its frequency, Cesarean section lags behind some other obstetrical operations, but when judged by its importance, the fascination of its history, and the drama of its technique, it commands the leading position. The operation consists of incising the lower abdomen, cutting into the uterus, and removing a child of viable (large enough to have a chance to survive) size.

Origin of Name

Pliny the Elder (A.D. 23–79) mentions the operation and states that it is the source of the surname of the Roman emperors, since "Caesar" is related to the Latin word for "cut," and it is romantically assumed that Julius Caesar (c. 100–44 B.C.) was "cut" from his mother's womb. It seems highly improbable that he was born in this way: first, because his mother survived his birth for many years, and Cesareans at this time were almost certainly never done on living women; and, second, because the ancients favored a very different origin for the name of their emperors. In the Punic language, *caesar* meant elephant, and since Julius once slew an elephant he was probably given this heroic sobriquet, which passed on to his successors.

Another improbable derivation for the term "Cesarean section" is the claim that at about 750 B.C., during the reign of Numa Pompilius, a law was passed which made it obligatory to open the belly of any woman who died near term in order to rescue the infant from its uterine grave. Originally codified as *lex regia*, under the emperors it became *lex caesarea*. It would have been a most remarkable law if it had been enacted in this, the earliest period of Roman history; however, its authenticity is highly questionable. And so it remains totally uncertain as to how the operation got its name.

History of the Operation

The early history of the operation is equally vague. What did Pliny know about it? Was it ever done in his day? Was there a law in antiquity in regard to post-mortem Cesarean sections? There are uncertain references to Cesarean sections in the Talmud, the book of Jewish post-Biblical law and lore written between A.D. 76 and about A.D. 200. Do these references in the Talmud to women who survived after being delivered by *"yoze dofan,"* a "cut in the side," mean that women actually lived after Cesarean section almost two thousand years ago?

It is somewhat apocryphally reported that in 1500 Jacob Nufer, a swine-gelder, wiped his butcher's knife on his Swiss Alpine trousers and before a gallery of thirteen midwives delivered his own wife by Cesarean section. Frau Nufer is said to have survived the operation and subsequently presented the bold Jacob with two more children born normally.

Post-mortem (Latin: "after-death") Cesarean section was probably freely practiced in antiquity; unquestionably it was widely used in the late medieval period and the early Renaissance.

The first detailed report of a Cesarean on a living woman was the account of an operation done in Germany in 1610.

Of the thirty-eight Cesarean operations performed in Great Britain from 1739 to 1845, a period of more than a century, but four women recovered.

According to the researches of the pre-eminent medical historian, the late Colonel Fielding H. Garrison, the first Cesarean section in this country was performed by Dr. Jessee Bennett in rural Virginia. The surgeon-husband did not publish a report of the remarkable feat, and several years later, when asked why, he replied, "No doctor with any feelings of delicacy would report an operation that he had done on his own wife," and added that "no strange doctors would believe that operations could be done in the Virginia backwoods and the mother live, and he'd be damned if he would give them a chance to call him a liar."

On January 14, 1794, in a frontier settlement of the Shenandoah Valley, Mrs. Bennett was confined in her first pregnancy. Labor was difficult because of a contracted pelvis, and neither her husband nor the consulting doctor was successful in the attempt at delivery by forceps. The choice lay between a destructive operation on the child, its death and piecemeal removal, and a Cesarean section. The patient chose the latter and, since the other doctor firmly refused to have anything to do with so dangerous a procedure, the unpleasant task fell to the husband. The patient, stretched on a crude plank table, was put under the influence of a large dose of opium. Assisted by two women, Dr. Bennett laid open the abdomen and uterus with a single, reckless stroke of the knife and rapidly delivered his daughter, who was still alive. He paused long enough to remove both of his wife's ovaries. As one of the witnesses declared, "He spayed her, remarking as he did so, 'This shall be the last one.'" The wound was closed with stout linen thread and, contrary to expectation, mother and child did well. The first Cesarean-section baby in this country lived to be seventy-three.

Before 1876 few women survived a Cesarean birth by many days, partly because of the crude surgery of that period and partly because the operation was reserved for desperately ill women—women who had labored for days and who were already profoundly infected. In that year Professor Edorado Porro of Pavia contended that it would be best to remove the whole uterus at the time of the operation, for with the removal of the large wounded organ the chance for postoperative hemorrhage and inflammation would be lessened. The wisdom of Porro's teaching soon became obvious; however, the great drawback to his technique was the fact that it rendered the woman permanently sterile. Today this type of Cesarean section, removal of the uterus after its incision to deliver the baby, is referred to as the Porro or Cesarean hysterectomy.

In 1882, twenty-nine-year-old, red-headed Max Sänger, then a lowly *Privatdozent* in Leipzig, published an epoch-making two-hundred-page treatise on *Der Kaiserschnitt* (The Cesarean Section). He called attention to the importance of sewing the uterine incision firmly together again after cutting open the uterus to deliver the baby. Of course it had always been customary to suture (sew) the wound in the abdomen, but previous to Sänger's contribution the unsutured uterus was dropped back in the abdomen, to remain there a constant source of danger— danger from hemorrhage and danger from growth of bacteria out of the open uterine wound into the abdominal cavity. An American, Harris, and others too, had suggested stitching the uterine incision together, but they did not suggest the orderly and thorough way which Sänger evolved and published. Since Sänger's operation was only a refinement of the old type of Cesarean section, and since it did not remove the uterus, it is referred to as either the classical or the conservative Cesarean section.

Because of dissatisfaction with the results of Sänger's operation if performed on women who had been in labor for several hours, Frank of Cologne brought forth the low cervical Cesarean section in 1907. Frank's new technique consisted of freeing the bladder from its filmy attachment to the lower portion of the uterus (the low cervical segment), then pushing the bladder out of the way, down in the pelvis, and incising the uterus through the area from which the bladder had just been dissected free. After child and placenta are removed, the wound in the uterus is sewn together, and then the bladder drawn up and tacked by sutures in its original position. This seals off the uterine wound from the abdominal cavity by plastering the bladder entirely over it. It is like putting a large rubber patch over an inflated ball whose edges had previously been cemented together.

Modern Results

The results of Cesarean section today are a far cry from those of eighty years ago or even twenty years ago. The procedure has become extremely simple, adding little if any extra time to the hospital stay, and above all it is as free of danger as any other uncomplicated operation. In our first 2500 Cesarean sections at the newly opened maternity Mount Sinai Hospital we had two maternal deaths associated with a Cesarean section, and in neither instance was the actual operation responsible. These figures are far from unique and can be duplicated or improved by many first-class obstetrical hospitals.

What has caused the improvement? Primarily the advance in general surgical technique with its great emphasis on asepsis (Greek: "not to make rotten"), prevention of bacterial contamination. Then, too, there is the growth in obstetrical knowledge. In the first years of the century it was observed that the earlier in labor the operation was done, the safer the outcome; in fact the very safest time was even before labor had begun. This was a radical discovery, for the pioneers in the field believed that a woman would bleed to death if operated on before the contractions of labor had set in. In the last decade the less safe type of classical section has been virtually abandoned, except in the face of a very acute emergency for child or mother, and the slightly slower technique of the lower segment operation substituted as standard routine. In explaining the dramatic improvement in the safety of today's Cesarean section one must mention enthusiastically expert anesthesia, as well as antibiotics and transfusion when indicated.

As far as the baby is concerned, Cesarean section offers it as good a chance as a very simple vaginal delivery, and a far better chance than a complicated vaginal delivery.

Indications for Cesarean Section

The most common indication for Cesarean section is pelvic dystocia— usually from a contracted pelvis. Less frequently dystocia is due to a pelvic tumor that blocks the pelvis, to a transverse lie of the fetus, to a malpresentation of the head, such as a brow, when a very unfavorable fetal diameter attempts to enter the pelvis, or to an infant of excessive size. Frequently the baby presenting by the breech, particularly a first baby, has a Cesarean birth. If the same child had been a vertex it probably would have been born vaginally. As I stated earlier, the head of a breech baby has no opportunity to narrow its transverse diameter by gradually molding during labor and therefore requires a roomier pelvis for safe delivery. Cesarean section is usually done in the treatment of the two serious hemorrhage complications of late pregnancy, premature separation of the placenta and placenta praevia. It is also occasionally performed to check a fulminating, severe toxemia which threatens to develop into eclampsia (childbed convulsions). Some clinics perform Cesarean sections on most women of thirty-five or more in their first pregnancy. Most, however, allow the elderly primipara a test of labor, remaining alert to the necessity of intervention by low-cervical Cesarean section if cervical dystocia or uterine inertia (inadequate pains) develop. To prevent fetal infection, usually pneumonia, a Cesarean is done if near term the membranes have been ruptured for twenty-four to forty-eight hours but delivery is not imminent because of no labor or poor labor. Modern obstetrics has relegated to the past long labors of more than eighteen or twenty-four hours. If after such a period the cervix is only partially dilated and many additional hours of labor are in prospect, more than likely a Cesarean will be done.

Repeat Cesarean Sections

"Once a Cesarean, always a Cesarean" is the terse dictum which means that if the uterus is once emptied by Cesarean section the operation must be repeated for the delivery of each succeeding pregnancy. This rule is based on the fact that a small percentage of those patients who have had Cesarean sections will rupture (burst asunder) the uterine scar in late pregnancy or labor. However, some authorities believe that it is usually unnecessary to repeat the section, unless the cause for the original operation, such as a small pelvis, is still present.

The decision whether or not to repeat the Cesarean section depends on several factors in addition to the indication for the original operation: the teachings and experience of the doctor; whether the patient has had a previous vaginal delivery in addition to a Cesarean section; whether the previous type of operation was classical or low cervical; and the position of the baby's head and the feel of the cervix near term.

In our own clinic, four out of five patients have a repeat Cesarean section for each subsequent delivery; in the country as a whole, I estimate, it runs nine out of ten.

Time Chosen for an Elective Section

If a repeat Cesarean section is decided upon it is usually done at a time predetermined in advance. Ordinarily the time selected is about ten days before the calculated date of confinement. However, a week or so before the date chosen the doctor will check things over to make as sure as he can that the baby is sufficiently mature. If he estimates that the baby will weigh less than six and one-half pounds he may postpone the operation for a week or longer. If labor comes on in the meantime his hand is forced and the operation is performed at once.

A primary Cesarean section if done for a contracted pelvis or a tumor blocking the birth canal is similarly scheduled several days before labor is anticipated.

Incidence of Cesarean Section

Cesarean section incidence has gradually risen until it is now between 6 and 7 per cent of all births. The operations are about equally divided between primary sections—first Cesareans—and repeat sections.

The increased incidence of Cesarean section follows quite logically its own increased safety. Statistically it once equaled and has now clearly surpassed in safety for both mother and child several alternative obstetrical procedures—notably, version, difficult forceps deliveries, and breech births through narrowed pelves. Naturally, in well-trained hands and minds, Cesarean section has all but replaced them. Then, too, its relative superiority to most other methods in the treatment of severe late bleeding complications has added to its frequency. The increased incidence of section parallels a decrease in perinatal mortality, stillbirths, and early infant deaths, in most clinics reporting.

How Many Cesarean Births?

People are curious as to how many Cesarean sections one woman can have. I know a patient who is well and strong after eleven, and I do not nominate her for the world's record. Patients are ordinarily sterilized by tying the tubes or removing the uterus at the third section, unless they desire more children. The logic of sterilization more or less routinely at the third Cesarean section is open to question, since ordinarily the third operation carried no more risk than the first, and the fifth no more risk than the third. However, each Cesarean birth is a major operation, which means a less comfortable convalescence than after vaginal delivery. Then, too, though the risk attendant upon a Cesarean birth is so magnificently low today, it is still two or three times that of normal birth. We encourage our patients to have more than three Cesarean births if their original family planning included more than three children. In a study we showed that it does not take longer to conceive following a Cesarean birth than after a vaginal birth.

Many think that the abdominal skin bears a scar for each operation, a sort of service stripe. Of course this is not true. The skin scar of the previous operation is cut around and the old scar excised, so that, at the time of closure, normal skin edges can be brought together.

The Operation

It requires about three-quarters of an hour to perform a Cesarean operation; either a longitudinal mid-line incision is made through skin, fat, and fascia (the tough membrane overlying the abdominal muscles) from just below the navel to the pubic bone, or a low, wide, transverse incision is made just above the pubis. This, the Pfannenstiel type of incision, is made in the area covered by pubic hair, so that when the hair grows back the scar is virtually invisible. Then the abdominal muscle fibers beneath the fascia are separated, revealing the peritoneum, the thin, glistening lining of the peritoneal or abdominal cavity. The peritoneum is opened longitudinally in the midline, which exposes the intact large uterus just beneath it. A small incision is made by a knife in the lower mid-portion of the uterus, and enlarged upward and downward to a distance of about six inches, if one elects to perform a classical Cesarean section. When the low cervical type is done, the bladder must first be freed of its attachments to the front of the uterus and pushed down in the pelvis beneath the pubic bone. Then a six-inch longitudinal or transverse incision is made in the lowermost portion of the uterus, that portion previously overlain by the bladder. The membranes usually rupture at this point, and a quantity of amniotic fluid wells forth. When the uterine incision is completed, the operator gently shoehorns the infant's head out of the incision and then extracts the rest of the child. The naval cord is clamped and cut and the child is turned over to an assistant. From the beginning of the skin incision to the delivery of the child is the shortest part of the operation, taking five or six minutes. The repair of the uterine and abdominal wounds takes many times longer. The placenta is manually removed from the opened uterus and an oxytocic drug given intramuscularly or intravenously to encourage the uterus to contract and remain contracted. Two or three rows of absorbable catgut sutures are placed in the uterus to close its incision, and then the abdominal cavity is mopped dry and clean of clots and blood. The abdominal wall is closed in its separate layers, also with absorbable sutures. Usually the skin sutures are of nonabsorbable silk and must be removed between the fifth and seventh days. Some operators prefer metal clips for skin closure; these too should be removed in a week or less.

Several anesthetics are satisfactory for Cesarean section. The most widely used and probably the best is spinal; in using conduction anesthesia of any type the operator can be more leisurely in delivering the infant than when a general anesthetic is used which crosses the placenta to the baby. Lumbar epidural conduction anesthesia is replacing spinal for Cesareans in some clinics to obviate the possibility of a spinal headache. Occasionally local anesthesia, the injection of the anesthetic agent directly into the abdominal wall, is used. It is common practice when using conduction or local anesthesia to put the patient lightly asleep with a general anesthetic after the baby is born. The general anesthetic removes anxiety by inducing light sleep. If the operation is done under general anesthesia nitrous oxide or cyclopropane are commonly used. To lessen the amount necessary, they are usually supplemented with intravenous pentothal and a muscle relaxant such as curare or succinylcholine.

The blood loss at Cesarean section is usually about a pint. If the patient has a borderline hemoglobin preoperatively, or loses more than a pint at operation, a transfusion while the operation is being concluded is more or less standard procedure.

Convalescence

Following the example set by the general surgeon in the early ambulation of abdominal cases, the obstetrician usually gets his Cesarean mother up the day after operation. If she is unable to void, sometimes the patient is gotten up the day of operation to avoid catheterization. Early ambulation reduces her hospital stay to about a week. Fortunately, the day of heavy postoperative dressings and abdominal binders is past, so don't feel cheated if you wake to find only thin gauze covering your incision. A liberal diet immediately after operation and the short stay in bed have almost abolished postoperative gaseous distention and weakness. There is no medical reason why a Cesarean mother should not nurse her baby. Physicians vary in their advice as to how soon it is safe to commence another pregnancy after Cesarean section. My observations lead me to believe that such a wound is as firmly and securely healed after three months as it is after three years; but ask your own doctor, since he is likely to dissent from my unorthodox opinion.

Forceps, breech extractions, versions, induction of labor, and Cesarean sections do not comprise all the operations employed by obstetricians, but these five are much the most common.

16

Convalescence after Childbirth

The puerperium (Latin: "having brought forth a child") is the period of several weeks that starts immediately after delivery and is completed when the reproductive tract has fully returned to its nonpregnant state. It is a period of rapid recuperation and readjustment from pregnancy to nonpregnancy. Physiologically it is distinguished by two conspicuous phenomena: the return of the uterus to its nongravid condition, and the appearance of milk in the breasts—though many less obvious alterations occur, such as diminution in blood volume and the loss of excess tissue fluid.

The Uterus Shrinks to Nonpregnant Size

When the puerperium begins, the uterus is a two-pound mass of muscle, and by the end of six weeks it has shrunk to three ounces. During the first few days of the puerperium it is a smooth, hard, gourd-shaped organ with its apex a few inches below the navel. By the end of the first week it weighs one pound and has descended to two inches above the symphysis (the bone forming the front of the pelvic girdle). By the tenth day its top can just be felt above the symphysis, and after this it sinks within the pelvis and can no longer be felt when one palpates the abdomen. The process of shrinkage (involution) progresses more rapidly in a woman who nurses. The diminution in size and weight continues, and after five or six weeks the uterus is once more the size and weight of a pear. This cycle of growth followed by involution, which the uterus repetitively undergoes in each pregnancy and puerperium, is unique in physiology. No other organ multiplies itself more than tenfold and then regresses back to its basic size. The growth is caused by a vast increase in the size of each individual muscle fiber forming the uterus, not by an increase in the number of fibers, and involution involves divestment by each cell of the additional cytoplasmic material.

Puerperal Vaginal Discharge

The puerperal vaginal discharge, called lochia (Greek: "pertaining to childbirth"), has a bright-red blood color for the first three or four days; from the fourth to the tenth day it becomes paler and pinkish; and from about the tenth day on it is yellow-white, often with a little blood admixed. Ordinarily all discharge disappears between the third and fourth weeks. The total fluid and tissue lost through the lochia has been collected and weighs eight to nine ounces. The lochia is often incorrectly called menstruation; the origin and constitution of the two are very different. Nevertheless the ordinary type of menstrual napkin should be worn; intravaginal tampons, such as Tampax, are forbidden until at least two weeks postdelivery.

Increased Urination

One of the most striking phenomena of the puerperium is the marked increase in urination which regularly occurs between the second and fifth days after delivery. Normal pregnancy is associated with retention of two or three quarts of tissue water. The puerperal loss through excess urine is simply a reversal of the process.

Return of Menstruation

True menstruation first returns at variable times after delivery. If the woman does not suckle her child, the menses usually reappear within four to eight weeks. In the woman who nurses there is the most extraordinary variability; the menses may return at any time from the second to the eighteenth month, the average being five months. One study found that 90 per cent of nonlactating women and 30 per cent of nursing mothers had a return of the menses within three months after childbirth. In both groups the amount of bleeding and the interval between the periods may be quite unusual for the first several months. In some, it appears that the rhythm-producing mechanism requires an adjustment period for complete regulation. Painful menstruation, dysmenorrhea, is almost always improved by a pregnancy; in many the pain, which may have been incapacitating, never returns.

Lactation

The breasts are prepared for the secretion of milk throughout pregnancy by the mammary-growth-stimulating hormones produced by the placenta.

These same chemicals prevent the pituitary gland from manufacturing its specific milk-producing chemical, the lactogenic hormone. With the abrupt withdrawal of the placental hormones, primarily estrogen and progesterone, concurrent with delivery of the placenta, their inhibitory influence disappears and the lactogenic hormone of the pituitary gland, prolactin, is promptly released. The immediate result is the marked increase in the amount of colostrum, the thin, sticky, colorless fluid secreted by the breasts, which changes to thin, bluish milk within sixty to seventy-two hours after delivery. Colostrum in some animals, notably cattle, is very rich in immunizing substances—antibodies—and unless the young partake of it they are likely to acquire a fatal infectious diarrhea. In cattle, as opposed to human beings, antibodies do not pass across the placenta from the mother's bloodstream to that of the fetus. Human colostrum also contains protective antibodies which probably offer immunity against some intestinal infections, and it also acts as a gentle cathartic. Synchronous with the establishment of lactation, on about the third postpartum day, the breasts suddenly become larger, firm, hot, and painful, the pattern of superficial blood vessels beneath the skin becoming more prominent. This phenomenon, known as breast engorgement, rarely lasts more than twenty-four to thirty-six hours. Now, on pressure, a small amount of bluish-white fluid—the milk—will exude from the nipple. At this time the patient may feel fatigued; she may have a headache, throbbing pains in the breasts, and a low-grade fever. If there is aberrant breast tissue in the axillae (armpits), as there is occasionally, she may develop painful lumps under the arms. As the engorgement subsides, the breasts soften, the pain lessens, and the milk becomes thicker, slightly yellowish, and more abundant.

Nursing mothers gain temporary relief with the sucking of the infant. In nonnursing mothers, a supportive brassière, codeine and aspirin, and occasionally the local application of ice bags are indicated. The day of tight breast binding, the use of a pump, and the restriction of fluids is past. Some physicians prescribe a single injection at the time of delivery of one of the milk-suppressing hormones or daily tablets of the same material for a few days, to inhibit lactation completely in those not planning to nurse. A popular technique is the intramuscular injection of estrogen and testosterone, the female and male hormones in combination.

Many substances taken by the mother promptly appear in the milk. This is particularly true of vegetable cathartics, antibiotics, sulfa drugs, sedatives, and alcohol. If alcohol is imbibed in large amounts, the child may be affected, since it appears approximately in the same concentration in the milk as in the mother's blood. Certain foods, such as onions, may give the milk a harmless pungency.

A woman's ability to produce milk cannot be gauged by physical examination or by laboratory tests. The size of the breasts or the amount of breast tissue seems to bear no relationship to this peculiar gift. The only index is the test of performance. As a rule, placid, emotionally stable women are better able to nurse than those who are tense.

A large number of preparations are sold as galactogogues (substances to increase the flow of milk), but none have any proved value. It used to be thought that large fluid intake, particularly of beer and porter, adds a favorable influence on milk production, but even this has recently been disproved. However, milk production is affected by several factors: emotional upsets diminish it, and moderate outdoor exercise increases it. The secretion of milk and the "let down milk mechanism" is stimulated by an Oxytocin-like hormone produced by the pituitary. When the infant starts to nurse, an immediate message in the form of a nerve impulse is relayed to the pituitary gland, which floods the body with the hormone. It, in turn, stimulates not only the mammary apparatus but the uterus as well. That is why nursing frequently causes uterine contractions and cramps, and that is why the uterus of the nursing mother involutes more rapidly than the uterus of a nonnurser. Linguets of Oxytocin placed under the tongue are being experimented with as galactogogues, milk stimulators.

The quality of the milk is dependent in part upon the food taken by the mother: a diet rich in protein increases the proportion of fat. A nursing mother does not have to stuff herself to feed her child adequately, but her diet should be increased and varied. She must supplement her well-balanced diet with a quart of cow's milk daily. The Food and Nutrition Board of the National Research Council issued pertinent dietary recommendations in 1968. For a five-foot-four-inch woman weighing 128 pounds it recommends 2000 calories per day when not pregnant, 2200 when pregnant, and 3000 calories while nursing. The daily grams of protein required are 55, 65, and 75 respectively. Calcium intake should be increased from 0.8 grams to 1.2 grams and 1.3 grams each day. Alcohol in small amounts—one drink—has no injurious effects either on the mother's milk or on the infant. Nicotine from cigarette smoking appears in the milk, but there are no hard data to show that it adversely affects the infant or the milk supply. However, there are many other health reasons to condemn smoking. Menstruation, contrary to some old wives' tales, exerts no serious effect on the quality of the milk. The child may become mildly upset during the days of menstruation, but since it returns to normal as soon as the menstrual period is over, there is no necessity to wean it. Nursing is a strain, and for this reason alone the infant should be weaned when a new pregnancy is diagnosed.

Conception during Nursing

During the first several months likelihood of reimpregnation is significantly less in a woman who nurses than in the woman who does not nurse, especially if she is still amenorrheic, i.e., has not resumed menstruating. However, lactation amenorrhea is no guarantee of sustained infertility. In a study of 500 pregnancies 9 per cent occurred before menstruation had returned. Therefore, in the absence of a readiness to be immediately reimpregnated, like the lady guinea pig or seal, to be safe, contraception should be used. The hormones in the birth-control pill reduce the milk supply in at least one-third of nursing women. Therefore, do not commence taking the pill unless lactation is well established and copious. Then, be prepared to stop if there is a significant decrease in your milk and to use another method of birth control. Hormones from the pill appear in the milk, but do not affect the baby. If you are not nursing you may start the pill as soon as you leave the hospital.

In a fertile stock of human beings who nurse their infants and use no contraception one may expect infants to be born on an average of twenty-four months apart. If the same group did not nurse, births would occur every nineteen months.

Weaning the Baby

When it is decided to stop breast feeding, weaning of the infant may be either gradual or abrupt. The former is accomplished by the progressive substitution of artificial feedings for the breast at one, then two, then three nursing periods during the twenty-four-hour schedule. When the weaning is carried out over a period of a week to ten days, it usually causes very little discomfort. Following completed weanings, the breasts continue to leak milk for several days. Within a week they should return to the nonpregnant status. There are occasional instances of women who harbor small amounts of milk in their breasts for years. Except for the inconvenience, it causes no harm. When weaning must be done acutely, a tight brassière is helpful. If the breasts become very hard and painful, ice bags may be applied during the interval the brassière is not worn. Also a dose of Epsom salts or citrate of magnesia, in addition to restricting fluids of any variety, helps. In cases of extreme discomfort, estrogen or testosterone, or a combination of both, may be given by injection or orally.

Weight Loss

The average patient one hour after delivery weighs about 13.5 pounds less than before. An additional 3.5 pounds is lost between the first postpartum hour and the twelfth day, much of it increased tissue water. At the sixth week postpartum the gain in total weight above the pre-pregnant figure is made up of fat and, in those who nurse, also of breast tissue.

Medical Care during the Early Puerperium

Rest and Quiet

From the doctor's point of view, the fewer the visitors during the complete hospital stay the better. In some progressive institutions visitors are restricted on maternity to the husband and parents. It should not be forgotten that the patient must recuperate from the last few uncomfortable weeks of pregnancy and the strain and fatigue of labor. Frequently the patient feels so well that she wants to see every person in the world; if permitted she is likely to pay for it by excessive weariness and a depressed, "let down" feeling. During the whole puerperium the period between two and four in the afternoon should be held inviolable for the sacred purpose of afternoon rest.

Diet

With the increased simplicity of modern deliveries and the period of enforced starvation in the labor room, most patients return to the postpartum floor with the question, "When do I eat?" The news is good news. Now, instead of starting off with unsatisfying liquids or soft mush, they are given a full tray with a general diet of about 3000 calories per day. Patients with rapid labors often pride themselves on not having missed a meal to have a baby. Of course, if a patient is nauseated postdelivery she will be given appropriate liquids by mouth, or intravenous fluids, until nausea disappears. If she is nursing, the postpartum diet includes three or four glasses of milk a day.

Getting Up

The length of rest imposed upon women after childbirth has varied widely from people to people, and from generation to generation. Among most primitive groups, it was customary for the woman to go about her regular duties the day of delivery or the day after. In the journal of the American explorers Lewis and Clark, it is recorded that an Indian woman with the expedition dropped out of the group to have her baby alone and within several hours the mother carrying her child caught up with the explorers. During the past several centuries it became general practice in the United States and in Europe for upper-class women to remain in bed for two weeks postpartum or longer. Despite this general practice, there have been several dissenters—among them Charles White of England in 1773, Goodell of Philadelphia a century later, and Kustner of Germany in 1899. They revived the practice of early rising in the puerperium, allowing patients out of bed on the third day, a practice termed early ambulation.

When I entered obstetrics forty-five years ago, patients remained in bed at least ten days postdelivery. This custom was rather generally adhered to until World War II. Then the first wide-scale modern experiment was forced upon England. During the Blitz it became practice to have the baby's bassinet near the mother's bed, and during an air raid each mother would grab her infant and make haste with it to the hospital air-raid shelter. It made no difference if the baby was a day or a week old. In preparation for such an eventuality, women were encouraged to get up on the day of delivery or shortly thereafter. Despite medical fears, observation proved that no harm resulted. Following notices in the *British Medical Journal* of the English practice, we allowed two hundred patients out of bed on the third and fourth days in the wards at the Sinai Hospital, Baltimore. No ill effects either immediately or after six weeks were found. Patients who had had babies according to the old rules enjoyed the innovation; they felt so much stronger than when they had gotten up after nine or ten days of complete bed confinement. Several other studies soon appeared, confirming and extending our preliminary published observations.

Today it is customary to allow patients out of bed the day of delivery if they desire. The only results accruing are good ones. We try to discourage walking about on the first day, but only too often, when making late-afternoon rounds, I would meet the patient I delivered that morning in the corridor. Daily shower baths are permitted, beginning the day after delivery. There is no conceivable harm in washing your hair in the shower or basin any time after the day of delivery.

Early ambulation has contributed to the short hospital stays of the modern puerpara (she who has borne). Many patients plan to stay in the hospital a week but feel so well by the fifth or sixth day that they plead for discharge. In many overcrowded hospitals patients are discharged after three days with no seeming ill-effects.

Cesarean-section cases ordinarily do not get out of bed until the day after operation, but by the fourth day they are usually as strong and vigorous as the others. It is customary to hospitalize them for a full week.

Exercises

With the patient going about normally so soon after delivery, the need for calisthenic exercises postpartum has disappeared. As a matter of fact, they have fallen in ill repute with some physicians, who now claim that chronic backaches may have their source in these exercises. Actually, I believe there are little data to show that they do any good or harm. The routine assumption of the knee-chest position for a few minutes twice a day during the early puerperium to prevent the uterus from assuming a backward tilt after delivery has fallen into the same disuse as postpartum calisthenics.

Afterpains

During the first few days of the puerperium most multiparas and some primiparas complain of afterpains. These usually begin soon after delivery but seldom last more than three days. They consist of painful contractions of the uterus, recurring irregularly and lasting about a minute. Afterpains are often initiated by the act of sucking, as noted earlier; whenever the child is put to the breast the uterus reacts by contracting, and such contractions may cause a spurt of lochia or the passage of a small clot. In most patients no therapy is required, but others must be repeatedly given codeine and aspirin or some other analgesic.

The "Blues"

"Postpartum blues," beginning a day or two after delivery and lasting several days, are frequently encountered. Periods of depression and crying without cause are common. If you are the victim of such a reaction, dismiss the family from the room and discuss it frankly with your doctor. He can reassure you that he has met postpartum blues many times in stable, well-adjusted, fundamentally happy people, whose depression cleared up in a few days without aftermath or treatment.

Baths

Many physicians allow patients to take full tub baths the day they return from the hospital; in fact, if the perineal stitches hurt or hemorrhoids cause pain, they may advise taking shallow, warm, unmedicated baths several times a day. The fact that a patient is still bleeding is no reason not to take a bath. However, bathing in the early puerperium is still sufficiently controversial to make it necessary to clear the matter with your own doctor before getting into the bathtub.

The Care of Special Areas

The vulva (entrance to the vagina). As soon as delivery is completed, a sterile sanitary pad is placed over the vulva and held in place with a sanitary belt. Usually the patient is supplied with a paper bag of sterilized pads, which she keeps in a bedside cabinet, and she changes them herself as need be. At least once daily, and after each defecation and before any local treatment or examination, the genitalia are bathed with soap and water or with a mild antiseptic solution. The day of messy irrigations and flushing of the perineum is a thing of the past. Episiotomy wounds and perineal tears require no special treatment unless they cause pain. Among the remedies for pain are: an ice-collar, warm salt or boric irrigations, alcohol or Epsom-salt compresses, dry-heat emanations from an electric-light bulb, and the application of various medicated ointments.

The bladder. Previous to our modern era of early ambulation it was not uncommon, particularly after a forceps or breech extraction, for a patient to be unable to void for several days. Today, with the almost immediate use of toilets or commodes instead of constraining bedpans, inability to void postpartum is an uncommon happening. In the rare instance that the patient cannot empty her bladder, she is catheterized every six to ten hours, or a permanent indwelling catheter is left in place for forty-eight hours or longer. If this becomes necessary, a prophylactic antibiotic is begun to protect against a urinary-tract infection.

The abdomen. It is a very old custom to swathe the abdomen after childbirth. It was believed that after the disappearance of the large abdominal mass, the woman's insides would rattle around in a dangerous fashion unless they were securely held in position. During the Renaissance a most elaborate ritual of swathing grew up, with resort even to the application of the skin of freshly killed sheep.

Ever since the time of Mauriceau, in 1668, the art of swathing has grown simpler and simpler, until now most obstetrical authorities have completely abandoned the use of postpartum abdominal binders and corsets. Their use in no way contributes to the restoration of the figure; in fact, there is pertinent evidence that they retard the process. I grant that this is difficult for all great-grandmothers and most grandmothers to accept, but I sincerely believe it.

As a result of the rupture of the elastic tissue fibers of the abdominal skin and the prolonged overstretching of the abdominal muscles from the large intra-abdominal mass, the belly wall remains soft and flabby for weeks after delivery. Usually, except for the pink skin stretch marks (striae), which fade and become silvery, the abdomen returns to normal. In some it may stay flabby and in others there may be separation of the two large abdominal muscles, creating a permanent narrow mid-line weakness—a longitudinal skin-covered fissure between the muscles. The greater the uterine distention, as a result of a very large baby or twins, and the shorter the woman's abdominal cage, the greater the likelihood of permanent abdominal changes. Resumption of activities, especially athletic pursuits, are advised as soon as feasible.

The bowels. With early ambulation and the virtual elimination of that awful contraption the bedpan, regulation of the bowels postpartum is far less of a problem than it used to be. Nightly cathartics may be used, and if necessary occasional enemas, unless the patient's perineal tear or episiotomy was extensive enough to involve the rectal sphincter or the rectum. Remember that a vegetable cathartic may purge a nursing baby.

Summary of Home Care after Leaving the Hospital

I have stated dogmatically my own rules for the management of pregnancy, and I do the same for the first few weeks after leaving the hospital. However, I again issue the sincere warning that if the rules which follow differ from your own doctor's, utterly disregard mine and follow his scrupulously.

On the day before the patient leaves the hospital I give her the following speech. It is meant only for the normal case who has had an uncomplicated vaginal delivery and in whom convalescence has been uninterrupted. The patient delivered by Cesarean section, or in whom there was some complication, receives different instructions.

Overhearing myself, I sound like this:

"Your case was delightfully normal. If you have a house, when you go home tomorrow, walk up the steps; more people are killed by being carried up than by walking up.

"Stay on the same floor for three or four days after getting home from the hospital, if convenient. If not, you may go downstairs once a day, perhaps for dinner; if you do, you might as well stay down for the evening. Rest for most of the afternoon, if possible sleeping for two hours.

"When you have been home three or four days, reduce the afternoon rest to two hours. If the weather is nice, go outdoors for a five-minute stroll. The next day you may go out a little longer; each day increase your activities. When you have been home ten days you may do nearly what you please—go downtown to the movies, go out to dinner, do light housework, et cetera. Don't assume unrestricted heavy household duties until the baby is at least two weeks old.

"You may ride in a car as soon as you go out, but don't drive it yourself until the baby is three weeks old.

"You may eat, drink, and smoke what you want. If you are breast feeding, you must drink a full quart of milk each day and go lightly on cigarettes and drinking, for both nicotine and alcohol are excreted in the milk—perhaps nature's attempt to build up tolerance early in life.

"You may take a full bath as soon as you get home, and bathe at least once a day. If stitches or hemorrhoids pain you, the more often you bathe the better. You may douche after the baby is three weeks old if you wish, but it is rarely necessary. If you decide to douche, use a can or bag and lie with your hips elevated in the bathtub. Use either two teaspoons of sodium perborate, three tablespoons of white vinegar, two tablespoons of salt, or some proprietary deodorant powder in an amount indicated on the label. I would not douche more often than every other day.

"In regard to clothing, wear any clothing which is comfortable. Do not wear a girdle constantly, since it acts like a splint to the abdominal muscles and retards them from getting their tone back.

"Make an engagement to see me at my office when the baby is about a month old, and it is wiser not to have sexual intercourse until I check you. Come alone—leave the baby at home.

"If any problems arise, telephone me as usual."

Occasional Complications after Delivery

Just as any disease can occur during pregnancy, it can also occur during the puerperium. I have seen patients with mumps, measles, chicken pox, scarlet fever, malaria, appendicitis, catarrhal jaundice, etc. The more frequent complications of the puerperium are: puerperal, or childbed, fever; mastitis, or infection of the breast; pyelitis, or infection of the uppermost portion of the tube which conducts the urine from the kidney to the bladder; abnormally excessive puerperal bleeding; a sore bottom, and anemia from excessive blood loss at delivery.

Puerperal, or Childbed, Fever

The term puerperal fever or puerperal infection includes the various complications which are caused by harmful bacteria that may infect the female reproductive organs during labor and the first few days of the puerperium. The majority of these disease-begetting germs are unwittingly introduced at this time from the outside by the doctor or the nurse, inanimate objects of the environment, or by the patient's own fingers.

Before the bacterial killers—the sulfa drugs, penicillin, and the various "mycins"—made their welcome debut, infection after childbirth was not only common but extremely dangerous. However, the picture has changed so completely that, as the director of an obstetric teaching service, I deplored today's absence of virulent, typical cases of puerperal infection to demonstrate to medical students, residents, and nurses, though I thrill at the lives saved and the illness spared. Today less than 3 per cent of deliveries are followed by infection, usually in a form so mild that the only evidence is the tell-tale thermometer.

The reason the incidence of postdelivery infection is so low is mainly the increase in measures for its prevention. The ordinary measures consist in the avoidance during late pregnancy of careless pelvic examinations and sexual intercourse, for fear these may introduce harmful bacteria, which will be lurking in the vagina ready to infect the woman during her labor or puerperium. (If harmful germs are introduced into the vagina several days before labor begins, they are normally killed off in time.) During labor, clean surroundings and carefully performed rectal and vaginal examinations are imperative. At the time of delivery, the preparation of the vulva with antiseptics; surrounding the vagina with sterile drapings; a physician properly gowned, gloved, capped, and masked; and the skillful conduct of delivery with the elimination of unnecessary operations, all reduce the chances of infection. Keeping the blood loss at delivery to the minimum, and, in case of excessive blood loss, a prompt transfusion, are important. After delivery, sterile perineal pads, fresh linens, and proper nursing care by intelligent attendants do much to prevent the disease. If a case of puerperal infection develops, its isolation is essential to prevent the spread of the infection to other freshly delivered women.

If a patient develops a rise of temperature to 100.4 degrees Fahrenheit (38 degrees centigrade) or above on any two of the first ten days postpartum, exclusive of the first twenty-four hours, she is presumed to have puerperal infection unless there is some obvious source for the fever such as an inflamed breast or bronchitis. Fever from puerperal infection commonly begins on the third day, although it may appear earlier or later. In mild infections the temperature usually remains below 102 degrees Fahrenheit. Severe cases may be accompanied by chills and high temperatures.

On the rare occasions that the temperature postpartum rises above 100.4 degrees for two readings of the thermometer twenty-four or more hours after delivery, bacterial cultures of the interior of the uterus, of the blood, and of the urine are taken, and wide-spectrum antibiotics are immediately begun. More than likely, by the time the bacteria have been grown and identified by the laboratory the patient's temperature is normal and she is entirely well. However, if the infection is still present and the temperature continues elevated, tests are run on the bacteria cultured from the particular case to find out to which of a half-dozen different antibiotics the organisms are particularly sensitive. This special drug is then given in adequate dosage, and in 99 per cent of the cases even the most resistant infection clears up dramatically.

Mastitis—Breast Inflammation

Mastitis, the development of localized inflammation of the breast, occurs uncommonly before delivery, but it occurs quite frequently in the puerperium. It is not to be confused with engorgement of the breasts or the normal caking which takes place on the third and fourth days after delivery, with the onset of lactation. True mastitis, inflammation of the breast, rarely occurs before the end of the first week and usually not until the end of the third or fourth week.

In the typical case of mastitis the patient develops a sudden and unexplained elevation of temperature, sometimes with chills, and a localized area of tenderness in one of the breasts. On examination, the tender area is found to be hard and red. The skin overlying it is hot. The site of predilection is the outer and lower quadrant of the right breast, though any area of either breast can be involved. It is believed the infant harbors the bacteria, usually *Staphylococcus aureus*, in its nose and throat and at the time of nursing the organism enters the breast through the nipple via a fissure or abrasion which may be quite small. It is doubtful that infection can enter through a wholly healthy nipple. The baby may have received the bacteria in the hospital nursery via the partially washed hands of nursery personnel or a thousand different sources. When mastitis is diagnosed, a drop of milk is expressed from the breast and sent for bacterial culture to identify the specific type of bacterium and for tests to determine the antibiotic to which it is specially sensitive. However, since most cases of mastitis are due to staphylococcus and the bacterium usually is sensitive to penicillin G, a dose of this drug is given in the meantime, unless the patient is allergic to it. If treatment is started early the whole miserable business can often be aborted in two days.

If the inflammation and temperature do not subside within forty-eight hours, an abscess usually forms—suppurative mastitis. The temperature goes higher, the area becomes more tender, and the skin above the abscess assumes a doughy consistency. The baby is now weaned completely. The deep, hard mass commences to soften, and when the center of the inflamed area feels as though it has become liquefied, the patient is completely anesthetized and the abscess evacuated and drained.

In the past breast abscess was relatively common, occurring perhaps once in about every hundred deliveries. Fortunately the highly successful modern treatment of the inflamed breast has made actual abscess formation uncommon. A localized breast inflammation is about four times as common in first pregnancies and is rarely seen after a woman has had more than two children. If operation becomes necessary, the average time for its performance is the thirty-ninth day after delivery. The average case is operated on eleven days after the onset of symptoms.

Cases may occur a year and even longer after delivery. The complication is far more frequent during the winter months, and apparently there is a definite association of the condition with the general prevalence of colds, bronchitis, sinus infections, and the high incidence of staph bacteria at these times. One breast abscess does not predispose to another in a future puerperium, so that the patient can nurse a subsequent baby with ordinary safety.

Prevention of breast abscess is the best treatment. Nursery personnel should have periodic throat cultures, and those having positive staph cultures must be excluded from any contact with mothers and babies. Proper care of the nipples is important. The nipples should be cleansed with mild soap and water before and after each nursing to remove encrusted flakes of dried milk which could irritate the nipple. When there is difficulty with the nipple, the patient complains of pain whenever the child sucks; and on inspection the nipple may look raw and deeply furrowed in one area, and a little bloody material exudes from the small wounds. Various treatments may be employed for this condition, but they are all planned to give the nipple a chance to heal through rest and the application of healing drugs. Many obstetricians take the child off the breast until the nipple is completely healed, and in the interim use either a breast pump or mere stripping of the breast with the fingers. Others allow the child to nurse through a nipple shield, a round glass rim which fits tightly over the area. The child nurses through a rubber nipple attached to the shield. This prevents the child's mouth from coming in direct contact with the nipple. Among the many healing drugs applied are tincture of benzoin, silver nitrate, castor oil and bismuth paste, balsam of Peru, and creams containing antibiotics. After a day or two the tender nipple usually heals and the baby can be put back on the breast.

Pyelonephritis and Cystitis

Bacterial infections of the urinary tract postpartum are less common now, since early ambulation has reduced the necessity of repeated catheterization. However, they still occur. Pyelonephritis infection of the collecting funnel within the kidney and some kidney tissue itself may cause acute pain and tenderness in the kidney region on the affected side, or the condition may be locally asymptomatic. Under such circumstances the patient runs unexplained fever but a specimen of urine carefully collected will show an excess of pus cells and bacteria on microscopic study. The right kidney is more likely to be involved than the left. Since the organism causing the infection is usually a bacterium called colon bacillus, antibiotics particularly lethal to this germ are prescribed. If the urine culture shows another type of organism to be the cause, the variety of antibiotic can be appropriately modified. Cystitis is a local infection of the bladder without involvement of the upper urinary tract. It ordinarily causes severe burning and pain on urination, with a marked frequency of voiding. It too can be successfully treated with antibiotics.

Excessive Bleeding

As explained earlier in this chapter, it is normal to have a bloody vaginal discharge for about ten days to two weeks after delivery. The bleeding may be irregular, and the passage of occasional clots the size of a quarter is not abnormal. However, the rate of bleeding should not exceed that seen during the menses, and the amount should gradually taper off.

In occasional cases, often around the seventh or eighth day, the bleeding may increase acutely, with or without the passage of large clots. If this occurs, call your doctor immediately. The cause for the abnormal bleeding may be either subinvolution—failure of the uterus to involute properly—or the retention of placental fragments. The latter is not due to the neglect or incompetence of the physician, as the layman is prone to imagine. In the third stage of labor, during the process of separation of the placenta, some isolated portion may be so firmly attached that when the placenta sheers itself loose the adherent tissue remains behind. Treatment of the excessive bleeding may be initiated at home or in the hospital, depending upon the gravity of the blood loss. Ergotrate is prescribed by mouth every three to four hours, for two or three days, to cause the uterus to contract; this may be supplemented by Oxytocin, ordinarily administered by intravenous drip. When necessary, a transfusion is given. If after approximately twelve hours the bleeding has not markedly diminished a curettage of the uterine cavity is carried out under general anesthesia. The scraping away of the offending tissue, whether it be portions of the pregnancy uterine lining which through faulty involution have not sloughed off or fragments of placenta, cures the condition.

Anemia from Blood Loss

Transfusions are given so frequently on an obstetric service that the staff views them as a commonplace procedure. Usually they are done merely to shorten convalescence or to forestall complications rather than to save a life. This is often misunderstood, and when the obstetrician suggests a transfusion patient and family become unnecessarily alarmed.

If a patient loses as much as a quart of blood at delivery, transfusion from a suitable donor is usually performed in the early puerperium. In addition, she is given some medicine containing iron, and liver is added to the diet. These measures are to stimulate blood formation in her own body.

Sore Bottom

Discomfort in sitting may be caused by the episiotomy or by hemorrhoids. Either is improved by frequent shallow, warm baths, and application of an ice-collar in between baths. Steeping gauze in iced witch hazel and applying it gives relief. Liberal use of aspirin or some other mild analgesic is also indicated. Sitting on a rubber ring is an old standby to reduce discomfort. Take heart; the pain always disappears, to be sure not as speedily as many would wish.

Postpartum Examination

A patient should be seen in her physician's office about one month after confinement for a thorough examination. This visit is an integral part of good obstetric care. It furnishes the physician an opportunity to take stock of his results, gives the patient the advantage of having any abnormality corrected, and offers patient and doctor a logical opening to discuss future pregnancies.

If at the time of the scheduled visit the patient is menstruating, it is preferable to make another appointment. Of course menstruation must be distinguished from abnormal nonmenstrual bleeding or staining, for if this is the case there is all the more reason to keep the date. When there is doubt the doctor can frequently differentiate the two over the telephone by the patient's description of the bleeding.

A pertinent history is taken, including ability to control urine and stool, pain in the perineal region, return of menses, lactation, etc. The doctor's nurse then takes charge of you.

After voiding, you undress, wrap yourself in a sheet, get weighed, and have your blood pressure checked. Then, properly draped, you lie on your back on the examining table. The doctor enters and examines your breasts and abdomen. When this is completed, your heels are placed in stirrups and you bring your buttocks to the edge of the table with knees spread wide apart. The doctor inserts his gloved index and middle fingers within the vagina and by downward pressure tests his perineal repair. More than likely he is quite proud of his seamstry. He then checks the uterus, tubes, and ovaries by bimanual examination. If he plans to fit you with a contraceptive diaphragm, it is usually done at this juncture. Then either the doctor or his nurse instructs you carefully in its insertion and removal. When this is completed, a two-bladed metal speculum is inserted in the vagina and manipulated so that the cervix is brought in clear view. If any raw area is visible on the lips of the cervix it is seared by a red-hot electric cautery tip. This sounds barbaric but, since the cervix is devoid of pain nerves, I promise you that it does not hurt; you may feel the heat, however. In a new development, cryosurgery, superficial cervical abnormalities are treated by a freezing technique. Frequently a rectal examination is made to check for the presence of hemorrhoids.

Finale

When you are dressed the doctor will discuss the results of the examination and offer any necessary advice. Some physicians make it routine to see all patients again six and twelve months after delivery.

The more than seven months of long, close acquaintanceship between doctor and patient are about to end. It is the unusual patient who does not feel gratitude and many express it. Most obstetricians remain life-long friends to the couples they have served. By being constantly associated in the parents' thoughts with the happiness and pleasures of parenthood, the accoucheur occupies a unique position in the medical hierarchy, a favorable position near the top.

Resumption of Sex Relations

If no abnormality is found at the postpartum examination, coitus may be immediately resumed, if it has not already been resumed. Undoubtedly some couples in the absence of bleeding, discharge, and perineal pain jump the gun. Among sins against health this ranks pretty low, probably below smoking. If cauterization of the cervix was performed, abstinence should be practiced for a week. If at the resumption of marital relations the scar of the perineal tear or episiotomy causes pain, this can be diminished by a preliminary hot bath and by both individuals lubricating beforehand with Vaseline or some jelly or cream. When pain or discomfort persists for more than four weeks after resumption of sexual relations, the patient should return to her doctor for treatment. The vaginal opening can either be stretched digitally or dilated with appropriate dilators.

And so we leave the puerperal woman, having followed her through both normal and abnormal convalescence. For most it is a happy period of adjustment to a new chapter in life. I realize that for a minority it is difficult and even threatening, particularly if some physical complication arises.

17

Twins and Other Multiple Births

How Many at a Birth?

We read in the works of Ambroise Paré, premier surgeon-physician of sixteenth-century France, that Lady Margaret, Countess of Hagenau, was brought to bed of 365 children at one and the same time in the year 1313. Milady's superfecundity came about in a miraculous way, through God's displeasure. It happened that, sometime the year before, the countess was walking through the gate of her walled palace when her skirt was plucked by a kneeling beggar woman who said, "My good lady, give me alms."

The countess, haughty and indignant, replied, "Why should I give you alms?"

The beggar woman answered, "Because of all the children I have begot."

The countess looked down upon her in disdain. "Fie upon you, you've had the pleasure of begetting them."

God in heaven overheard, we are told, and he was wroth. The next year the countess was lain in with 365 children, one for each day in the year. There were 182 females, all baptized Elizabeth by the good Bishop of Utrecht, and 182 boys, all baptized John. There was one "scrat" (hermaphrodite), who pathetically remained unnamed and unbaptized. In reporting the same case a hundred years later, Mauriceau said it was either a "miracle or a fable"; we are inclined to the belief that it was a little of both.

Other fabulous cases are recorded, such as "Dorothy, an Italian who had twenty at two births, at the first nine and at the second eleven, and she was so big . . . her belly . . . rested upon her knees."

When we descend to the number seven it becomes impossible to know whether we are dealing with fact or fable. In the German town of Hamelin, which the Pied Piper made famous in 1248, we find the following tablet attached to the front of a house in Emmenstrasse: "Here on this spot dwelt . . . Thiele Romer, and his helpmate Anna Byers. It came about that in the year 1600 . . . at three o'clock in the morning on the ninth day of January, she was delivered of two small boys and five small girls. . . . All peacefully died by twelve o'clock on the twentieth of January and were given the beatitude which is guaranteed to those who believe." That is all we know about the possible, perhaps even probable, Hamelin septuplets.

We come now to undisputed facts outside the realm of the fabulous and the pseudo-fabulous. There are quite a few authentic cases of sextuplets, one reported in 1969, in which all six survived.

Quintuplets are reported every few years, but so infrequently that it is impossible to state the mathematical frequency. The first set of quintuplets ever to survive in history were the Dionne sisters of Canada in 1933—not even a single quintuplet had ever survived before.

Natural and Artificial Multiple Births

In the early 1960s, the situation in regard to the frequency of multiple births was radically altered by the introduction by Dr. C. A. Gemzell of Sweden of the hormone gonadotropin recovered from human pituitary glands collected at autopsy. Unlike gonadotropin made from other animal pituitaries, the human material on injection made the ovaries of infertile, nonovulating women ovulate. However, the effect of this new hormone could not be accurately controlled, and, in many instances, it caused several Graafian follicles to mature and ovulate simultaneously. In the forty-three deliveries Gemzell reported among the first hundred nonovulating women whom he treated, there were twenty single births, fourteen twin births, and nine births of triplets or more children.

A series of seventy-eight ovulation-induced pregnancies reported from the Tel-Hashomer Hospital in Israel resulted in forty-seven single births, twenty-three pairs of twins, five sets of triplets, two sets of quadruplets, and one set of sextuplets. A chemical compound, clomiphene, was discovered to have similar properties to Gemzell's human pituitary substance. In general, about 16 per cent of human-gonadotropin births give rise to more than one baby and at least 10 per cent of clomiphene-induced deliveries. Since multiple ovulations are produced, each baby comes from a separate egg. So far as I know, the largest multiple birth resulting from ovarian stimulation has been octuplets, eight. No octuplets or septuplets have as yet survived. To keep the record straight, I think drug-induced multiple births should be termed "artificial multiple births," and the spontaneous variety "natural multiple births." The statistical data given in this chapter refer only to natural multiple births.

Frequency of Natural Multiple Births

Hellin in 1895 stated that twins occurred once in 89 births, triplets once in 89^2 (7921) and quadruplets once in 89^3 (704,969). Actually, Hellin's so-called law is wrong on two counts. A sufficiently close mathematical relationship does not exist between the different orders of multiple births so that squaring and cubing the twinning frequency will accurately give the frequency of triplets or quadruplets. Hellin also failed to recognize that the incidence of multiple births varies markedly in different population samples.

In an analysis of the 80 million births which occurred in the United States between 1928 and 1955 I found that quadruplets occurred once in 490,000 pregnancies, triplets once in 9300, and twins once in 90.

What Chance Have You for Twins?

I cannot answer without knowing your race, age, parity (number of children you have conceived), and whether you or your husband have a family tree studded with two apples for each blossom (inaccurate metaphor; these would only be one-egg twins).

What about your race? In vital statistics throughout the world, marked differences are found in the incidence of multiple births among black, white, and yellow populations. In this country twins occur once in 73.2 nonwhite births (96 per cent of which are black), and once in 93.2 white births; triplets once in 5800 and 10,200 births respectively. In Japan twins occur once in 154.4 pregnancies, triplets once in 17,200. You have the best chance for twins if you are black, the poorest chance if you are Oriental, and an intermediate chance if you are white.

What about your age? White women under twenty have a very low twinning incidence—1 in 167 births. After twenty it steadily rises, the peak frequency being recorded for the age group thirty-five to forty, when its occurrence is 1 in 59. The frequency then declines, so that women over forty-five have the same poor chance as girls under twenty.

What about your parity? Parity, the number of children already begot, exerts an influence independent of age, but usually the two go hand in hand, for younger women ordinarily have fewer children and older women more children. If you are a white woman of thirty-five to forty in a first pregnancy, you have 1 chance in 74 of bearing twins, but if you are thirty-five to forty having your seventh pregnancy, your chance is increased to 1 in 45.

What about your heredity? A tendency to multiple births is inherited in some families, and it affects both the men and women of these stocks. In other words, not only the women bring this gift as part of their dowries, but the men as well. Such families are distinguished by the fact that their trees have several instances of twinning on almost every branch, not just an occasional sporadic pair, as almost all of us can find if we scan family horizons diligently. The tendency to twinning does not skip a generation; it is expressed in succeeding generations.

Types of Twins

There are two types of twins. One variety originates from a single fertilized egg which divides into two very early in its development. In these circumstances, one egg is fertilized by one sperm, and the germ plasm of the two offspring is therefore identical. Consequently they must be of the same sex and exactly alike in skin, hair, and eye color. They also bear a striking resemblance to each other in body build and facial features and possess exactly the same blood factors. Such twins are termed identical, one-egg, or monozygotic.

The other type of twinning results from the fertilization of two different eggs by two separate spermatozoa. The eggs may come from the same ovary or from opposite ovaries. Twins of this variety, known as fraternal, two-egg, or dizygotic, are simply a litter of two and bear no greater resemblance to each other than brothers or sisters at exactly the same age. They may be of the same or opposite sex and may or may not have the same blood types. As we stated, all artificial twins and even all artificial octuplets are of this type.

Can You Tell One-Egg from Two-Egg Twins at Birth?

If they are boy and girl, they necessarily must be from two eggs, non-identical. If they are of the same sex, your doctor can get either a definite answer or a strong hunch from careful inspection of the placenta. If the two children have a single placenta, and examination of the membranes at the point where the two sacs surrounding the fetuses come in contact to form a partition wall demonstrates only two thin membranes, one can be certain that the twins are identical, from one egg. On the other hand, if each twin has its separate placenta, or examination of the partition wall in the single placenta demonstrates three or four membranes instead of just two, there are nine chances in ten that the twins, though of the same sex, are not identical but fraternal and from two eggs. An absolute decision in such cases must await further tests.

One of these tests can be carried out at birth, a study of the two bloods. The two bloods must be exactly alike in all respects: Rh, major groups (A, B, AB, O), and minor groups such as M, N, Kell, etc. If the blood groups differ even in the slightest, one can be sure the twins are not identical. If the blood groups are exactly alike, ordinarily final decision must await physical-resemblance studies when the twins are a few years old. To be identical the two must have the same coloring and same body builds, and must be so alike that they are difficult to distinguish. However, a final and absolute test to establish the identity or non-identity of a pair of like-sexed twins is the use of reciprocal skin grafts. If the twins are from one egg, a small piece of skin grafted from twin A to twin B will "take" as perfectly as though the graft were taken from A and grafted to A. If they are from two eggs, the graft will wither and be rejected. This viability of grafts from one identical twin to the other member of the pair has been utilized in transplanting one kidney from a healthy twin to his co-twin dying from kidney failure. The great majority of identical twin kidney transplants have succeeded.

Frequency of the Two Types

In the United States, among whites, 34 per cent of all twins are identical, while 66 per cent are fraternal; among nonwhites 29 per cent are identical and 71 per cent fraternal. In direct contrast, the yellow populations studied have all shown the majority of their twins identical.

From this it becomes obvious that those racial groups with a high frequency of twinning have a large proportion of fraternal, two-egg twins; while those groups with a low incidence of twinning have a relatively small proportion which are two-egg. Further study has shown that one-egg identical twinning occurs with the same fixed frequency in all people, irrespective of race, age, parity, and family history. The variable, the factor which affects both the frequency of twinning and the proportion between the two types, is the occurrence of two-egg, fraternal twinning, which is highly sensitive to race, age, parity, and family history.

Triplets, Quadruplets, and Quintuplets

The same factors influencing the occurrence of twins similarly affect the production of triplets, quadruplets, and quintuplets.

One or several eggs may be involved in the creation of multiple pregnancies of the greater magnitudes. Quintuplets, for example, may come from one, two, three, four, or five eggs. On the basis of physical-resemblance studies by a group of Canadian scientists, the Dionnes are known to have arisen from one egg. The proportion of the various egg combinations has been studied for triplets. In six out of every ten cases, two eggs are involved (a pair of identical twins plus a singleton); in three, all come from one egg (identical triplets); and in one, three eggs are fertilized (fraternal triplets).

Siamese Twins

Siamese, or conjoined, twins are always one-egg twins whose misfortune was that the embryonic area failed to split completely, so that the ovum only partially divided. The undivided portion is that part of the body that the conjoined twins have in common; the divided portions are those parts of the body that are separate in the two individuals.

Conjoined twins are predominantly female, and the commonest variety are twins joined back to back in the regions of the sacrum, called pygopagus. They ordinarily have many vital structures in common, including the rectum and, in females, the vagina.

Between 1927 and 1965 twenty-one surgical separations of Siamese twins were attempted. In five cases in which the infants were united by tissues around the navel (omphalopagus), all ten children survived; in five cases joined by the scalp and the deeper cranial tissues (craniopagus), eight survived; in two cases joined in the breast-bone area (xiphopagus), four survived; of six pairs joined by the chest (thoracopagus), there were eight survivors; and of three pairs joined by the soft tissues overlying the sacrum and involving the vagina and rectum (pygopagus), four infants left the hospital alive.

It is obvious that sophisticated physiologic studies must be done to determine which cases are operable. For example, if only one heart or one pair of lungs serves both twins a successful operation is out of the question. Experience dictates that the operation should not be performed until the twins are at least two months old, and then the procedure requires a large, well-rehearsed, expert surgical team.

I made the rounds at the Texas Children's Hospital in Houston in 1965 when the Bay City twin girls who were joined in the chest area were being studied preoperatively. At eight weeks old they were charming little girls, each lying about three-quarters on her back and seemingly oblivious of the presence of the sister who was part of her. How complex the preoperative procedures were for the successful surgical separation of these twins is indicated by Dr. Luke Able, the senior Baylor surgeon involved in the operation: "A supporting team of anesthesiologists, operating-room nurses, pediatricians, physiologists and their monitoring crews, photographers, and medical artists was assembled. Practice sessions in the operating room were carried out, first on manikins and finally on the thriving twins."

Conjoined twins are an obstetrical rarity, probably occurring once in

50,000 to 100,000 births—slightly more often than one in a thousand twin births. Many are stillborn, frequently quite prematurely. Occasionally they are diagnosed by X-ray late in pregnancy. I have seen the X-ray films of one such case. In all the X-ray exposures, no matter what the position of the mother, the twin skeletons maintain a fixed close relationship to each other. Since the tissue of union usually involves soft parts, most of the term Siamese twins were delivered vaginally without great difficulty. One twin slides out ahead of the other, greatly stretching the soft-tissue union. Today, with Cesarean section having become so safe and so common, diagnosed conjoined twins at term are usually delivered abdominally.

There have been many famous pairs of Siamese twins; their lives have elicited much curiosity, which has resulted in complete biographies of several. The stories of two such cases follow.

Eng and Chang were born in Siam in 1811, the fourth pregnancy of a half-Siamese, half-Chinese mother by a Chinese father. The boys were united by a pliable bridge of tissue four inches in diameter, reaching from the lower end of the breastbone to the navel. As the connecting link allowed much freedom of movement, they were both able to face for ward if they tired of looking at each other. They were not identical in health, strength, or temperament. Eng, the right twin, was the stronger and healthier of the two and had the better disposition. When eighteen, they came to America and soon fell under the golden direction of the great showman P. T. Barnum, who made them rich and famous.

After amassing financial competence, the twins retired to North Carolina, where they raised tobacco and children. Eng's wife, Sally, had twelve children, and Chang's wife, Adelaide, ten. The wives were sisters, daughters of a Virginia clergyman, and delivered their first children within three or four days of each other. Things went well until the wives, resenting the unnatural intimacy forced upon them, began to quarrel, compelling the two families to take up separate abodes a mile and a half apart. Eng and Chang arranged to spend three days in one home and then three days in the other. The one whose home they occupied was complete master over their joint destiny for the three-day period.

The Civil War destroyed their property, and when nearly fifty-five the Siamese twins had to take to the road again. In 1872, when sixty-one years old, Chang had a paralytic stroke which so incapacitated him that his healthy brother had to half drag the paralyzed victim about for the two years they survived. On the day of death Eng awoke and tried to arouse Chang; not succeeding, he called for one of his sons, who also failed to awake the twin. Terrified, the son called out, "Uncle Chang is dead!"

Eng sighed and exclaimed, "Then I am going also!" Soon he complained of suffocation and asked to be propped up. He became weaker and weaker, and a little more than two hours after he discovered his brother's death he died.

The dead twins were transported by special train to the University of Pennsylvania, in Philadelphia, where an autopsy was performed before the most distinguished group of physicians that had hitherto gathered in America. Chang, the autopsy report shows, died of pneumonia. The pathologist reported Eng was frightened to death, since both his testicles had ascended high up into the inguinal canal, thought to be the benchmark of extreme fright. The twin's band of union, it was found, could easily have been severed even in 1874, as the only organ they had in common was a pencil-sized bridge of liver tissue.

Rosa and Josepha Blazek, Bohemian twins born in 1878, were united at the base of the spine and had a common rectum and vagina, though separate uteri. As far as I know, they are the only female pygopagi to bear a child. It is stated that the two had one husband. At the age of thirty-two Rosa gave birth to a normal son after a very short labor. Josepha did not experience the pains of labor, and both women were equally able to nurse the infant. They died a few hours apart in Chicago during the influenza epidemic of 1918.

Superfetation–Conception during Pregnancy

Superfetation means conception during pregnancy. One of the medical worthies of yesteryear phrased it very succinctly—"a reiterated conception." In some cases the interval between conceptions is thought to be several months, so that a term child is born with an immature fetus as co-twin. This presupposes ovulation during pregnancy, the passage of spermatozoa through the pregnant uterus into the tube, fertilization of the second egg, and its downward passage into the uterus, where it must implant alongside its co-twin, which has had a several-week or several-month start. This is theoretically possible until the fourth month of pregnancy, when the uterine cavity is completely sealed off by the enlarging fetal sac. After such an obliteration of the uterine cavity, it is theoretically impossible for spermatozoa to ascend.

The evidence in favor of superfetation is of two kinds. The first is the simultaneous birth of two fetuses with great disparity in size and birth weight. Cases have been reported with both twins born alive, one weighing 3110 grams (6 pounds, 14 ounces) and the other 420 grams (14½ ounces). This extraordinary difference could be due to superfetation or to inequalities of nutrition during intrauterine existence, so that one twin was luxuriously nurtured, while the other, due to an abnormal insertion of the cord or some other placental factor, was grossly undernourished.

The second evidence in favor of superfetation is the birth of living twins many weeks or even months apart. A case reported from Australia tells of the birth of a twin of 3 pounds, 10¾ ounces, and the delivery of its co-twin, 5 pounds, 14¾ ounces, fifty-six days thereafter. Both twins survived, the first having reached the weight of 6 pounds when the second was born. It is almost an infallible rule that when twins are born more than seventy-two hours apart, the mother has a rare abnormality, a double uterus with a gestation in each. One uterus goes into labor, and the woman bears a premature infant; a few months later the other uterus empties itself of a term-sized co-twin. The birth, then, of living twins many weeks apart is no real evidence of superfetation.

Despite the fact that superfetation has apparently been proved for the rat, its proof for the human remains uncertain. Until such proof is adduced, we feel that superfetation is simply a theoretical possibility.

Superfecundation

Superfecundation is the fertilization of two ova within a short period of time by spermatozoa from separate copulations. It is distinguishable from usual two-egg twinning only if the female has had coitus with two males with diverse physical characters, each passing his respective traits to the twin he fathered, or when the study of the blood groups of the mother and the twins demonstrates that one man could not have fathered both. Superfecundation is commonly recognized in animals and has also been observed in the human. One of the early authentic cases was reported by John Archer of Maryland in 1810. In this case, the white mother gave birth to a white child with a mulatto as co-twin. On questioning, it was determined that she had had coitus with her white husband and with a black man within a few hours.

Fertility of Twins

There is an old canard that twins are less fertile than singletons. This probably has its source from the fertility difficulty that the heifer co-twin of a bull calf is likely to encounter. In 95 per cent of such cases, the female litter mate, termed a freemartin, has no uterus and ovaries, and has an underdeveloped vagina. In cattle twins of opposite sex the testes of the male twin develop before the ovaries of the female twin, and the male passes some of the hormone testosterone, which its fetal testicles secrete into the circulation of the female. This is possible because of a unique type of placenta in cattle, in which even two-egg twins have a very extensive connection of blood vessels from one placenta to the other. The transfusion with hormones from her brother's testes inhibits in the heifer the development of ovaries and of the whole female generative tract. There is no such phenomenon in the human, whether a two-egg twin pair are of opposite or same sex. As early as 1839 the famous Scottish obstetrician Mathews Duncan submitted the fertility of human twins to statistical analysis and found it no different from that of those singly born. I may point out that one-egg human twins, always of the same sex, transfuse blood to each other freely while in uterine residence.

The Causes of Twinning

A consideration of the causes of twinning brings out more clearly than anything else the inherent differences in the biology of one- and two-egg twinning. The one-egg variety is simply a biologic phenomenon that occasionally occurs in all mammals, including subhuman primates. There is suggestive evidence from comparative biology that deleterious influences exerted upon the ovum just after fertilization increase twinning and other forms of pathologic tissue doubling. It is likely that in man the most frequent deleterious influence is the temporary reduction of maternal oxygen through one of several theoretical mechanisms.

Two-egg twinning is a very different phenomenon, resulting from, of course, a double ovulation. It is simple to explain the hereditary transmission of the tendency to produce two-egg twins through the female. In such cases we must either postulate an abnormal tendency to double ovulations in the stock, or an unusual ability to have fertilized and to implant and develop every egg ovulated. To explain the hereditary tendency through the male is not so simple. One must either hypothesize spermatozoa of great potency which are so utterly normal that all ova are fertilized and develop, or that the spermatozoa of the particular family have been endowed with an uncommon ability to fertilize a polar body—a by-product extruded from the normal egg just before it is ripe for fertilization. The polar body contains the twenty-three chromosomes cast off by the egg to halve its number of chromosomes before fertilization from forty-six to twenty-three. Both of these hypotheses are purely conjectural, particularly the latter, since we lack proof that a polar body is ever fertilized.

Diagnosis of Twins

Twins are diagnosed before delivery in about seven out of ten cases, those undiagnosed being as great a shock to the doctor as they are to the patient. The larger the infants and the nearer to term the pregnancy, the less likely it is for twins to be missed. If either twin weighs 5½ pounds or more, there are four chances in five that the diagnosis will be made during pregnancy.

The following observations by the physician create in his mind suspicion of twin pregnancy:

1. A uterus, appreciably larger than is usual for the duration of pregnancy, which continues to grow at an accelerated rate. Twins must be differentiated from hydramnios (excessive amniotic fluid), fibroids (uterine muscle tumors), hydatidiform mole (replacement of the pregnancy by abnormal grapelike structures), and a very large single child. The doctor's suspicions are likely to be aroused by increased uterine size during the sixth month.

2. Excessively rapid weight gain in the absence of apparent increasing obesity, edema (watery swelling of the tissues), or hydramnios.

3. A small presenting part in the pelvis on vaginal examination, with the cervix markedly shortened and already partially dilated, four weeks or more before term, without evidence of labor.

4. The complaint by the patient of excessively pronounced fetal movements, especially if she has had children and compares fetal movements in the current pregnancy with others.

The doctor can be sure that twins are present if the following conditions prevail:

1. He can feel two heads or two breeches on abdominal examination.

2. He can distinguish a fetal heartbeat in each of two separate areas of the abdomen. The rates should differ by ten beats or more per minute. The observation is best made by two persons, each counting one of the heartbeats. If the two heart rates are nearly alike, one fetus may be stimulated by deep palpation of the abdominal wall; the stimulated fetus will react by an increased cardiac rate, which then differs from that of the co-twin. Two fetal heartbeats may be picked up any time after the fifth month, but usually are not detected until the seventh or eighth month. A fetal electrocardiogram with two different rates in different uterine areas is absolute proof of twins. Diagnostic tracings can be noted as early as the twelfth week.

3. Twins have been diagnosed by ultrasonography, using the Doppler ultrasonic technique discussed on page 39. Ultrasonograms as early as six or seven weeks will sometimes demonstrate two fetal sacs. Later, two heads can be vividly recorded. A report from Queen Charlotte's Hospital in London states that in a case of quintuplets five fetal sacs were identified by ultrasonic technique during the ninth week and five fetal heads at thirty weeks. The mother, hospitalized at twenty-three weeks, delivered five living infants at thirty-one weeks.

4. Formerly X-ray was used routinely to confirm or refute the presence of suspected twins. Today, with appreciation of the theoretical danger to the fetus from intrauterine exposure to X-ray, the other diagnostic methods are given preference. If X-ray is used, two fetal skeletons may be apparent by the eighteenth week or earlier, but the presence of a

second skeleton cannot be completely ruled out until about the twenty-fifth week.

Length of Pregnancy

In our study of twinning we found that the average length of pregnancy was 257.8 days—that is, labor occurred twenty-two days before the calculated date of confinement.

Discomforts of Pregnancy

I truly sympathize with the woman pregnant with twins; the minor discomforts are doubled just as much as the number of fetuses. Breathlessness, varicose veins, hemorrhoids, insomnia, and swelling of the legs and even of the vaginal lips are all too common.

Complications of Pregnancy

Certain complications are particularly frequent in multiple pregnancy. Prominent among them is hydramnios, which makes the already distended abdomen even more distended. The excessive water usually involves only one of the two fetal sacs and is seen in one-egg twins more commonly than in two-egg twins. Treatment consists of bed rest and sedatives when necessary to relieve discomfort; in very extreme cases the uterus is tapped with a needle and some of the fluid withdrawn. Pre-eclampsia and eclampsia, the two specific high-blood-pressure conditions associated with pregnancy, show an increased frequency. Since two fetuses are present, and either one excessively large placenta or two placentas, the unknown factor that causes such blood-pressure complications, perhaps produced by the placenta, probably also occurs in excessive quantities. Anemia occurs more frequently when a woman carries twins, since there are two fetuses which parasitically deplete maternal iron stores. Weight gain is likely to be excessive. Part of the excess is due to the additional fetus, placenta, and amniotic fluid (ten pounds), and part to an excessive retention of tissue fluids. This can be observed in the greater tendency of the patient with twins to develop dependent edema (swelling of the lower limbs).

Conduct of a Multiple Pregnancy

The doctor's special care of a woman pregnant with twins revolves around two main considerations: her greater likelihood of premature labor, and her increased liability to toxemia.

When twins are diagnosed, the pregnant woman is advised to avoid physical strain by stopping work at twenty-four weeks instead of the usual thirty-four weeks. She also must give up travel, not only because a twin gestation may possibly make premature labor more likely, but because, since labor may come on at any time without warning, absence from her home city may be hazardous as well as inconvenient. The patient should take long afternoon rest periods. Coitus should be eliminated during the last three months because of the possibility of a prematurely dilated cervix or the early onset of labor. The patient is placed on a low-salt diet. The frequency of prenatal visits is also increased to facilitate detection of incipient pre-eclampsia. Since anemia is so common in multiple pregnancy, iron is usually prescribed.

If on vaginal or rectal examination the doctor finds that the cervix is materially shortened and partially dilated, and pregnancy is not yet far enough advanced to assure two good-sized babies, he may recommend complete bed rest in the hope that it will forestall labor's onset.

Labor

Most twin labors are satisfactory. Because of the smaller size of the fetuses and the fact that the cervix frequently is partially dilated before labor begins, the ordinary plural labor is shorter than the ordinary single labor. Yet there is a greater proportion of unsatisfactory, sluggish labors among plural births than among single births, due in the main to an increased incidence of uterine inertia and poor, inadequate contractions. The overdistention to which the uterus is subjected is probably the cause. False labor is more frequent in multiple than in single pregnancy.

The membranes are more likely to rupture before the onset of labor in multiple pregnancy (29 per cent) than in single pregnancy (12 per cent).

In regard to fetal position in twins, one finds all the possible combinations and permutations for two fetuses, either of which may assume any of three positions—head, breech, or transverse. One presenting head first, the other breech, is the most frequent combination; although both presenting as cephalic is almost as common.

Since labor complications are increased in multiple pregnancy, whenever possible such deliveries should be conducted in a hospital. Furthermore, while in labor, each patient with a multiple gestation, when possible, should have matched blood held in readiness. Almost certainly it will not be used, but having it available gives the doctor a relaxed feeling—just in case.

If rupture of the membranes occurs before the onset of labor, the patient is likely to be hospitalized and may be put on prophylactic antibiotics. Because of the frequently small size of the fetuses, a twin labor must often be conducted with a minimum of analgesia, since the respiratory center of the small fetus is more easily depressed by drugs.

Conduct of Delivery

The best fetal and maternal results are obtained in multiple births when the least operative interference is employed.

If the first child presents as a vertex or a breech, delivery is carried out as if it were a single child. An episiotomy is done routinely unless the vagina is relaxed and the infant small. The clamp on the placental end of the cord is doubly checked, for in single-egg twins hemorrhage from the severed cord of the twin already born might be fatal to the twin still undelivered. Today, five to ten minutes are allowed to elapse after the birth of a first twin before commencing the delivery of the second. The obstetrician inserts his hand into the vagina and determines the presenting part of the second twin and, by combined vaginal-abdominal examination, its exact presentation. If the head or breech is over the pelvis, the second sac is ruptured and the presenting part guided into the pelvis by the vaginal hand, as the abdominal hand makes downward pressure on the uterus. If the second fetus lies in the oblique or transverse, frequently it can be maneuvered into a longitudinal presentation, and then the membranes are ruptured. After the presenting part of the second child engages in its longitudinal axis, pressure on the uterus usually causes the head or breech to descend rapidly to the pelvic floor, as the delivery of the first fetus just minutes before has dilated the soft parts so that they offer no resistance. After the head or breech of the second child descends, it can be delivered either spontaneously or by simple operative means. If the second fetus cannot be manipulated into its longitudinal axis, an internal podalic version and extraction must be performed. The operator introduces his hand into the uterus, grasps the feet of the infant, turning the baby from its oblique or transverse position, and at once proceeds to extract it as a footling breech birth. If the first twin presents as a transverse in labor, a Cesarean section is the safest solution.

Anesthesia

Some physicians prefer conduction anesthesia, usually saddle-block, for twin deliveries; while the majority, with which I align myself, claim better results with general anesthesia.

Postdelivery Care

Care after delivery of the mother who delivers twins does not differ essentially from the care of the woman who gives birth to a singleton, except that during the first few hours she is watched with special vigilance to detect and treat a tendency of the uterus to relax and bleed excessively. Early ambulation is allowed as with a singleton. Lactation is normal. A mother of twins has a difficult time no matter how she decides to feed. Women who have breast-fed twins claim one advantage over the bottle is in being able to feed both simultaneously, one on each breast. It is not uncommon to find that each twin prefers his own special side to nurse from. Giving way to such preference is not regarded as overpermissiveness.

The Babies

One twin pregnancy in twenty terminates so prematurely that the fetuses each weigh from 14 ounces to 2 pounds, 3 ounces, and only one single fetus in two hundred has a birth weight in this range (400–1000 grams). In nine twin pregnancies out of twenty the larger of the twin babies weighs between 2 pounds, 3 ounces, and 5 pounds, 8 ounces (1000–2500 grams); in single pregnancies the chance of such an occurrence is one in twenty. In one-half of all twin pregnancies at least one child has a birth weight of 5.5 pounds or more. In 93.7 per cent of single pregnancies the newborn weighs at least 5.5 pounds.

The average birth weight of single babies is 7½ pounds; the average birth-weight of twins, 5 pounds, 5 ounces. The disparity in size is due to two factors: the usual earlier termination of multiple gestations, and the relatively unfavorable nutritional environment twins suffer while in the uterus. Twins grow more slowly *in utero*. When a single baby and a twin baby are carried the full nine months, there is an average difference in birth weight of 1½ pounds. The difference in body length is less marked, being about three-quarters of an inch. Not all twins are small at birth. In our series of 1000 twin infants, 3 per cent weighed 8 pounds, in contrast to approximately 20 per cent of single births; 0.4 per cent weighed over 9 pounds, in contrast to 6 per cent of singletons. The largest twin of our series was 9 pounds, 2 ounces; the heaviest pair totaled 17 pounds. This hardly competes with a pair reported by Holzapfel in 1935; the twins together weighed 20 pounds, 4 ounces.

Difference in Birth Weight between Twins

There may be a tremendous difference in the birth weight of a pair of twins, two or three pounds not being extraordinary. The difference is likely to be greater in identical twins than in fraternal twins. In our study the average intrapair difference in identical twins was 14 ounces, while in fraternal twins it was 6 ounces. There is no rule as to which twin, the heavier or lighter, will be firstborn. When a pair of twins are of opposite sex, the male averages 3 ounces heavier.

Sex Ratio

Of 126,328 pairs of twins born in the United States, 42,923 were both male, 42,557 male and female, and 40,848 both female. The total of 128,403 male twins and 124,253 female twins produces a sex ratio of 101.6 males per 100 females, instead of the usual 106-to-100 ratio in singletons. Very likely, relatively fewer female twins die between conception and birth.

Results to the Babies

Twins face a four times greater mortality risk than do single infants. The factor responsible is the relatively large proportion of twins weighing less than 4½ pounds.

When both twins are born alive there is no consistent difference in survival between twin number one and twin number two unless the second twin weighs less than 4½ pounds, when its chances for survival are less than that of its co-twin born first, even if its weight is the same or even slightly less.

Since ordinarily at the same birth weight twins have a greater gestational age than single fetuses (have spent more days or weeks in the uterus), the twins fare better than the premature singletons. In other words, a twin born alive weighing 3 pounds has a greater chance for survival than a single baby weighing 3 pounds.

Congenital malformations are slightly more common among twins. Two-egg or fraternal twins never show the same malformation except through sheer coincidence. On the other hand, it is rare for an identical twin to suffer from a defect not shared by its fellow. Such identity of abnormalities may appear on the same side of the body of each twin or, through the biological mechanism of mirror-imaging, common in one-egg twins, may occur on the opposite side. This same process of mirror-imaging is responsible for the high frequency of opposite-handedness found in adult pairs of identical twins. In 30 to 45 per cent of identical twin pairs, one twin is right-handed, the other left-handed.

18

Family Planning

Throughout history the human animal has attempted to control the number of persons for whom he must provide food and protection. Before the recognition of the sexual origin of life infanticide was the method used, not infrequently selective infanticide, eliminating mainly females since they were not hunters. In the more hostile environment in parts of the Arctic, female infanticide was common well into the first quarter of this century. The existence of the practice is supported by statistical data compiled in 1932. As an example, among the Netsilik Eskimos the ratio of females to males in the age group up to eighteen years was 48 to every 100 males in the population, and in the Barren Grounds area the ratio was 46 to 100. The sex ratio at birth was probably the usual 100 females to 106 males.

It is uncertain when man discovered that impregnation resulted from insemination. According to Hartland, it is relatively recent in terms of *Homo sapiens'* two-million-year existence. The basis for this judgment is threefold. First, the cave man, and even those who followed him lacked means of measuring time much beyond sunrise to sunrise. He had no calendars, nor did he think in terms of weeks or months. Therefore, to associate a birth with an occurrence several seasons before was an impossibility. Secondly, intercourse with females before sexual maturity was the rule, and since no baby resulted from such intercourse, the act could not be easily identified as the source of new life. Furthermore, coitus was a mundane, casual thing in the category of eating and sleeping, and man sought a far more dramatic event to explain the momentous gift of life. He believed that such ephemeral phenomena as lightning or the foam from the sea fathered babies—not men. The third source of puzzlement was the observation that some women and men copulated throughout their lives and still no pregnancy resulted; for there are sterile members in all families of the vegetable and animal kingdom, and primitive man was almost certainly no exception.

Early References to Contraception and Abortion

When the Babylonian Code of Hammurabi was drawn up in about 1800 B.C., abortion was important enough to be discouraged through the penalty of death by crucifixion. Among the medical treatises written on papyrus by the priest-physicians of the ancient Pharaohs 4000 years ago, seven of which survive in part or in whole, three are gynecological works which contain contraceptive and abortifacient recipes for ladies of the court. By the time that the first book of the Old Testament, Genesis, was written about 1500 B.C., contraception by coitus interruptus was sufficiently widespread among the early Hebrews that four valuable verses (Genesis xxxviii: 7–10) were devoted to its interdiction through the parable of Onan.

Which Is Older, Abortion or Contraception?

It remains unresolved—and probably will remain so forever—whether abortion or contraception is the older form of family planning. The early hunters slew pregnant mammals and saw the uterus and the fetus within. No doubt some of his pregnant females had their bellies ripped by marauding beasts and he must have witnessed the residence of the unborn fetus. Did he attempt to evacuate it forthwith? Or did he learn first that externalized semen is sterile? It may be stated categorically that few if any people throughout history have bred or breed to their full capacity. Some method of family limitation—continence, often through taboos; abortion or simple methods of contraception—is employed. The average woman who commences her sex life at seventeen and makes no attempts at family limitation will produce thirteen liveborn children. Today and in yesteryear this degree of unrestrained fertility is met only occasionally. At present it is seen largely in unusual religious sects, such as the Hutterites in this country.

Evolution of the Birth-Control Movement in the United States

Previous to 1873 there were no laws in the United States concerning contraception and contraceptives, although in some areas contraception was sometimes sporadically forbidden under existing obscenity laws. However, in 1873 Anthony Comstock, Secretary of the New York Society for the Suppression of Vice, persuaded the United States Congress to pass a federal anti-birth-control law. He then persuaded many state legislatures to pass their own anti-birth-control statutes, "little Comstock Acts." The laws were enforced, particularly postal prohibitions, and poor families in America were without access to birth-control information or supplies, except for the condom since its primary function in the eyes of the law was to prevent disease, not pregnancy. The legal ban on contraception had many critics. Among the medical profession two of the foremost were Doctors Abraham Jacobi and Robert L. Dickinson. Prohibition of contraception was opposed by many laymen as well, the more vocal being socialist radicals, like Emma Goldman and Big Bill Haywood. However, these opponents were occupied with other causes and vocations, opposition to the blue laws against birth control being of lesser importance.

Margaret Sanger

The first full-time American evangelist to fight for the liberalization of birth control was a trained nurse, the mother of three children, Margaret Sanger. She had had good training in fighting for causes on the picket lines of the I.W.W. and woman's suffrage. Her focus of interest was concentrated on birth control through her experiences while nursing among Jewish and Italian immigrants in the slums of lower Manhattan. There she saw at first hand the misery resulting from unplanned and unwanted pregnancies, which led to either life-threatening abortions or a plethora of ill-provided-for children. In 1912, at age thirty-three she defied the United States postal-department regulations by writing articles on birth control for the *Call*, a socialist paper widely distributed by mail. When indicted she fled abroad, where she used her self-imposed exile to study birth control in England, France, and Holland. When she returned to the United States she brought with her the knowledge and appreciation of the usefulness of the diaphragm. Mrs. Sanger's motivation in the espousal of birth control, a term she coined, was singleminded —prevention of unwanted conceptions among the married poor. This ideal was not influenced by efforts to limit population growth, for then there was no problem in the United States or elsewhere of excessively rapid population growth. Mrs. Sanger opened the first birth-control clinic in th Western world in the slums of Brooklyn in October 1916, which immediately led to her arrest—the first of eight. Under her leadership federal and state anti-birth-control statutes were eroded by public and judicial opinion. In November 1921 the dispersal by the police on the order of Cardinal Hayes of a public meeting which she was to address in New York's Town Hall brought the American press to her side.

Legal Emancipation of Birth Control

In 1936 there was a landmark decision by the New York Circuit Court of Appeals in the case of *The U.S.* vs. *One Package,* the package being three diaphragms imported from Japan. The favorable opinion of the three-judge court legalized prescription of contraceptives by the medical profession for health indications. The final blow against the statutory ban on birth control was the United States Supreme Court's decision in 1965 declaring the prohibitory law of Connecticut unconstitutional, largely as invasion of privacy. Beginning in 1966, federal funds have been increasingly allotted to both domestic and foreign voluntary birth-control programs. Currently the United States government is an active partner with health agencies in expanding the knowledge, availability, and practice of birth-control techniques. Its main voluntary-agency partner in the United States is the Planned Parenthood Federation of America (Planned Parenthood–World Population), and its overseas partners are several foreign governments and the International Planned Parenthood Federation (IPPF) established in 1952 and based in London. The IPPF has grown from eight to seventy-nine member nations.

Birth-Control Organizations

The first birth-control organization in the United States was the National Birth Control League founded in 1915. It was succeeded in 1921 by the American Birth Control League, which through several name changes has become Planned Parenthood–World Population (PPWP). This national organization with its headquarters in New York has affiliates in 190 United States cities. Slightly more than 150 of these operate 640 clinics while the remainder carry out only educational activities. In addition to giving contraception to 409,000 patients in its clinics in 1970, PPWP furnished community leadership and service in the wide area of conception control. Many of its affiliates provide male sterilization, abortion counseling and referral, sex education, infertility service, and genetic counseling, and several in New York State are equipped for the performance of abortion. The aim of PPWP is each child wanted joyfully by responsible parents. To further this aim it feels that no one who seeks contraceptive advice should be denied it, irrespective of age or marital status. It favors removal of abortion from the criminal code and making termination of pregnancy a medical decision between patient and doctor. Further, it recognizes sterilization as an excellent technique for permanent contraception and one that should be readily available and freely employed after proper counseling.

Contraception vs. Abortion

Soranus, the most famous gynecologist of antiquity, in Chapter XIX of his *Gynecology*, written in about 130 A.D., examines the tissue as to which is the better method to control conception, abortion or contraception. He concludes that it is safer to prevent conception than to eliminate it. This conclusion I heartily endorse on both physical and psychic grounds.

Induced abortion was discussed fully in Chapter 10. Although a recognized form of family planning, it should not be viewed as the first line of defense against unwanted conception. The first line of defense is effective contraception. Abortion is a second-line measure to be used for failed contraception or for failure to use contraception. When contraceptive methods improve, when all obstacles against the prescription of contraceptives, such as age and marital status, are removed, and when we introduce family-life education in our schools, including contraception, it is hoped the need for abortion as a family-planning measure will greatly decrease.

Indications for the Use of Effective Contraception

1. Whenever coitus is practiced in or out of marriage, unless a child is earnestly desired, effective contraception should always be employed.

2. The availability and use of effective contraceptives is essential to accomplish family limitation. Each couple should be given the means to tailor the size of the family to suit personal desires and plans. Since 96 of 100 babies born alive in the United States reach adulthood, young married people should be offered the opportunity to plan with reasonable assurance the number of children they want to rear. The number of children is a personal decision. There is no over-all idea family size because the ideal varies from couple to couple affected by age, health, income, social and religious mores, and emotional needs for parenthood.

3. Ability to space pregnancies according to plan is one of the great gains accruing from the effective use of contraception. The best infant results are seen with a minimum of one year and a maximum of two to three years between childbirth and the initiation of another pregnancy. There is no scientific data showing that the health of a normal woman is adversely affected by short intervals between births.

4. The excessively rapid growth of United States and world population underscores the necessity for man to curtail severely his inborn fertility. Since the world is a finite space everyone admits that some day growth of population must halt. This can be accomplished only if births equal deaths. There is difference of opinion in assessing the urgency of

this problem. The fact that there are about 130 million births in the world each year and only 60 million deaths demonstrates that the attainment of population stabilization at equilibrium is far off and therefore the effort must be now. Even with a vigorous population-control program several decades will pass and billions will be added to the world census before growth is checked. A second disagreement revolves around the implementation of a population-curtailment program. Can it be accomplished through voluntary means, wide latitude of individual choice, or must it be coercive, through governmental intervention and edict? The answer may be different in different parts of the world. In the United States, with freedom of choice, there has been significant slowing of the birth rate over more than a decade, which if it continues will make coercive measures unnecessary. What happens in the next two decades will furnish our answer.

If voluntarism is to succeed a large educational effort must be made. Beginning in the schools the facts and threats of population growth must be taught. Individuals must be made to feel that a decision to add another child must be weighed not only in terms of responsible behavior to the family unit, but to the local and world community as well. Small families must be encouraged by training women for useful careers other than childbearing and setting up day nurseries so that they can practice the careers for which they have been trained. Young couples must be relieved of the multiple social pressures which sometimes seduce them unwillingly into parenthood, and the social status of the childless couple and of the bachelor and spinster must be upgraded.

Successful voluntary population control requires widespread diffusion of contraceptive knowledge and materials. Contraception must be taught in the schools with the pragmatic point of view of promoting responsible sexual behavior. All restrictions, such as age or marital status, on the prescription of contraceptives must be totally removed. In addition, large sums of money and scientific talent must be expended to improve current birth-control methods through basic research.

Medical Factors Associated with Planning a Family

There are several considerations worth mentioning, if for no other reason than to give emphasis. First, youth is a respected ally of successful pregnancy and delivery. Second, no physical harm has been proved to result from having children close together. Third, having borne many children and being relatively advanced in reproductive age are both factors that penalize the efficiency and safety of childbirth. Fourth, if one is unfortunate enough to have a child born with a serious congenital abnormality it is imperative to seek highly competent genetic counseling before another pregnancy is undertaken to get expert opinion on the risk of repetition. After the degree of risk is spelled out a couple can then make a knowledgeable decision about future childbearing.

Special factors may place a woman in an individual category, so that a doctor may feel it necessary to offer specific advice rather than generalities. Some of the commoner conditions which make advisable a short interval between the termination of one pregnancy and the beginning of the next follow:

1. A woman starts her family at the age of thirty-five or more and wants several children.

2. Fibroid tumors of the uterus are present and their removal is not contemplated. Since the speed of their growth is unpredictable, one had better make hay while the sun shines.

3. When pregnancy has just resulted in a spontaneous abortion, a stillbirth, or the death of the newborn, it is psychologically imperative for most women to conceive at once. No substitute will eradicate their sense of frustration.

4. The couple for whom it required several years to achieve a pregnancy cannot afford to wait, as it is impossible to know whether relative infertility will thwart them again. Usually it does not.

On the other hand, there are conditions which argue strongly in favor of the lengthy postponement of a new pregnancy. For these patients time must elapse so that one may evaluate the effects of the completed pregnancy and newly acquired parenthood on the physical abnormality.

1. Malignancy, particularly breast. No pregnancy should be undertaken for five years after the breast operation.

2. Heart disease, more than slight.

3. Active or recently active tuberculosis.

4. Persistently high blood pressure.

5. A psychiatric disturbance during pregnancy or the puerperium.

Neither list is intended to be complete; each indicates medical thinking in this area.

Cesarean section, diabetes, pre-eclampsia, and eclampsia do not appear above. Their omission is purposeful, since I do not feel that any of the four should affect the time interval between pregnancies.

Methods of Contraception

There are many methods of contraception, some relatively new, some antedating written records. Even the two newest, the pill and the intra-uterine device (IUD), had their progenitors in the deep past. The Talmud, more than 1500 years ago, recommended a "cup of roots" to prevent pregnancy. One such prescription was to dissolve in beer Alexandrian gum, alum, and the bulb of the crocus and "to drink thereof." All folk people have a particular plant reported to diminish fertility. The American Indians made tea from *Lithospermum ruderale*, which grew on the western slopes of the Rockies, and each spring the squaws and braves who sought no pregnancy drank it. Temporary lodgement of a foreign body in the uterine cavity, an IUD, was first used by sixteenth-century Arabs to prevent their camels from becoming pregnant. A long, hollow reed loaded with a small stone was introduced through the vagina and cervix and a stone blown into the uterine cavity. When pregnancy was desired, it is said the stone was milked out.

I propose to create a schedule of contraceptive methods classifying them into six groups on the basis of relative effectiveness, Group I being the most effective, and Group VI the least effective. However, before doing so, I want to state that contraceptive effectiveness depends on three factors of equal importance: intrinsic value of the method, consistency of use, and proper application. An inferior method used with complete consistency is far better than an effective method used irregularly. Therefore the couple must choose a method which possesses high acceptability for them both. On these grounds there is no best method of contraception, but there is a best method for the individual partnership. The tremendous psychic component in sexual satisfaction makes it unwise for a couple to choose a contraceptive method in which they lack confidence, or fear because of side effects, or which is unesthetic or objectionable to either partner, no matter the reason.

Probably many experts will not agree completely with my assessment of relative effectiveness.

Group I—Pill
Group II—IUD (intrauterine device)
Group III—Condom; Diaphragm
Group IV—Coitus Interruptus (withdrawal); Intravaginal Foam; Rhythm using basal body temperature (BBT)
Group V—Nonfoaming intravaginal creams, jellies, and tablets; Rhythm using calendar
Group VI—Douche

The Birth-Control Pill

The pill if taken as directed is the most effective contraceptive known. Its active ingredients are two hormones, estrogen and progestin, both synthetically produced. These manufactured hormones are similar to, but more potent than, naturally occurring hormones and exert their contraceptive affect by four physiological actions. The primary action is inhibition (prevention) of ovulation; absence of an ovum makes impregnation impossible. The way it works is that when the two hormones are present in sufficient concentration they prevent the hypothalamus (a specialized area on the underside of the brain) from sending a signal to the pituitary gland to mobilize the two gonadotropic hormones, F.S.H. (follicle-stimulating hormone) and L.H. (luteinizing hormone), which trigger ovulation. A secondary action of the pill prevents the cervical mucus from entering its midcycle profuse, watery phase, a phase which creates a perfect fluid medium for penetration by sperm cells. Instead, under the influence of the pill the cervical mucus remains scant, viscid, and relatively impenetrable to sperm. Another action affects the lining of the uterus, the endometrium. For a fertilized egg to implant successfully the endometrium must present a very specific pattern of cells, glands, and blood vessels. The pill alters the endometrial pattern materially. Then too it may affect the transport of the egg down the tubes. These four antifertility actions combine to prevent pregnancy and if one is lacking the action of the others will suffice—accounting for the pill's unparalleled contraceptive effectiveness. If the pills are taken precisely as prescribed, without omitting a single dose, theoretically there should be no more than 0.1 unplanned pregnancy per year per 100 women using the pill (1 per 1000). However, the practical pregnancy rate (use effectiveness) is 0.7 unplanned pregnancies per 100, the higher rate stemming from careless use.

Administration

The pill (in reality a tablet) is begun on the fifth day of the menstrual cycle, counting the first day of menses as day number one, and taken once daily, preferably at the same hour, for twenty-one days. Then no medication is taken for one week, or if easier for the patient to monitor, she takes a different-colored, inert, placebo pill daily for seven days before recommencing the twenty-one-day (birth-control pill) regimen. Many women find it easier to take a daily pill rather than going through the mathematical routine of twenty-one days yes and seven days no. There are about twenty different brands of birth-control pills being marketed in the United States. The majority combine estrogen and progestin in each of the twenty-one active pills and therefore are known as "combined" pills. A second type is known as "sequentials." For the first fifteen or sixteen days the woman takes a pill containing only estrogen, which is followed by five daily combined pills. The sequential type of administration is not quite as effective, yielding a use effective rate of 1.4 (failure rate) per 100. However, some women who have unpleasant side effects with the combined type of pill tolerate sequentials.

About seventy-two hours after taking the last birth-control pill vaginal bleeding commences, which can be considered a menstrual period. In actuality it differs physiologically, since pill bleeding is from a different type of uterine lining than normal menses. A pill menses is usually briefer and scantier than a true menses and is almost always free of menstrual cramps. In approximately 3 per cent of pill cycles no bleeding episode occurs after the last pill. This makes no difference, and despite absence of bleeding the woman starts her new twenty-one-day cycle precisely one week after the conclusion of the previous pill cycle. If there is no bleeding for two successive cycles, it is wise to consult a physician to rule out the unlikely possibility of pregnancy.

If for some reason one wishes to postpone the bleeding for a trip or participation in an athletic contest, there is no harm in taking the pill continuously for thirty or forty days instead of twenty-one. However, it is deemed unwise to take the pill continually for an indefinite period, since the creation of cyclic bleeding mimics nature's normal pattern and probably maintains the reproductive tract in better condition.

Extreme youth is no bar to use of the pill, nor is an approaching menopause.

Contraceptive protection is given in the first cycle if the pill is started on Day 5, but if it is started later than Day 5, additional means of contraception should be used through the first cycle.

There is no time limit on how long the pill can be used. There is no need to discontinue it after two or three years and substitute another contraceptive method for a few months before resuming its use. Such a pill "vacation" is not medically indicated.

If one forgets to take a pill for two or more successive days or for two separate days during the month, either abstention during the rest of that cycle or the use of another contraceptive is advised.

Effect on Subsequent Fertility

In most individuals there is no effect on subsequent fertility. At first it was thought that the pill increased fertility by granting physiological rest to the ovaries and pituitary, but there are no hard data to confirm this theory. Ordinarily, true menses—not the immediate withdrawal bleeding—resume four to six weeks after abandoning the pill. About 30 per cent report initiation of pregnancy within three months after stopping the pill. A small percentage of women (0.75 per cent) have amenorrhea (absence of menses) associated with sterility for six months or longer after terminating the pill. If the menses are not re-established after nine months, Clomid, one of the two ovulatory drugs, is ordinarily given and usually, though not always, triggers normal ovulatory cycles. If Clomid fails, treatment with human pituitary gonadotropins (Pergonal) is likely to succeed. Spontaneous return of menstruation has been observed as long as seventy-two months after stopping the pill.

Side Effects

The pill is a powerful drug, so powerful that it should be taken only on a doctor's prescription and under medical supervision. Before starting to take the pill a preliminary breast and pelvic examination should be done including a cervical Pap smear. Blood pressure and urine should also be checked. There are a few contraindications to the pill: among them, lactation unless well established and copious; previous malignancy of reproductive organs, including the breast; history of phlebitis or embolism; recurrent jaundice during pregnancies; scant and irregular menses; high blood pressure, and diabetes. The two latter do not rule out the pill, but call for specially careful medical supervision. If there is aggravation of either condition the pill is discontinued.

Side effects of the pill are classified as minor and major, the minor ones being unpleasant, but not threatening health or life, as major side effects may. Most of the minor adverse reactions associated with hormonal contraceptives are thought to be related to estrogen and are similar to the usual complaints of early pregnancy. These commonly include nausea, vomiting, painful breast swelling, and irregular spotting or bleeding. Less common complaints are weight gain, headache, dizziness, and occasionally chloasma, areas of darkened skin on the face, particularly over the cheekbones. Most side effects, except for chloasma, either diminish or disappear by the second or third pill cycle. If not the doctor is likely to switch the patient to another brand of pills. If there is no improvement, the woman is probably prescribed another method of contraception.

The only proved serious side effect of the pill is an increased tendency in occasional patients for the blood to form clots. This serious problem has been extensively studied in England and the United States. In England among women aged fifteen to forty-five who are not on the pill and who have no predisposing cause for clots, such as recent surgery, the rate of those admitted to a hospital per year for a blood-clot difficulty is only 1 in 20,000, but for women of the same age group on the pill the rate of hospital admission is 1 to 2000. Infrequently a fragment of a clot (thrombus) breaks off and is carried by the blood flow to a vessel of smaller caliber (embolus), which the clot plugs up (thromboembolism). If the plugged vessel is in a vital organ such as the lung, grave illness or death may result. According to British data, the risk of death is as follows:

In the age group twenty to thirty-five, the annual death rate from clots traveling to the lung (pulmonary embolism) and from clots formed in arteries of the brain (cerebral thrombosis) is 0.2 per 100,000 women not on the pill and 1.5 for those on the pill; in the age group thirty-five to forty-five the comparable death rates were 0.5 and 3.9, respectively. The published reports point out that automobile accidents claim more lives per 100,000 women than the pill, as do cigarettes associated with lung cancer and heart disease. Furthermore, in both age groups pregnancy and childbirth have a mortality risk more than ten times that of the pill.

There are some strange findings concerning the relation between thrombo-embolism and the pill. Its incidence seems to have no correlation with how long the individual has been taking the pill or with other factors except for age, as the previously quoted mortality figures indicate, and perhaps for the amount of estrogen in each daily pill. The data involving estrogen dosage was sufficiently suggestive to prompt the governmental drug regulatory authorities of the United States and England to advise strongly that pills containing no more than 50 micrograms of estrogen be prescribed. Previously the standard amount of estrogen in each pill was 80 to 100 micrograms. Both United States and British research workers are collecting additional data to determine whether lowering the estrogen component truly lessens risk of thrombo-embolism as hoped and anticipated.

The two unproved major side effects are cancer and damage to one or more of the body systems. Giving large amounts of estrogen continuously —or in some instances one of the progestins—can cause increased incidence of breast tumors in certain experimental animals but not in others. This is particularly true for certain strains of mice and beagle dogs, both of which have a relatively high incidence of spontaneous breast tumors. Similar studies in monkeys have been completely negative. More than a decade after the introduction of the pill there is no evidence that cancer of the reproductive tract in the human female is increasing or that its incidence is affected in any way by the use of the pill. Cancer experts warn that the whole story is not yet told because in humans the latent period between the cancer-causing insult and its clinical appearance may be as long as twenty years. Therefore they claim that whether or not the pill is carcinogenic cannot be finally determined until 1975 or 1980. It is important to note that in animal experiments the hormones are given continually rather than cyclically and that the dose per pound of body weight in experimental animals is much more than that taken by a woman in birth-control pills.

Some women on the pill show symptomless changes in the chemistry of the body such as increase in blood triglycerides and cholesterol (blood lipids), abnormal sugar tests (glucose tolerance), and changes in the metabolism of water and sodium. However, the alterations are often transitory and all usually revert to their previous status when the pill is discontinued. There is no evidence that any of these temporary drug-induced changes are hazards to health.

All this leads to the conclusion that the pill should be taken under medical supervision. Any departure from health should be reported to the prescribing physician. It is important to report promptly any swelling of the leg, protracted or unusual headache, blurring of vision, excessive nervousness, or depression.

Should You Take the Pill?

Both the United States Food and Drug Administration and the British Committee on the Safety of Drugs feel that the advantages of the birth-control pill, its almost complete protection against an undesired conception and its great acceptability because it permits spontaneous intercourse without preliminary contraceptive preparations, outweigh the infrequent hazard to health. This is also the verdict of the American public. The pill has become our most popular method of birth control and probably nine million women are now using it. Following the Nelson Senate hearings on the pill's safety there was a temporary decline in pill use, but by late 1970 its popularity was largely restored. Almost 40 per cent of married couples who were using contraception in 1970 were relying on the pill. Some pill-users switch to other contraceptive methods, and some discontinue it to achieve pregnancy. The continuation rate is about 80 per cent after twelve months and slightly over 70 per cent after twenty-four months.

In my opinion the pill has a special advantage in early marriage. Properly used, it guarantees postponement of pregnancy until the couple is ready for a family and it enhances good adjustment by permitting wholly spontaneous sexual behavior. For older women, particularly those who have borne children, the IUD or the diaphragm may have advantages.

The Morning-after Pill

"The morning-after pill" is based on the experimental observation made many years ago that if mice or rats are administered a large amount of estrogen after mating, pregnancy does not occur. In the early 1960s this technique was reinvestigated on monkeys by Morris and Van Wagenen at Yale University. They artificially inseminated thirty-five fertile females during the ovulation phase of the cycle, a procedure which normally results in a 50 per cent pregnancy rate. As in rodents, if a large amount of estrogen was begun within seventy-two hours of the insemination the monkeys did not become pregnant.

This interesting observation has been applied to the human, at the moment without the permissive benediction of the Food and Drug Administration. At Yale University 1500 cases have been observed by the Student Health Service, and 1000 at the University of Michigan. All the students had experienced unprotected coitus in mid-cycle and all were prescribed 250 mg of stilbestrol taken over a five-day period, beginning within three days of the sexual intercourse. At one institution a nightly 50-mg dose of stilbestrol by mouth was given for five days, and at the other, 25 mg twice a day for five days. A paper published on the Michigan study reported no pregnancies and, according to a personal communication from Yale, only one pregnancy occurred in their series. In the absence of therapy probably no less than 125 pregnancies would have occurred in two groups comprising 2500 young women with unprotected mid-cycle exposures.

Such a large dose of stilbestrol, however, may cause severe gastrointestinal upset and, theoretically, perhaps even long-term toxicity. I stress "theoretically" because long-term observations have not yet been possible, and therefore such toxicity cannot be ruled out. Many physicians have substituted 2.5 mg of ethynyl estradiol twice a day for five days with equally good effectiveness and less vomiting and nausea. Others are using Premarin, on two successive days intravenously.

Postcoital estrogen is not recommended as a routine contraceptive because of the possible severe side effects. It should only be viewed as an emergency measure after rape or unpremeditated coitus. Then, too, more research is required to say definitely how truly protective it is.

Undoubtedly the high-dose-estrogen technique does not prevent fertilization. It may alter the contractions of the tubes so that the zygote reaches the uterus at a time when implantation cannot occur; or perhaps it modifies uterine contractions sufficiently to disturb implantation; or it may change the chemistry of the endometrium (lining of the uterus) so that it is rendered inhospitable to a newly fertilized ovum. In the opinion of some it causes early abortion, but others feel that there can be no abortion unless the ovum has implanted.

Intrauterine Devices (IUDs)

Modern intrauterine devices are fashioned either from molded plastic or chemically inert stainless steel. They are made in many configurations and shapes, some quite artistic. The one most extensively used in 1971 was a loop made of slender, solid, polyethylene tubing in the form of a double S, about one-and-one-half inches long and one inch across. Since the loop is open-ended and made of molded plastic, it can be stretched into linear form and inserted into a hollow plastic tube called an introducer, resembling a soda straw. One end of the tube loaded with a loop is placed through the cervix into the cavity of the uterus. When extruded from the introducer by a plunger the loop again assumes its double-S shape within the uterus. Another popular form of IUD is the safety-coil, which resembles a pair of coiled ram's horns. A new and excellent plastic

IUD, the Dalkon shield, is elliptical in shape, measuring one by four-fifths inches, and has short plastic fins, or spikes, protruding on the two sides, which help anchor it in position. For introduction the Dalkon shield is notched into place on a special metal probe, which is passed through the cervix to the apex of the uterine cavity, and is then disengaged and withdrawn, leaving the shield behind.

Metal devices are less popular than plastic IUDs since they give rise to more side effects and have a tendency to imbed in the muscle wall of the uterus, sometimes making removal difficult. Almost all IUDs have a nylon thread attached to the lower end, a few inches of thread being allowed to protrude from the mouth of the cervix into the upper vagina. This serves a dual purpose. The protruding thread permits self-examination to make sure the device is still in position, not having been unknowingly expelled. Also, the thread can be easily grasped by the physician and the IUD simply removed by traction. Ordinarily neither insertion nor removal of any of the IUDs is painful and no anesthesia is required. All are inserted with sterile technique by the physician to minimize chance of infection. In some foreign countries where physicians are in short supply, nurse-midwives are specially trained to insert IUDs. I have seen them do it expertly in Ghana and Barbados.

The way an IUD works is still not entirely understood. Perhaps fertilization does occur, but the zygote is prevented from implanting. Some people believe that preventing a fertilized egg from implanting is abortion but, for most, abortion occurs only after the ovum has been implanted within maternal tissues and is dislodged from the site where it began to develop. Another possibility is that the presence of an IUD causes chemical changes in the uterine fluid that adversely affect spermatozoa, preventing fertilization. Microscopic tissue studies show a mobilization of scavenger-type white blood cells in the uterine lining where the IUD rests. Confirmation of the importance of the white blood cells is furnished by interesting experimental IUDs. In Chile many heavy metals were tested to determine whether they possessed contraceptive properties. Only two, copper and zinc, gave positive results. The additive effect of copper has been incorporated in some plastic IUDs, one such device called the T because it is shaped like the capital letter "T," and another called the Cu 7, Cu being the chemical symbol for copper, and 7 because it looks like the numeral "7." Two hundred square millimeters of nascent copper wire are wound around the upright stem of the T device or the longitudinal arm of the Cu 7. For eighteen months, while sufficient copper ions are being released into the tissue which lines the uterus, the contraceptive value of the device is markedly enhanced. It has been demonstrated by microscopic study that copper ions increase the concentration of scavenger cells. Neither the T nor the Cu 7 device can now be prescribed in this country under F.D.A. restrictions. They are being monitored in carefully observed experimental studies in which tests for possible toxic effects of the copper are being conducted. It is anticipated that the tests will be negative and IUDs incorporating copper will soon be released for general use. The initial reports of effectiveness and tolerance by patients are impressive.

Effectiveness of IUDs

Two or three unplanned pregnancies can be anticipated each year in 100 women wearing the usual all-plastic IUD. If pregnancy occurs the presence of the IUD does not interfere except for the risk of abortion, which is somewhat increased. When pregnancy does occur, the IUD lies outside the fetal sac and is pushed aside by the developing fetal membranes. It never makes contact with the fetus. In such pregnancies followed to term there is no increase in fetal malformations. In early pregnancy, it is possible, but not necessary, to remove the device by traction on the cervical thread. Later in pregnancy it is not removed and the IUD is expelled with the placenta and membranes.

Insertion

Although it may be inserted at any time, an IUD is best inserted during the waning days of the menses. The advantages during the menses are that one can be sure that at that time no early pregnancy already exists and that the canal of the cervix is more open at that time, making insertion technically easier. Studies are being conducted on insertion after delivery, while the patient is still on the delivery table, and also immediately after abortion.

Insertion is ordinarily performed by the physician in his office. The cervix is exposed by a vaginal speculum and usually grasped by a clamp to steady it. With sterile technique, the introducer, after being loaded with an IUD, is threaded through the cervical canal into the uterine cavity and the device is deposited in the uterus.

Side Effects

The minor side effects of the IUD are expulsion, pain, and irregular bleeding, or profuse menses. During the first year about 10 per cent expel the IUD, usually during the course of a first, second, or third menses. If retained beyond the third period the likelihood of expulsion is greatly reduced. If an IUD is reinserted, about 50 per cent retain it the second time. Cramps during the first twenty-four hours are not unusual and can ordinarily be tolerated with the aid of simple analgesics, such as aspirin. If pain lasts beyond forty-eight hours the doctor should be consulted, and he may decide to remove the device. Staining or mild bleeding after insertion is usually transitory. Profuse menses or irregular bleeding during the cycle may be sufficiently worrisome to dictate discontinuance. The cases of pain and of bleeding account for about 11 per cent of removals of IUDs during the first year, less frequently thereafter.

Age and the number of children both modify the effectiveness and tolerance of standard IUDs—plastic loops and coils. Older women, thirty and above, with two or more children, experience fewer pregnancies as well as fewer side effects, especially expulsions. However, the Dalkon shield and the experimental T device have shown excellent results in young women who have never been pregnant. Both also, in all patients, demonstrate low pregnancy rates, infrequent expulsions, and relatively few discontinuances for side effects.

The only major side effects of IUDs are pelvic infection and perforation of the uterus, with extrusion of the IUD into the abdominal cavity. Pelvic infection is rare and may or may not be associated with insertion of an IUD. It can almost always be successfully treated with antibiotics without disturbing the IUD. Perforation of the uterus which does not cause pain is reported once in 2500 insertions. Either the doctor realizes it at the time of insertion, or days or weeks after insertion the nylon thread can no longer be located protruding from the cervix. The patient has either unknowingly expelled the device or it has been lost in the abdominal cavity. X-rays will furnish the answer. If the device is intra-abdominal it may be left alone or removed at laporotomy. The decision is usually made by the physician after conferring with his patient. Two to three deaths per 100,000 users per year occur from pelvic infection.

There is no evidence that an IUD causes uterine cancer or that it has any systemic effect.

Acceptability

Like the pill, the IUD has the great psychological advantage of being disassociated from the act of intercourse. The IUD is in place and no preparations have to be made or care taken to prevent pregnancy, thus allowing spontaneity of coitus. An IUD is used by one to two million women in the United States. In clinic populations 75 per cent continue to use the IUD after one year, and 60 per cent after two years. The newer IUDs, such as the shield and the T device, may improve these figures.

The Condom

The techniques in Group III (page 274), the condom as well as the diaphragm, are known as mechanical contraceptive devices, since they interpose a physical barrier that prevents the union of sperm and egg. The failure rate for methods in this group varies from 5 to 15 per hundred couples per year, depending on the care of usage.

Early History of the Condom

The derivation of the word is uncertain. It is claimed without strong evidence that a certain Dr. Condom was attached to the court of the seventeenth-century English king Charles II, who perhaps holds one of the world records for creating royal bastards. Dr. Condom is said to have invented the sheath for the welfare of his monarch, who had become alarmed by the number of illegitimate offspring he had fathered. For the relief his device supplied, it is said, Dr. Condom was knighted by his grateful sovereign. Doubt is cast on this intriguing story by the evidence that animal bladders were probably used as penile sheaths in the days of imperial Rome and that, as early as 1564, an Italian physician, Guy Fallopius, in his poem on syphilis, mentions the value of a linen penile sheath in the prevention of venereal disease. The less romantic but more likely etymology of the word "condom" is its derivation from the Latin *condus*, meaning "a receptacle."

In the late eighteenth century, condoms made of finely spun linen were advertised for sale in the London *Times*. In the mid-nineteenth century rubber condoms became available after the vulcanization process was introduced. Currently most condoms are of molded latex. Animal-membrane condoms made of sheep's intestine are preferred by a small minority who claim that this type affords improved sensation by both partners. These condoms must be softened by soaking in water before use unless they are packaged in a fluid medium.

Modern Use

Shaped like the finger of a glove, condoms are placed on the erect penis before intercourse and receive the man's ejaculation during orgasm. They can be purchased without prescription in drugstores and elsewhere. When used properly and regularly, they will provide a very high degree of protection against unwanted pregnancy.

Condoms are relied upon by 9 per cent of married couples currently practicing contraception, and are probably used more frequently outside of marriage. Their popularity is explained by the fact that they are harmless, simple to use, and easy to purchase, and do not require medical advice.

If the American male does not learn about condoms during adolescence, he may become familiar with their use in the armed forces, where instruction is given as part of the program to control venereal disease. For, in addition to their contraceptive value, condoms also prevent the spread of venereal infection from an infected sexual partner to an uninfected one. The annual United States production of condoms is estimated to be one billion or more.

The upper, open end of the condom, usually one and three-eighths inches in diameter, is surrounded by a rubber ring; its closed end may be plain-ended or have a pocket or teat, in which the semen can be trapped. The teat-ended variety, which is supposed to be less likely to burst after ejaculation, is more popular in Europe than in the United States. Condoms are about seven and one-half inches in length and are made of such thin material that each weighs only one-twentieth of an ounce. They are packed rolled in aluminum foil, cardboard boxes, or metal containers in quantities of three to a dozen. Some latex condoms that are packed singly in fluid are said to increase enjoyment. Packaged condoms have a shelf life—the period of time during which a packaged product can be kept before it deteriorates—of at least two years.

Improvements in manufacturing permit automated production of condoms, which are virtually free of defects. Testing procedures instituted by the manufacturers themselves now utilize electronic methods which can pick up even minute flaws. A single worker is able to check more than 2000 per hour. A few years ago I watched an electrical testing machine at work in the family planning headquarters in Stockholm, which acts as the national purveyor of contraceptives in Sweden. A technician was check-testing a mixed batch of British and American condoms, which had had their initial tests in the country of manufacture. The lot was so perfect that after several minutes the demonstrator had to stick a pin in a condom to demonstrate how the machine automatically rejects a condom with a flaw.

Improvements in manufacture have made obsolete instructions formerly given to pretest a condom immediately before use by inflating it with water or cigarette smoke.

Condoms provide a very high degree of protection against conception, but accidents can happen. The major cause of failure is rupture of the condom during use, which occurs approximately once in 150 to 300 occasions. Two steps may help to forestall this. First, if the condom is the usual plain-ended American variety, it should be unrolled on the erect penis with a half-inch of space or overlap left at the end to accommodate the ejaculate. Second, if the natural moisture in the woman's genital tract is scant, the outside of the condom should be lubricated to prevent tearing on insertion. The best lubricant is one of the many commercial contraceptive jellies or creams. Vaseline or other oils should not be used since they cause rubber to deteriorate.

Failure may sometimes be caused if the condom slips off when the penis is being withdrawn after orgasm. When this happens, some semen may be spilled into the vagina. This can be avoided if the man does not dally and securely holds the ring at the top of the condom to prevent spillage as he withdraws.

Despite these precautions, however, accidents can occur. If this happens, the woman should immediately insert an applicator full of contraceptive aerated or nonaerated cream or jelly into her vagina. If such equipment is not available, immediate douching is second best. Plain water acts as a spermicide, and, since time is of the essence, it is unwise to delay by preparing a douche solution. It is ill advised to insert the erect penis into the vagina before adjusting the condom, as there may be loss of pre-ejaculatory secretion containing perhaps sufficient sperm to impregnate.

Despite the popularity of the condom, some couples don't like to use it for a variety of reasons. One objection is that love play must be interrupted to put the condom on, but imaginative couples have found this presents no difficulty: it becomes a part of the pleasurable preparation for intercourse with the wife undertaking its placement as a signal of her readiness. Some men claim that the condom interferes with normal sexual response by dulling sensation, and others tend to ejaculate prematurely while placement is being made.

On the other hand, there is ample evidence that many husbands and wives find condoms perfectly satisfactory and use them throughout their married lives.

It should also be pointed out that there are medical situations in which the condom would be the preferred contraceptive method, as for example, when the wife has vaginitis, an inflammation of the vagina usually associated with a copious vaginal discharge and itching. Not infrequently the husband has acquired the condition, the causative organism being harbored in his prostate gland. Usually a cure can be obtained only if the physician treats wife and husband simultaneously. Until both are unquestionably cured the couple may be counseled to use a condom during coitus.

Some couples prefer the condom for essentially psychological reasons. If a woman finds it distasteful to use a diaphragm, it is undesirable to prescribe one; and if she also rejects the idea of the pill or IUD, the condom might well be indicated. Likewise, many couples find the condom reassuring because they can see clearly that it works by preventing semen from entering the vaginal canal. This may be particularly true for couples whose knowledge of sexual anatomy and physiology is limited and who therefore feel less security with other contraceptive methods. Certainly for promiscuous sexual encounters a condom has special relevance. It prevents the acquisition of a venereal infection. No other contraceptive does this.

The Diaphragm

It has long been known that when semen is ejaculated into the vagina pregnancy cannot result if an obstruction prevents the seed from entering the cervix. In preliterate societies gums, leaves, fruits, and seed pods were used for this purpose. The Hebrew Talmud, compiled in the fifth century, recommends stuffing wool in the upper vagina. None other than Casanova suggests that a half lemon, squeezed of its contents, be inserted over the cervix as an obstructive cup.

One hundred and fifty years ago a German physician created a removable, individually molded cap for his patients to insert over the cervix. Ninety years ago a Dutch physician published a study on a vulcanized-rubber, domed cap attached to a circular watchspring, which not only occluded the cervix but the upper vagina as well. Known as the vaginal diaphragm, it was prescribed virtually routinely in all birth-control clinics in the days before the pill and IUD.

Today the diaphragm is made of soft rubber or latex in the shape of a shallow cup, with a metal spring forming the circular rim. It comes in a variety of sizes measured in millimeters, ranging from 50 to 105 mm (two to four inches) in diameter. A diaphragm must be fitted to the individual woman by a doctor who is trained in this field. He then designates to the druggist the size required. Most physicians advise insertion of the diaphragm with the dome up, the concavity down. About a teaspoonful of a contraceptive cream or jelly is squeezed from a tube onto the surface of the diaphragm that will have contact with the cervix. At the same time, some cream or jelly is smeared about the rim of the diaphragm to make insertion easier and to create a protective seal between the edge of the diaphragm and the vaginal wall.

A diaphragm is designed to fit snugly beneath the bone forming the forward part of the pelvis—the symphysis—and against the vaginal tissues covering the end of the spine—the sacrum. This distance varies considerably in different women. If an improper size is chosen the likelihood of failure will be increased because the diaphragm cannot carry out its function of forming an impenetrable dam between the upper third of the vagina, where the cervix is located, and the lower two-thirds of the vagina in which semen is deposited. If an improper size is worn, sperm can get around the edges of the diaphragm and enter the cervix. When a diaphragm is too small or too large, moreover, it can be more readily displaced by the penis during intercourse.

Furthermore, Doctors Masters and Johnson in their studies on human sexual response point out that in a multiparous patient even an accurately fitted diaphragm is very occasionally displaced during extremely active coitus. This is much more likely to occur if the woman is in the superior position, astride the male. The vagina normally alters its shape during sexual excitement, enlarging in all diameters. Vaginal size changes less with sexual excitement in women who have never had a pelvic delivery, for the tissues forming the vaginal walls are unstretched by parturition and hence are relatively rigid; in such women the diaphragm almost always retains its inserted position. Doctors Masters and Johnson, on the basis of their work, advise prescription of the largest diaphragm a patient can comfortably accommodate. After the first vaginal birth a woman always requires a larger diaphragm from the stretching of her soft tissues. Virgins after the honeymoon may have to be refitted with a slightly larger size.

Most women can be taught to insert a diaphragm easily with their fingers, but some prefer to use a specially designed inserter. Inserters are made of plastic or metal and come in the form of a slightly curved rod with a series of notches along the shank, corresponding to various diaphragm sizes. The diaphragm is attached to the inserter, which is then pushed as far back into the vagina as possible. A slight twist of the inserter releases the diaphragm. The inserter also has a short blunt hook on one end, which can be used to grasp the forward rim of the diaphragm to remove it. This device is generally advised for patients with short, stout fingers who find it difficult to position the diaphragm manually, and for those who are squeamish about self-handling. It is also useful in proper placement of the diaphragm in a woman whose uterus is tipped back (retroposed).

In addition to the circular diaphragm, which is suitable for nine out of ten women, there are diaphragms designed with unusual shapes for women with various anatomical difficulties or with greatly relaxed vaginal tissues following frequent childbirth.

If the diaphragm is well fitted and inserted properly a woman will not be aware of its presence. If she is, she should check its position immediately, and, if the feeling persists, she should return to her physician for a refitting.

One should get into the habit of inserting the diaphragm each night when getting ready for bed. Then there will be no need to interrupt love play in order to insert it if intercourse is desired.

Whenever an additional act of intercourse is going to take place within several hours after inserting the diaphragm, squeeze another teaspoonful of jelly or cream into the vagina beforehand but leave the diaphragm in place.

Do not remove the diaphragm until at least *six hours* after the last act of intercourse. If you wish, it may be left in place for twenty-four hours.

No douche should be taken until you are ready to remove the diaphragm. A douche is not required and is entirely optional. Modern physicians discourage douching under almost all conditions. If a douche is taken (six hours after intercourse or later), half of it may be taken while the diaphragm is in place, and then after the diaphragm is removed, the douche is completed.

After removing the diaphragm, wash it carefully with mild soap and water, and dry it with a towel. Powder it lightly with any kind of powder or corn starch and put it back in its box or container. A diaphragm which is properly cared for lasts for years.

For women who do not find insertion too irksome and who have the determination to use it regularly, the diaphragm is a highly reliable and useful contraceptive method.

The cervical cap designed to cover only the entrance to the cervix is a small cup, made of plastic, metal, or rubber, which fits securely over the cervix, much like a tight thimble on the finger. The cervix itself is a round projection, about an inch in diameter and an inch in length, located in the upper part of the vagina. If the cap fits snugly, remaining undisturbed during intercourse, it acts as effectively as a diaphragm.

Like the diaphragm, a cap also must be fitted carefully by a trained physician. Unlike the diaphragm, however, self-insertion and placement are a difficult procedure for some women because the cervix is located so deep in the vagina. Though this difficulty tends to limit the cap's usefulness, for those who can master the technique of placement it may be an ideal method, as the cap can be worn for days or even weeks at a time without being removed, and thus provides an ever-present form of protection. Some doctors instruct the woman to insert the cap after menstruation and leave it in place for almost the whole cycle between menses, removing it only a few days before the next period is due. If it is fitted accurately and placed securely, it cannot be moved by the penis during intercourse. A cervical cap is used infrequently in the United States. Occasional males claim that during coitus they are conscious of the presence of a diaphragm or cap and dislike the sensation. If so, a different method of contraception should be sought.

Coitus Interruptus (Withdrawal)

The failure rate of the methods in Group IV is in the order of 10 to 20 per hundred couples per year again depending on care in application. The first method discussed in this group is coitus interruptus, which has many synonyms, including withdrawal and "taking care." As mentioned earlier, it is very likely the oldest method of birth control, and perhaps the one still most extensively used in the world. It is given main credit for making possible the decline in European birth rates during the eighteenth and nineteenth centuries. In several modern Catholic countries, such as Italy and France, coitus interruptus and illegal abortion have made possible their relatively slow population growth. In the United States less than 5 per cent of contracepting couples use it as the sole method of birth control, although 18 per cent use it occasionally.

Withdrawal is a simple method requiring no equipment or preparation before the sex act; it costs nothing and is always available. And though it requires intercourse to be terminated rather abruptly by the male, it permits full contact between the sex organs of the partners. However, withdrawal has had a poor reputation among doctors, and some physicians still attribute many male and female ills to this technique.

What are the accusations? First, that sexual intercourse cannot be enjoyed in a relaxed mood by either partner if the uppermost thought is withdrawal in time. Second, that reliance on withdrawal for a prolonged period will cause some men to ejaculate prematurely. Third, that in women slow to achieve orgasm, pre-ejaculatory withdrawal by the male gives the female even less than normal opportunity to achieve orgasm. This, in turn, is said to cause congestion of blood in pelvic organs, resulting in chronic pelvic pain and other female complaints.

The absence of substantial evidence to support these accusations makes it difficult to assess them. Many now believe that the charges stem more from an author's personal dislike of the method than from his professional observation. Perhaps I lean toward this view because of the old phrase "Fifty million Frenchmen can't be wrong"—and by the evident fact that happy, sexually well-adjusted American, as well as European, couples find this method of conception control satisfactory.

Withdrawal is a legitimate method of contraception and should be considered by couples in deciding which method to employ. If it has been used with complete satisfaction for both partners, there is little reason to change. It is probably more satisfactory in later marriage, when husband and wife have established a consistent pattern of sexual response, and the man is better able to control and anticipate ejaculation. Obviously the cause of failures in this technique is reluctance by the man to withdraw before ejaculation has started. Spilling even the initial drop of semen in the vagina is dangerous since it has been demonstrated that the first portion of the ejaculate contains the greatest bulk of the spermatozoa, the latter part being mainly a diluent. This method, therefore, places a great responsibility on the husband. Another source of failure is reputed to be the pre-ejaculatory loss of a drop or two of semen.

Chemical Contraceptives

Among the chemical contraceptives listed on page 274 in Groups IV and V, those in Group V have about 20 failures per hundred couples per year. Vaginal contraceptives rely for their effectiveness on both their chemical and physical properties. The chemical ingredient is intended to immobilize and kill the sperm cells promptly on contact, without irritating or damaging vaginal tissues. The vehicle carrying the chemical is also intended to act as a physical barrier to obstruct entry of the sperm cells into the cervix. Therefore, the better vehicles are all either gelatinous, oily, or foam-producing.

Vaginal contraceptives come in the form of jellies, creams, tablets, foams, or suppositories. The suppositories, which have a soap, gelatine, or cocoa-butter base, are solid at ordinary temperatures, but readily liquify when inserted in the vagina and exposed to body temperature. The chemicals employed in vaginal contraceptives are basically quinine, boric acid, lactic acid, chinosol, hexyl resorcinol, ricinoleic acid, or formaldehyde. All such vaginal contraceptives must be inserted a few minutes prior to the coital act to afford them an opportunity to distribute themselves throughout the vagina. If coitus is postponed for an hour or longer after insertion of the chemical contraceptive or if the act is repeated, a new application is required.

The only vaginal chemical contraceptives I place as high as Group IV in my scheme of effectiveness are the foams; all the others I relegate to Group V. This means they are decidedly better than nothing, but not sufficiently protective to be relied upon if there is urgent reason that pregnancy should not take place.

The advantage of the aerated foams which earns them a place in Group IV is that, in addition to the spermicidal agent, the effervescent mass creates a relatively dense physical barrier that obstructs the entrance to the cervix. Then, too, a foam readily distributes itself evenly throughout the vagina, the distribution being aided by the motion of the penis.

Foam tablets (Group V) are less effective than aerosol foam creams, in which a butane propellant is added to an effective spermicidal cream. Aerosol foams are packaged in a bottle or small cylindrical metal container. To use them, the protective cap over a release valve is removed and a special transparent applicator is placed over the uncapped top. Pressure on the applicator triggers the release valve, and a measured column of white, aerated cream, resembling foam shaving lather, is forced into the syringe, pushing out the plunger. The foam-loaded applicator is unscrewed and the applicator introduced to the top of the vagina. The plunger is pressed inward slowly as the applicator is being gradually withdrawn. Douching is unnecessary, and is inadvisable until at least six hours after intercourse.

The Rhythm Method

The two types of rhythm method in Groups IV and V are practiced by about 5 per cent of American couples. Calendar rhythm has a failure rate of at least 16 per 100 women per year. Rhythm using basal body temperature (BBT) has a failure rate of at least 7 when medically supervised and correctly followed.

Normally a woman ovulates once each menstrual month. The egg cell survives for about twelve hours, during which it can be fertilized. A man's sperm has a fertile life of forty-eight to seventy-two hours following ejaculation into the female reproductive tract.

These facts form the basis for the rhythm method of birth control, also known as the safe period. They lead to the simple conclusion that a woman can be impregnated during only about eighty-four hours each menstrual month. If this three-and-a-half day period can be determined accurately and if sexual relations are avoided during this time, pregnancy will not occur. Aside from total abstinence, the rhythm method—which is really timed abstinence—is the only technique of birth control declared licit by the Pope. It requires no special equipment and is therefore without cost, and it is physically harmless. No doctor's prescription is needed, although, as we shall see, the guidance of a physician experienced in calculating ovulation may indeed be useful in increasing the chances of using the method successfully.

The three-and-a-half days during which a woman can become pregnant are the three days before ovulation and the half day after it. In order to utilize the rhythm method, therefore, it is necessary to figure out exactly when ovulation is going to take place, and that is where the trouble starts.

For, unfortunately, as yet we have no certain way of knowing when a woman is about to ovulate or is ovulating. No definite sign is given at that time, or at any time beforehand—there is no easily demonstrable chemical change in such body fluids as the urine or saliva. Instead of having precise information from which to calculate when a woman will be fertile and when she won't, one has to rely on estimates.

A normal woman usually ovulates twelve to sixteen days *before* her next menstrual period begins. If a woman menstruates every twenty-eight days, she should ovulate halfway through the cycle—on the thirteenth to the seventeenth day after menstruation begins. Similarly, if her cycle were regularly thirty-three days, her ovum would be released between the eighteenth and twenty-second days after the first day of menstruation.

The difficulty, of course, is that few women ovulate or menstruate with clocklike regularity. In most women the cycle can—and does—vary considerably, and then too, ovulation does not always occur precisely fourteen days before the next menses.

To make allowances for irregularities, it is necessary to lengthen the period of abstinence to provide a few days' margin of safety before and after the day on which it is believed ovulation will take place. To figure out the safe period by the calendar technique:

1. Keep a written record of the menstrual cycles for twelve consecutive months. Count the first day of menstruation as the first day of the cycle, and the day before the next period as the last day of the cycle. At the end of twelve months, choose the shortest and longest cycles for that year.

2. Subtract eighteen from the number of days in the shortest cycle. This determines the first fertile, or unsafe, day of the cycle.

3. Subtract eleven from the number of days in the longest of the twelve cycles. This determines the last fertile day of the cycle, or the day on which the safe period begins. For example, Jane Doe's shortest cycle was 27 days and her longest 30. 27—18=9 and 30—11=19. No intercourse should take place between 9 and 19, inclusive.

The "eighteen and eleven rule" will help a woman determine with some degree of accuracy which days of the month are "safe" and which are fertile. It is as accurate as any special calendars, slide rules, wheels, and other assorted devices produced as "aids" to calculate the safe period. As each month is ended, substitute its length for the same month last year. This keeps the twelve menstrual intervals current and permits for physiological changes in cycle length caused by age and other factors.

A far more accurate means of practicing rhythm is the use of BBT (basal body temperature, discussed on page 311). This depends on the fact that during the first half of the monthly cycle, the days preceding ovulation, a woman's temperature is relatively low and with the occurrence of ovulation it rises about six-tenths of one degree Fahrenheit, remaining elevated until just before menstruation. If pregnancy ensues, the temperature remains elevated and does not show the premenstrual drop. The reason for the temperature rise is that ovulation causes a wound in the ovary with the rupture of the follicle; the wound is immediately filled in by a rapid growth of cells forming a new gland,

the corpus luteum, which promptly manufactures the chemical progesterone, a thermogenic substance causing the temperature to rise.
Therefore in the absence of any other cause for temperature elevation
in mid-cycle, such as a cold or sore throat, it is safe to assume ovulation
has occurred.

To use the BBT rhythm method the woman takes her temperature
each morning on awakening, before getting out of bed—or even before
rousing her husband so that he can catch the 7:48. After the
thermometer is kept in for the necessary three minutes, she can put it
aside to read at her leisure. She charts the temperature daily, preferably
on widely spaced graph paper, and when she notes that the temperature
has risen a half-degree or more and that it remains elevated for three
consecutive mornings, she can be relatively certain ovulation has
occurred and intercourse is very unlikely to result in impregnation. A
bad cold or tonsillitis makes the method useless for the time being.

Special thermometers that are calibrated only from 96° to 100°, so
that the tenths-of-degree marks are more widely spaced, make the BBT
technique easier; also rectal temperatures are more reliable than mouth
temperatures, though if care is taken mouth temperature is satisfactory.

Using BBT is far superior to the calendar technique, but it usually
restricts the days for intercourse to the last ten or eleven days of the
menstrual month, no intercourse being permitted during the entire
month before the third day of elevated temperature. In the grouping
of contraceptive effectiveness which I made earlier in this chapter, I
placed rhythm by BBT in Group IV and rhythm by calendar computa-
tion in category V. There is that much difference.

The great hope for improving the rhythm method lies in development of simple procedures which will enable a woman either to predict when ovulation will take place, or to cause it to occur at a given
time. There is evidence that such procedures are scientifically possible.

Approximately 15 per cent of women menstruate with such irregularity
that they cannot use rhythm at all. Moreover, this method is not
recommended during the months immediately after childbirth since
the first several postpartum menstrual periods may be very irregular. It
is probably safe to apply the "eighteen and eleven" formula only after
the third menstrual cycle following childbirth.

For the 85 per cent of women who can use it, however, the rhythm
method is far more effective than no contraceptive method at all,
although less effective than the pill, IUD, condom, or diaphragm.

It has always been a puzzle as to why some couples fail so consistently
in preventing pregnancy when using rhythm correctly. Perhaps Masters
and Johnson have given the clue. Through laboratory observations they
discovered that a very small percentage of women, like the female rabbit,

cat, and ferret, ovulates out of cycle, after orgasm. Such rabbitlike behavior is uncommon in the human female.

The Contraceptive Douche

All alone in Group VI—the least effective of common contraceptive techniques—is the postcoital douche, which has a failure rate of 25 to 30 per 100 users per year. Its progenitor is probably the bidet, which was introduced in France during the eighteenth century. Robert Knowlton, who received his medical degree at Dartmouth in 1824 and who published in 1832 the first American book on contraception, entitled *The Fruits of Philosophy*, claims to have invented the postcoital douche. Knowlton was rewarded for his pioneering publication by three months in jail at hard labor for authoring obscene literature. Knowlton prescribed a solution of alum " to which in winter a little spirits is added" to prevent freezing. It makes one shiver to contemplate the uncomfortable state of the poor New England wife who resorted to a postcoital douche, scantily clad in winter with no inside plumbing.

The chief advantages of the douche are its inexpensiveness and availability. Its chief disadvantage, apart from its poor rating for effectiveness, is a psychosexual one, for it places the entire burden on the woman, compelling her to spring out of bed immediately after intercourse.

There are two main types of douching apparatus, the bag (or fountain) syringe and the bulb syringe. The latter has a shield, or flange, which when pressed against the opening of the vagina keeps the water from flowing back out until after the vagina has been distended. The bag syringe may be suspended from a wall hook or shower rod so that it is a few feet above the level of the hips—a height that allows the water to flow in gently. The douche is repeated several times. With either the bag or the bulb syringe, it is best to take the douche sitting astride a toilet seat.

Three important rules should be followed in using the contraceptive douche:

1. Use a nonirritating, but if possible a spermicidal, solution.
2. Distend the vagina by slight pressure.
3. Douche *immediately* after intercourse.

The douche should be at a comfortable temperature. Complicated chemical formulas are unnecessary. The following solutions are safe:

Lemon juice or vinegar: two tablespoons per quart of water.

Alum: three tablespoons per quart.

Castile or white soap: dissolve a half-inch cube, or two tablespoons of white chips, per quart.

In every survey of contraceptive methods, the douche is least effective on the list. I hasten to add, however, that it still provides more protection against unwanted pregnancy than no effort at contraception.

Research Leads

Research into better methods of contraception—less cumbersome, devoid of side effects, and at least as effective as the birth-control pill—is going on in many countries. It is being funded by pharmaceutical concerns, by the United States government through the National Institutes of Health and the Agency for International Development, and by the United Nations through its Fund for Population Activities, as well as by private foundations. The funding is insufficient considering the importance of the quest in terms of the consequences of the unbridled growth of world population. Studies are being conducted on progestins alone since the estrogen component of the pill is judged the cause of its blood-clot complications. Progestin is being given by mouth, by the vaginal route, and by implantation of progestin-filled silastic capsules beneath the skin. Steroids are being given experimentally by injection, and by mouth in a once-a-month pill that permits them to be absorbed by the body fat and given off in equal daily increments. Perhaps the most interesting is employment of the prostaglandins, a group of fourteen body chemicals with many functions, including initiation of labor or abortion, as discussed on page 150. Currently, suppositories impregnated with one of the prostaglandins when inserted vaginally give promise of initiating menstrual-like bleeding in pregnant women two to seven days beyond their menses. This would be a postconceptual type of contraceptive. Immunizing women against pregnancy is making progress, albeit slow progress. There is no contraceptive pill for the male on the horizon, though studies leading to hormonal control of male fertility are being conducted.

It is fair to conjecture that one or several methods of better contraception will be in common use within the next five years.

Contraceptive Sterilization

Sterilization as a contraceptive measure is any therapeutic procedure that permanently prevents the union of sex cells. Removal of either the ovaries or the testes would be a method of sterilization, but it is rarely done for this purpose because of its undesirable castration effects. In some instances, particularly if the uterus is diseased or if the woman is older than forty, a hysterectomy may be done to accomplish sterilization. The vast majority of sterilizations are performed simply by interrupting the pathways of the sex cells. In the male an operation on the *vas* eliminates all sperm cells from his ejaculate and in the female an operation on the tube creates a physical barrier for downward passage of the egg and upward passage of sperm. These operations interrupting the pathways of the sex cells are accomplished without removal or disturbance of the testes or of the ovaries or uterus.

I repeat, today the common sterilization operation for either men or women leaves the sex glands intact and has no effect on the secretion of hormones which physiologically determine an individual's sexual behavior. *Modern sterilization is thus not a desexing operation,* and sexual activity should not be affected. In fact, because it completely eliminates the chance of pregnancy, it may produce a more spontaneous and wholesome marital relationship in those seeking the guarantee that coitus will never again result in impregnation.

Women sometimes fear that the operation will bring on menopausal symptoms, but if the procedure simply consists of tying or severing the Fallopian tubes this will not happen. Menstruation will continue each month, the ovaries will ovulate each month, and sex hormones will continue to be secreted in normal amounts. If the uterus is removed, menstruation ceases; but if at the time of hysterectomy one or both ovaries are left behind, no change other than the absence of menstruation is likely to occur.

Legal Status

There is confusion among doctors, lawyers, and laymen on the legality of sterilization in the United States. There are no federal laws on the subject, but there are sterilization statutes in some states, most of which are concerned only with *compulsory sterilization* of feebleminded and insane inmates in mental institutions, or of recidivist sexual criminals. These so-called eugenic-sterilization laws were enacted when the science of heredity was in its infancy and were designed to prevent the transmission to succeeding generations of hereditary mental defects and antisocial behavior. In 1927 the legality of compulsory eugenic sterilization was confirmed by the United States Supreme Court in the now famous case of *Buck* vs. *Bell*. It was in this case that Justice Oliver Wendell Holmes created the memorable epigram "Three generations of imbeciles are enough." As a result of advances in the science of human genetics, enthusiasm for compulsory eugenic sterilizations has decreased significantly: in 1943, 2818 were performed and twenty years later the total was reduced to 467. Today, I believe the number is even smaller. Our concern is not with mandatory procedures, but with sterilization when it is chosen voluntarily by a couple, either to safeguard the woman's life or health, or as the preferred means of limiting family size.

With the absence of specific restraining state statutes, voluntary sterilization is legal on medical or social grounds in every state.

It is common practice not to perform sterilization unless signed permission is given beforehand by both husband and wife, or by the individual if he or she is unmarried. In the case of a minor or a mentally incompetent adult, signed permission of the nearest relative or a court order is required. Coercive sterilization, as opposed to voluntary sterilization, is illegal except in some jurisdictions on eugenic grounds or for chronic aggressive sexual offenders. For example, it is illegal, as well as unjustified, for a court to order the mother of several illegitimate children sterilized.

Medical Attitudes

Sterilization policies vary from community to community, from hospital to hospital, and from doctor to doctor. Some hospitals have staff committees which must validate each case of female sterilization since the operation is normally done as a hospital in-patient procedure while others have remitted the decision to the doctor and his patient. Then other hospitals play a number game: to comply with its rules the number of living children multiplied by the mother's age must exceed a certain number, for example, 120. If she is thirty years old, four children suffice to qualify for sterilization, but if she is twenty-nine, five children are required. For male sterilization, which usually is performed in the privacy of a doctor's office or clinic, such restrictions are unenforceable. More and more hospitals are rescinding rules about sterilization, leaving the decision to doctors and their patients who frequently request sterilizations after two or three children. Catholic hospitals do not permit sterilization operations per se, but do permit the removal of diseased tubes or ovaries, or a hysterectomy of a pathological uterus—a procedure in which sterilization is a secondary effect, a by-product as it were, rather than its primary cause.

No doctor has been judged guilty by a court for performing a contraceptive sterilization, nor has any physician received a civil judgment against him, if before the operation he has secured a properly signed consent form.

When Should Sterilization Be Considered?

Although there has been success in re-establishing fertility in some men and women who have been sterilized, the odds for such an achievement are not better than 50 per cent. Therefore it is wise to view sterilization as nonreversible. This makes the decision to be sterilized difficult—one which should be made only after consultation with a qualified physician and full discussion of its implications with one's spouse. Both husband and wife must weigh the reason for the operation against unknowns—the possibility of death of existing children, divorce and remarriage, and other unlikely occurrences which sometimes cause a man or a woman to regret having been sterilized. Because this is a decision—and a commitment—which should be taken only by the individuals concerned, I never attempt to persuade a reluctant patient to undergo the operation. The operation should be freely chosen and earnestly desired by both marital partners.

By the same token, sterilization should never be considered as a remedy for conditions with which less permanent means of birth control can equally cope. It should only be considered if the couple is positive that they have produced all the children they will ever desire and also have found other contraceptive methods onerous, objectionable, or undependable. An important indication for sterilization is a chronic physical or emotional illness which pregnancy may aggravate. It also may be highly advisable if a previous birth produced a child with serious genetic abnormality likely to recur. In some instances preventive sterilization may be in order, as in the case of a female member of a hemophiliac family about to marry. A gravely retarded child approaching reproductive age who is not institutionalized should also be evaluated as a candidate for sterilization. If the child is a subnormal female it allows her greater freedom, perhaps leading to employment away from home, since if her vulnerability should lead to ill-advised sexual relations, the catastrophic resultant of pregnancy would be avoided. At times sterilization has its place in the rehabilitative regimen of a mentally subnormal male. If the disability is serious but not severe enough to justify institutionalization, through sterilization he is protected from having the responsibility of parenthood added to his other difficulties.

Undoubtedly sterilization is most frequently done to one member of a couple which considers its present family complete and seeks permanent protection against pregnancy for the rest of the childbearing years. Most often, this is desired by mature couples in their middle or late thirties who feel that regardless of what might happen to existing children they would not wish to begin a family anew at this stage in their lives. I firmly believe in the justification of such a decision.

When a couple decides that its family is complete and sterilization is indicated, the next step is to determine which one should undergo the operation—wife or husband. This is not an easy decision; certainly it should not be based only on the fact that the operation on the male is simpler and less costly. The total family picture should be evaluated by the couple in consultation with a physician.

Incidence

There has been a sudden upsurge in the number of sterilizations performed during the past few years in the United States and England, particularly vasectomies (male). In 1970, 750,000 vasectomies and 250,000 tubectomies (female) were performed in the United States. The reason for this marked increase is comprised of many factors, perhaps the most important of which is the availability of the procedure. The medical profession has suddenly released its prohibitions against voluntary sterilization, and private practitioners, as well as clinics, throughout the United States are doing vasectomies. For example, in 1969 only one Planned Parenthood affiliate conducted a vasectomy clinic, in 1970 vasectomies were performed in ten cities by Planned Parenthood affiliates, in 1971 twenty, and no doubt the number will increase to fifty. Men and women pleased with the results inform friends and thus demand soars. Hospital rules regarding female sterilizations are being rapidly liberalized. Instead of the antique numbers game, many hospitals have eliminated their requirements and place the decision wholly in the hands of the physician and his patient. The basic philosophy toward an individual's reproductive capacity has shifted. Instead of an individual's fertility being regarded as a vested interest of State or Church it is now held to be his or hers to control as he or she deems best. The curtailment of family size through sterilization is no doubt influenced by the public's interest in ecology, pollution, and overpopulation.

Female Sterilization

For pregnancy to occur a woman must have at least one functioning ovary, one Fallopian tube open throughout its five-inch course, and a uterus. Therefore, if both ovaries are removed, or if both tubes are removed, or if the canal in each tube is interrupted so the egg cannot pass down and the sperm cannot pass up, or if the uterus is removed, a woman cannot become pregnant. All sterilization procedures are based on these basic facts.

Most procedures intended to achieve sterilization are carried out by operations on the Fallopian tubes. Tubal operations for sterilization are termed tubectomies or, more technically, salpingectomies. Sterilization may be accomplished by the total and complete removal of both tubes or by a much simpler operation which consists of interrupting the passage through the tube. Today this is usually done by the Pomeroy operation.

The Pomeroy Technique

A Pomeroy operation consists of raising a knuckle of tube in its mid-portion and placing a tie around the base of the knuckle. The portion of the tube included in the knuckle is then cut off, the tie at its base having been tightly drawn so that the severed ends of the tube are squeezed together. A catgut tie is used because it remains intact for only four or five days and unlike silk or cotton is then digested by body juices or fluids. As the tie gives way, the two severed ends of the tube spring apart, since they are under tension. The patient has no sensation from this event. If such a patient has another operation months or years later, the surgeon finds the two cut ends of the tube lying an inch or more apart, the severed ends sealed closed by scar tissue.

The Pomeroy operation is rapid and an experienced gynecologic surgeon can carry out the technical procedure involved in thirty to sixty seconds for each side. Infrequently there is failure—at a rate of 1 in 250 operations. For reasons not clearly understood, failures are more common when sterilization is carried out at the time of Cesarean section, the rate then being about 1 failure in 55. If sterilization is done immediately after vaginal delivery or while a woman is not pregnant, the failure rate is 1 in 350 operations.

The second most common method of female sterilization is removal of the uterus, hysterectomy. This is not done in younger women unless the organ is diseased. The abnormality most commonly met is fibroid tumors. If fibroid tumors are present and sterilization is to be done, it is wise to extirpate the uterus since later the removal of the fibroid-studded organ is likely to become necessary. Occasionally a history of profuse menses may lead to the removal of the uterus as the best method of sterilization.

If the uterus is removed, the tubes and ovaries ordinarily are left. Today hysterectomy usually includes removal of the cervix, which will then serve no purpose and if unremoved remains a potential source of danger. Cancer of the cervical stump occurs with the same frequency as if the uterus had not been removed, and elimination of the useless cervix prevents its occurrence.

Female sterilization can be carried out at three different periods. First and most common is puerperal sterilization—sterilization almost immediately after childbirth. One to twelve hours following delivery is the best time to carry out puerperal sterilization. The early postdelivery period is favored because the operation is technically simpler at this time; since the uterus is still greatly enlarged a small incision beneath the navel is sufficient to expose the tubes, which are high in the abdominal cavity. Furthermore, if done promptly after childbirth, the operation adds little time to a normal hospital stay.

A second period at which sterilization can be carried out is at Cesarean section. As soon as the uterus has been cut into, the baby removed, and the incision in the uterus stitched, the surgeon performs sterilization on both tubes. Occasionally, Cesarean section is combined with hysterectomy.

The third is sterilization performed on nonpregnant women, known as interval sterilization. Unless done post-delivery, sterilization is delayed until three months or more after childbirth because if done earlier there is a tendency to increased bleeding. Interval sterilization can be done either abdominally or vaginally. An incision through the vault of the vagina permits the uterus to be brought down into the operative field and the tubes can be tied by the Pomeroy technique. Vaginal hysterectomy is also an excellent interval-sterilization technique.

Puerperal sterilization is sometimes done under the anesthetic used for delivery; this is possible if spinal anesthesia has been given and the surgery can be performed before it has had time to wear off. Ordinarily, since the operation is done between one and twelve hours after delivery, the anesthetic will have worn off and a new one is administered. I prefer sodium pentothal, an intravenous anesthetic, for so simple a procedure —the operation from skin to skin (surgical jargon for from skin incision to skin closure) takes only fifteen or twenty minutes.

An interval sterilization requires a longer abdominal incision because the uterus is then a small organ deep in the pelvis and the surgeon has to insert his hand into the pelvis to bring the uterus up into the area of surgery. The skin incision can be made longitudinal or transverse, the latter sufficiently low so that the scar is obscured by the regrowth of the shaved pubic hair.

Modern surgery has progressed so remarkably that there is minimal risk and discomfort associated with sterilization. In such simple procedures, a patient is usually allowed out of bed on the day of operation or the day thereafter.

Laparoscopy and Culdoscopy

Two new and promising methods of interval sterilization have been developed. Under general anesthesia a laparoscope, a metal tube with a magnifying lens and electrical illumination at its end, is inserted through a tiny incision below the navel and above the bladder or an incision on the rim of the navel. The abdomen is then distended by carbon dioxide gas introduced through the tube which pushes the intestines aside. An excellent view of the abdominal cavity is obtained including the pelvic organs. An electrocautery is introduced through the same instrument and the mid-portion of each tube coagulated. A biopsy forceps is used to sever the tube through its coagulated portion. The same procedure can be carried out through the vault of the vagina by a similar instrument termed a culdoscope.

The advantage of sterilization by laparoscopy or culdoscopy is that either can be done as a hospital-outpatient procedure making overnight stay unnecessary. The patient comes in without breakfast and is discharged as soon as the general anesthetic has worn off. Some physicians perform culdoscopy without anesthesia, but with analgesia, pain-deadening drugs.

Reversal of Female Sterilization

Occasionally a woman who has been sterilized by a tubal operation seeks restoration of fertility. This requires an abdominal operation, excision of the scarred part of the tube and a recoupling of the two severed ends. It is delicate surgery and if possible should be undertaken by a very experienced gynecological operator. Chance for success is no greater than 50 per cent.

Male Sterilization

Vasectomy

Sterilization of the male for permanent contraception is carried out by vasectomy, which is a simple operation. Since there are two testicles the operation must be done on both sides. Vasectomy consists of blocking the duct which leads from the testicle, where sperm are manufactured, to their point of exit, the penis. Blocking is accomplished by cutting out an inch or an inch-and-a-half from the passageway, the *vas deferens.*

Vasectomy is simple surgery since no body cavity is entered; hence it carries no appreciable risk. One would venture the guess that having a tooth pulled is as risky as vasectomy. The procedure is done either in a doctor's office or in a clinic or hospital. It is ordinarily performed by either a genitourinary surgeon, a so-called G.U. man, who specializes in male reproductive and urinary problems, or by a general surgeon. Occasionally general practitioners perform vasectomy.

A local anesthetic, a cocaine derivative, is injected into the operative site to eliminate pain. Some physicians or patients prefer a general anesthetic.

A small incision, about an inch in length, is made in the upper and lateral region of the scrotum, directly over the large tube called the spermatic cord. The cord carries within it not only the much smaller duct, the *vas deferens,* but also blood vessels and nerves. The incision is extended about a quarter-inch downward from the skin until the cord is reached; then the cord itself is incised and the *vas deferens* isolated from other structures within the cord, much like isolating the largest wire in a coaxial cable. Two ligatures, frequently of silk, are tied around the *vas deferens* an inch and a half apart and the intervening portion cut out.

The skin incision is closed with one or two sutures and a dressing is applied. The man is advised to wear a suspensory to support the testicles so they don't make traction on the wound, which might be painful. The operation requires fifteen or twenty minutes, most of the time occupied in injecting the local anesthetic. If the operation is performed in the hospital, the patient is discharged twenty-four hours later. If done in the doctor's office, or in an outpatient clinic, the man is kept under observation for an hour and then is allowed to go home and advised to refrain from strenuous activity for forty-eight hours. The skin suture is usually removed five or six days after operation.

In ninety-nine cases out of a hundred, the operation is completely successful. Tying and cutting the vas deferens stops the upward progress of sperm cells from the testicles. The 1-per-cent failure is attributed to the fact that the two severed ends of the *vas* find each other and grow together again, forming a new canal. Since the seminal vesicles act as reservoirs for the sperm cells, even in successful cases, spermatozoa do not disappear immediately from the ejaculation. Therefore it is cautioned that contraception be carried out for several weeks after vasectomy, or until at least six ejaculations. It is then advisable to take a semen specimen to the physician for microscopic examination. If he finds complete absence of sperm, he will allow intercourse without contraceptives. If recanalization of the *vas* occurs, it is likely to happen within the first six months. It is therefore advisable to have a semen specimen checked approximately every six weeks during this period. After six months such precautions are no longer necessary.

This simple procedure does not change a man's coital performance. Since sperm cells make up a negligible portion of the semen, the volume of semen is not even appreciably diminished. Apart from the absence of sperm in the ejaculate, there are no other physiological effects. Sperm continue to be produced after the operation, but with their exit blocked they disintegrate and are then reabsorbed by the body.

Vasectomy should have no effect on a man's virility—except perhaps subconsciously. Some men are so fearful of impregnating their wives that the fear diminishes sexual enjoyment and enthusiasm. The fact that after vasectomy they can have intercourse without chance of impregnation may greatly revivify the sexual activity of such worriers.

Emotions can be tricky and there is the occasional man who claims that sexual activity is adversely affected by sterilization. There is no chemical or physical basis for this. Since, however, the subconscious plays such an important role in everyone's sex life, it is conceivable that the operation could have an adverse effect in individual cases. This is more likely if a man has feelings of guilt, again perhaps subconsciously, about having had vasectomy. Therefore no doctor or wife should persuade a reluctant man to be sterilized.

Reversal of Male Sterilization

Only about half the attempts to restore fertility in vasectomized men have been successful. The reversal procedure is accomplished by exposing the operative site, finding the two severed ends of the *vas*, cutting out the scarred areas, and coupling the patent portions with sutures. According to a report from India by the late Dr. G. M. Pfadke and his son, in seventy-three attempts to restore fertility after vasectomy 55 per cent were successful, pregnancies following the corrective procedure. One of the successful operations was performed fifteen years after the vasectomy.

An operation to restore fertility after vasectomy requires skillful surgical technique and the odds for success are too small to depend on. Therefore one should view vasectomy as permanent, not temporary, and the decision to have it performed should be based on certainty that no more children will be wanted, no matter what happens.

Because of the uncertainty of reversibility some men are buying fertility insurance by storing preoperative ejaculates in a semen bank at −195° centigrade. Then if they change their minds about "no parenthood," the semen is thawed and artificial insemination performed. This makes sense, but important unknowns still exist. Do all semen specimens withstand freezing equally well, and how long does frozen human semen retain its high fertilizing potential? To date we lack answers to these questions.

Experimental work is being done to perfect a 100-per-cent-reversible technique, which would further increase the popularity of male sterilization. In one project in Korea a nylon suture is threaded through an inch of the *vas* canal to obstruct it; the suture is anchored in place but can easily be withdrawn to restore fertility. In India work is progressing with a small, removable tantulum clip to compress the *vas*. In a New York clinic a tiny gold pipe with a closed screw valve is being placed in the *vas* canal experimentally. The valve can be opened later by turning a lever much like a fire hydrant. Unfortunately incision is necessary to reach the lever, so it lacks the convenience of allowing the wearer to turn it off and on himself.

Summary Figures

A 1970 representative sample in the United States shows the correlation of sterilization with the wife's age. The survey revealed that 17 per cent of all marriages had been rendered infertile by sterilization of either the husband or the wife—that is, one couple in six. In 5 per cent the husband had vasectomy, in 5 per cent the wife had had a contraceptive tubectomy, and in 7 per cent sterilization was a by-product of indicated gynecological surgery. When the wife was less than twenty years old no couple had been sterilized; with wives in the age group 20–24, 2 per cent had been sterilized; 25–29, 9 per cent; 30–34, 21 per cent; 35–39, 29 per cent; and 40–44, 33 per cent.

19

Infertility

To include a discussion of infertility in a book on pregnancy and birth may have seemed irrelevant in previous editions, but now that a thorough discussion of family planning has been added, its relevance can no longer be questioned. Moreover, I have learned that *Pregnancy and Birth* was read by many people before they married and had even contemplated pregnancy. It was particularly rewarding to hear that earlier editions of the book were recommended in many college courses. Therefore, I assume that many readers of this book have not tested their fertility. What are the prospects of an infertile marriage? How long should a couple be thwarted in their attempt to initiate pregnancy before being concerned, and how long before being seriously worried? What type of specialist should be consulted and how does one locate a competent doctor in the field of infertility? What tests are performed to diagnose the cause, or causes, of an infertile mating? If such and such an abnormality is found, what treatment should be tried? It is hoped that this discussion will answer these and other questions.

The Chances of an Infertile Marriage

It has been estimated that about one in ten married couples in the United States are unable to have a child. There seem to be no inherent social, economic, or racial group differences affecting the ability or inability to create a baby. Existing group differences in family size are probably dependent upon the employment or lack of employment of contraception. Years ago it was believed that the smaller families of professional and white-collar workers compared to blue-collar workers and laborers were occupational. I assume the greater use of the brain was supposed to syphon off some mysterious fertility prowess from areas below the waist. Research has shown that couples with more money or education than average resort more frequently to measures for both limiting family size and deferment of the first pregnancy. Studies have proved that medically sanctioned methods of birth control do not cause the slightest impairment of fertility subsequent to their use, except for the infrequent case (1 per cent) in which normal menses are not resumed for six months or longer after stopping the birth-control pill. The prolonged use of contraception, however, may postpone attempts at conception beyond the age of highest fertility.

Effect of Age and Coital Frequency on Conception

As previously stated in this book, youth is the greatest ally of successful reproduction. Two studies to determine the percentage of childless unions were made of couples who used no birth control in marriage but married at different ages, one sample from the province of Quebec and the other from England and Wales. When the women married before age 20, 4 per cent remained childless; 20–24, 6 per cent; 25–29, 10 per cent; and 30–34, 16 per cent. Other studies differently constructed show little decline in the fertility of the woman before age 30, but declining fertility thereafter.

Little attention has been paid to the relationship of a man's age to his fertility, perhaps because it is difficult to separate the age factor of the man from his wife's since their ages are usually closely correlated. However, MacLeod has reported on the relationship of the husband's age and his ability to cause his wife to conceive in six months or less. Of men less than 25 years old, 75 per cent impregnated their wives in six months or less; 25–29, 48 per cent; 30–35, 38 per cent; 35–39, 26 per cent; and 40 and over, 23 per cent.

The only other general factor in addition to age which seems to influence fertility is frequency of intercourse. As a rule, couples having sexual intercourse four times and over per week are far more likely to achieve pregnancy in less than six months than couples practicing coitus once or less often per week. Since coital frequency is correlated to age, perhaps these two modifying factors of fertility are in large part one and the same.

Usual Time Required to Initiate Pregnancy

Of 5574 couples whom we studied who achieved pregnancy, one-third succeeded the first month, and more than half within the first three months. Fifteen per cent required four to six months; 13 per cent, seven to twelve months; and 8 per cent, one to two years. More than 6 per cent of those who eventually had a baby took more than two years to initiate pregnancy. The median time, or most usual time required, was about two and one-half months.

When to Seek Medical Help

I feel that young couples—those in which husband and wife are less than thirty-five—should wait a full year before consulting a physician. On the other hand, if either is above thirty-five, they should see a doctor after six months of unsuccessful attempts.

Whom Should One Consult?

The choice of the doctor is important. Treatment of infertility is a relatively new and complicated field, and many family doctors have not had the training to manage it. However, the family doctor can refer the problem to the specialist of his choice or to a clinic. Most infertility specialists are members of The American Fertility Society; names of members in a specific geographic area can be obtained by writing to the Office of the Director, Dr. Herbert H. Thomas, 1801 Ninth Avenue South, Suite 101, Birmingham, Alabama 35205. Then too, a first-rate local hospital, especially a teaching hospital, can refer an inquiring couple to qualified members of its staff. Furthermore, there are fertility clinics in many cities of the United States. If you are unable to locate such a clinic in your community, write for help to the Planned Parenthood Federation of America, 810 Seventh Avenue, New York City 10019. In the New York area, the world-famous Margaret Sanger Research Bureau, 17 West 16th Street, is available for consultation.

The Physician's Examination

The physician will first examine both partners in an infertile marriage for their general health. Sound health enhances fertility. I recall two men who were partners in sterile marriages who came to me for help. One suffered from unsuspected leukemia, and the other from undetected diabetes. After appropriate treatment the diabetic fathered children. Sometimes the fertility level of one or both members of a childless couple can be elevated to the point at which pregnancy will occur by improving nutrition, possibly for weight loss or gain, by correcting anemia, by changing conditions that may be causing fatigue, or by adjusting glandular disturbances. Relieving nervous tension by taking a relaxing vacation or simply through the feeling of confidence engendered by a sympathetic, knowledgeable physician or a clinic may work miracles for the childless.

The Medical Record

A second step is the compilation of a medical history of both husband and wife by interviews with each. Many facts may be relevant. For example, involvement of the testicles as a complication of mumps in the male may offer a clue. Among women, previous abdominal surgery sometimes leaves scar tissue which may create an obstacle. As mentioned earlier, gonorrhea, if not promptly treated in either sex, may create similar difficulties.

The doctor will seek to learn, ordinarily in separate talks with husband and wife, about the couple's sex knowledge and sexual activity: what is the frequency of intercourse and if the couple can pinpoint the most fertile portion of the month in the wife's cycle for intercourse. Does the wife find intercourse painful or unpleasant, and does she get up to douche, wash, or void immediately after relations? Then, some couples use certain kinds of lubricants, such as Vaseline, which may injure sperm cells and reduce the likelihood of conception.

Tests for Husbands

After gathering the pertinent historical data, the specialist proceeds with a series of tests. He usually starts by examining the sperm content of the husband's semen. The specimen is collected directly into a wide-necked, dry, clean bottle or jar, and the man must be very careful none is lost, as the first few drops of the ejaculation contain the bulk of the sperm cells. If the first few drops are lost, a normal specimen may test as defective. It can be collected at home either by masturbation or withdrawal, and taken within a few hours to the doctor's office, where it is tested to determine whether it meets certain requirements. To be normal it must be about a teaspoon in quantity and have a sticky, but not a ropy, consistency, and under the microscope there must be 60 or more million sperm cells per cubic centimeter, of which 80 per cent must show a progressive type of swimming movement in the seminal fluid. Then, too, at least three-fourths of the cells must appear normal in form when stained and studied.

If the first specimen tests below normal, it is likely additional specimens will be checked. If the results are consistently deficient but still not so woefully deficient that improvement by therapy is impossible, the physician will suggest treatment. His efforts include measures aimed at improving general health: better diet, physical exercise, or sports, etc. If a glandular deficiency is found—for example, in the thyroid gland—corrective medication can be given. Unfortunately, to date, the various pituitary-hormone injections have proved very disappointing.

If sperm cells are completely absent from the semen specimen, two possibilities present themselves. Either no spermatozoa are being produced in the two testicles, or they are being produced but their egress through the penis is blocked so that they cannot appear in the ejaculation. Such blockage usually occurs in the tiny tubules of the epididymis, where the testicle joins the vas deferens, the conducting tube which conveys the sperm cells upward. A biopsy, the removal of a fragment of tissue from the testicle for microscopic study, will determine whether the absence of spermatozoa is due to failure of their formation or to blockage. If sperm cells are being formed, a bypass operation around the point of blockage is successful in about one-third of the cases.

Occasionally, surgical elimination of a hydrocele, a cystlike collection of fluid outside the testicle, improves poor semen, as may ligation of large varicose veins of the scrotal sac. Close-fitting jockey-shorts, which may raise the intrascrotal temperature, should be abandoned in infertility cases.

Tests for the Wife

There are several requirements for fertility in the wife: normal ovulation (egg production); proper functioning of the tube for picking up the egg; unobstructed passage through the tube for the ascent of spermatozoa and descent into the uterus of the fertilized egg cell; and implantation of the early conception into the lining of the uterus, specifically prepared by naturally occurring hormones.

The occurrence of ovulation can be determined by several tests. One is the relatively simple method of taking and recording the temperature daily under standard basal conditions—called the basal body temperature, BBT. Though referred to in a previous chapter, we repeat it here for the reader's convenience. The temperature is taken each morning, immediately on awakening, before the slightest activity, and recorded throughout the month on a piece of graph paper. The BBT is relatively low during menstruation and for a week or so thereafter. Then it rises five- to eight-tenths of a degree, either in one jump or in steps over two or three days, and remains elevated at this new level until twenty-four hours before the next period. Such a sustained temperature rise during the second half of the menstrual cycle is proof of ovulation. If the BBT is constantly erratic, with no clear-cut period of relatively low temperature during the first half of the cycle and of higher temperature in the second half of the cycle, one can assume ovulation did not occur that month.

Another test for ovulation involves an endometrial biopsy in which minute pieces of the uterine lining are removed, with virtually no discomfort, just prior to menstruation or during the first twelve hours of the flow. These fragments are studied microscopically; if ovulation has occurred that month, the resulting corpus luteum will cause the tissue to show a so-called "secretory pattern," which is the body's preparation for the reception and implantation of an egg. If ovulation does not occur and therefore no corpus luteum is formed, the uterus omits this chapter of its story and characteristic secretory changes are absent.

Other tests less often used to detect ovulation are frequent examinations of the mucus of the cervix to determine whether during mid-cycle it goes through a "watery" phase, and observation of daily vaginal smears to seek for "cornified" or mature cells, which are found only during a month in which ovulation takes place. Still another way is to identify chemically the presence of the substance pregnanediol secreted by the corpus luteum through the laboratory analysis of twenty-four-hour collections of urine.

If examination of the biopsy specimen shows a secretory lining, but of poor quality, taking progestin hormones in the latter half of the cycle is said by some authorities to increase the secretory state sufficiently to support normal implantation of the fertilized egg.

When ovulation is proved consistently absent for several months, your physician will treat you with clomiphene or human pituitary gonadotropin (Pergonal). The latter is either extracted from pituitary glands collected at autopsies or from the urine of women past the menopause. Clomiphene is given in daily doses of 50 mg for five days and, if unsuccessful, a second course doubling the dose is given six weeks later. A favorable response is monitored by checking the BBT for a rise of 0.5 to 1.0 Fahrenheit. Seventy per cent of nonovulators ovulate with clomiphene therapy, and 30 per cent become pregnant. Treatment with human pituitary gonadotropin is preceded by another hormone, chorionic gonadotropin. This double therapy is followed by a 50-per-cent conception rate. Both treatments lead to a much higher incidence of multiple births than normal. Ten to 16 per cent of ovulation-induced pregnancies, according to different reports, have more than one fetus, the maximum number reported being eight. Each fetus comes from a separately ruptured Graafian follicle and a separate ovum, so the infants are fraternal, not identical. The current epidemic of quadruplets, quin-tuplets, etc., is the result of the ovulatory drugs, a kind of overcorrection.

Occasionally, failure to ovulate after drug therapy, particularly when menstruation is also absent, is associated with a thickening of the normal membrane on the outer surface of the ovaries and can be cured in properly selected cases by surgery. This condition is known as the Stein-Leventhal Syndrome.

The underactivity or overactivity of the thyroid gland may be associated with infertility, sometimes of ovarian origin. A basal-metabolism test or determination of the PBI (protein-bound iodine) can be used to assay accurately thyroid function. The patient with abnormal thyroid function can be rendered euthyroid (neither high nor low) by appropriate drugs.

Tests and Treatments for Blockage of the Tubes

If tests indicate normal ovulation, the next step is to determine whether the ovum is being blocked in the tube during its passage downward from ovary to uterus, and sperm cells in their journey upward. Fallopian tubes which have no obstruction in their four- or five-inch length are termed "patent." Patency, or lack of patency, is demonstrated either by the Rubin test or by hysterosalpingography.

Rubin Test

The Rubin test (named after its originator, the late Dr. I. C. Rubin, my mentor several decades ago at the Mount Sinai Hospital), or insufflation test, introduces the gas carbon dioxide into the uterus under pressure. When there is a clear passage from the uterus through the tubes into the abdominal cavity, the gas escapes freely into the relatively large and capacious abdomen from whence it is rapidly absorbed. If both tubes are closed, the gas cannot pass upward into the abdominal cavity and the pressure quickly builds up because it is being introduced into a small closed system from which it cannot escape. The physician, observing the pressure recorded on a gauge, can thus determine the absence or presence of tubal blockage of the gas. Blockage does not necessarily mean that both tubes are closed, since a temporary muscle spasm of the tubes may occur and produce, in effect, a false result. The expert physician will generally make this test several times during various phases of the cycle before concluding that the tubes are truly sealed closed by scarring, adhesions, or some congenital defect.

Often the Rubin test itself corrects a minor blockage, perhaps by straightening out a kink, destroying minor adhesions, or dislodging a thick plug of mucus, and thus may be therapeutic as well as diagnostic.

Hysterosalpingography

The name of this second test for tubal patency is derived from three Greek words meaning uterus-tube-picture. A radio-opaque fluid, instead of a gas, is injected into the uterus, and an X-ray picture is then taken of the lowermost portion of the abdomen. If the tubes are open, the fluid flows freely out into the abdomen; if they are obstructed, the picture shows the point of blockage. Hysterosalpingography, like the Rubin test, occasionally has curative value, since the fluid injected may correct a minor tubal obstruction.

With modern X-ray equipment, the amount of radiation delivered to the target area is minimal and virtually without danger to the ovaries. The test is usually performed a day or two after the cessation of the menses, in order to avoid radiation of a newly fertilized egg or the dislodgement by the injected fluid of an egg in the process of implanting.

If the tubes are proved nonpatent, surgical correction may be possible in cases appearing favorable for such a procedure on X-ray. Plastic surgery may release adhesions or bypass an obstructed area. Sometimes closed fimbria at the ovarian end of the tube may be teased open, or, if not, the fimbriated end can be amputated and an open tube restored.

Hysterosalpingography can reveal only the approximate state of closed tubes. "A look and see" through a small, surgical abdominal incision or by culdoscopy will reveal the exact situation. Culdoscopy consists of inserting a periscope-like, lighted, visual apparatus through the vagina into the pelvic cavity. The patient is given analgesic drugs and placed in the knee-chest position. She lies on her stomach, shoulders resting on the table; the knees are then drawn up toward the breasts with the buttocks pointing skyward. The apex of the vagina is pierced by a large-caliber, hollow metal tube allowing air to enter the abdomen which pushes the intestines away. The culdoscope is then inserted. An operator experienced in the use of the culdoscope can see the pelvic organs perfectly. Culdoscopy is usually a hospital procedure. If findings on culdoscopy indicate the wisdom of performing an operation, it is usually not done through the culdoscope, but through an abdominal incision under anesthesia. Some gynecologists prefer to use the laparoscope to view the pelvic organs. Laparoscopy was discussed earlier, in the section on tubal sterilization. It is normally performed in a hospital under general anesthesia.

The P.C. Test

The initials stand for post-coital (after intercourse); the test is also frequently referred to as the Sims-Hühner, named after the two physicians who popularized its use. For even if normal ovulation occurs and the tubes are proved patent, pregnancy cannot result unless the husband's sperm cells can make the four- or five-inch journey to the trysting site, the mid-portion of the tube, where fertilization takes place. Since conditions in the woman may prevent passage of the sperm, the physician checks this possibility. The woman comes to the doctor's office shortly after intercourse without use of contraception. Samples of fluid from the vagina and mucus from high up in the cervix are aspirated into separate glass tubes and examined under the microscope. Live, motile sperm cells in the vaginal sample are not highly significant, but they should be plentiful and actively moving in the sample of cervical mucus. Because the ability of spermatozoa to penetrate cervical mucus and enter the cervical canal varies in different phases of the menstrual cycle, p.c. tests are usually made about two weeks before the next expected period when the mucus is at its optimum for sperm penetration. If only dead sperm cells are found in the cervical mucus on repeated tests, it is likely that the woman's cervical secretions are hostile to the man's sperm cells. Treatment with antibiotics and hormones may alter this unfriendly situation. The possibility that such immobilization of sperm cells may be due to complicated immune reactions is being studied.

Then, too, an abnormal anatomic position of the cervix—the fact that it points too far forward or too far back—may decrease the likelihood of impregnation. Varying position during intercourse, the man below or behind, may change a negative to a positive p.c. test. If not, some surgical procedure, such as the abdominal suspension of a markedly fixed, tipped-back uterus may be indicated.

Surgery as Applied to Infertility

In the Male

1. Very infrequently the urethra, the excretory tube leading through the penis, has an opening at the base of the penis instead of its tip (hypospadias) and therefore the semen is delivered externally. A plastic-surgical procedure will close the defect, allowing the semen to exit from the tip of the penis.

2. Bypassing an obstructed epididymis is sometimes surgically feasible, a procedure termed epididymovasostomy.

3. If the testicles are retained in the abdomen, either hormonal or surgical correction must be carried out before puberty, as described on page 11.

4. If a male with a poor semen specimen has a hydrocele or large scrotal varicose veins, either of these two conditions is usually eliminated surgically.

5. If the man has been sterilized by vasectomy (a tie or ligature placed around the *vas deferens* on each side and a small segment removed) the procedure can be undone surgically in about 50 per cent of the cases.

In the Female

1. Attempts to restore patency of the Fallopian tubes are successful in 50 per cent of the cases if only adhesions are responsible, but in only 10 to 15 per cent of the cases if the tubes are scarred closed from disease.

2. Surgical removal of fibroid tumors of the uterus, if they are deemed responsible for failure to conceive or repeated miscarriage, yields a high success rate in cases favorable in all other respects.

3. Surgical correction of a congenitally malformed uterus. This may involve combining two small uteri, as found in the occasional patient, into a single organ, or the elimination of a partition which either completely or partially divides the uterus into two chambers. Success rate high.

4. An operation to constrict the point of union between the uppermost portion of the cervix and the lowermost portion of the uterus. From 60 to 70 per cent of patients who have had repeated late miscarriages (eighteen to twenty-six weeks) are enabled by this type of surgery to carry the baby to eight or nine months. This was discussed in the chapter on spontaneous abortion.

5. If the capsule of the ovary is thickened and neither ovulation nor menstruation occurs, either peeling the ovary or splitting it to remove a central wedge of tissue and then sewing the split halves together causes ovulation in most cases. This is not done until trial has first been made with the two ovulatory drugs, clomiphene and Pergonal, and they have failed to produce ovulation.

6. If the woman has been sterilized by a tube-tying operation (neither uterus nor tubes removed) she has 50 per cent likelihood of having her fertility restored.

7. Suspending a uterus which is tipped back in a fixed position. Rarely indicated, success unpredictable.

Psychological Factors

It is very difficult to assess accurately the importance of mental and emotional factors in infertile matings. Of course, sometimes they are obvious. For example, if the husband is either incapable of maintaining a firm erection or ejaculating, or if conscious or subconscious factors cause the vagina to clamp closed at the time of attempted intercourse so that it is too painful for the wife to permit entry. Such difficulties with intercourse are almost never physical. Obviously, these are serious problems because they prevent not only pregnancy but also satisfactory marital relations. In such situations an experienced gynecologist should be consulted and if he feels the problem is outside his competence he is likely to refer the couple to a team of experts in this complex area. Dr. William Masters and Dr. Virginia Johnson in St. Louis pioneered the field and have described the therapeutic regimen and results in their book *Sexual Inadequacy*. Many teams of therapists have been trained by Masters and Johnson and now practice in other parts of the country.

How often mental and emotional factors are responsible for barrenness when sexual intercourse is normal and all tests in husband and wife are negative is a question that cannot be answered categorically. It seems to happen. Everyone who has written on infertility points out the fact that long-standing cases are cured when the husband and wife cross the threshold of a well-known specialist or a highly regarded clinic. Pregnancy often occurs even before routine tests are completed and advice is given. Since pregnancy is not contagious, the only influence at work under such conditions is thought to be a reduction in tension through replacement of anxiety by confidence. The supposed association between child adoption, in cases in which all hope of having one's own child is given up, and the prompt occurrence of pregnancy is similarly explained—reduction in tension and anxiety. Perhaps relief of psychic factors explains some cases, but the matter of coincidence or happenstance should at least share the credit.

Many physicians feel so strongly that psychic infertility is a real entity that they refer patients to psychiatrists routinely when other forms of infertility treatment have failed.

Artificial Insemination

If the wife has been found apparently fertile and her husband irremediably sterile, or if delivery or reception of the husband's fertile-appearing sperm cells is impossible through intercourse, conception may still occur through artificial insemination, sometimes called therapeutic insemination. The lay press refers to a child conceived by artificial insemination as a "test-tube baby" for reasons unclear, since ordinarily no test tube is used in the procedure.

There are two types of artificial insemination: homologous, when the husband is the semen donor (A.I.H.) and heterologous, when the semen is donated by someone else (A.I.D.). A.I.H. is only performed if intercourse is impossible, if the husband suffers from uncorrected hypospadias, or if his semen is subnormal, and it is thought that giving the sperm cells a two-inch boost on their five-inch journey might accomplish fertilization. Occasionally, A.I.H. is done if the mucus in the woman's cervix seems ill suited to act as a ladder for ascending sperm cells.

Donor insemination, sometimes referred to as semi-adoption, offers potential advantages to actual adoption. The wife and husband have all the experiences of pregnancy and delivery. Then, too, genetically the child is at least half theirs.

Very infrequently, A.I.D. is performed for a reason other than substituting fertile semen for the husband's sterile seed. This reason is genetic. For example, if the woman is Rh negative, the husband Rh positive, and the woman so highly sensitized that a live child is impossible, then by using A.I.D. from an Rh-negative donor, a normal pregnancy results. Occasionally, if husband and wife each have a recessive genetic defect that has expressed itself by a particular abnormality in their child, the substitution of another biological father by A.I.D. virtually eliminates the likelihood of such a defect. It is impossible to say how many births occur each year in the United States as the result of donor insemination but a fair guesstimate is seven to ten thousand.

Donor insemination is not morally acceptable to all and was officially condemned by the Catholic Church by Pope Leo XIII (in 1897). Pius XII in 1951 also condemned artificial insemination from the husband. There are few pronouncements concerning artificial insemination by United States Protestant groups. In 1962 the Presbyterian Church bestowed its sanction. Orthodox Judaism forbids donor insemination, but if a couple transgresses their prohibition the resulting child has been ruled legitimate. Conservative Judaism has taken an ambiguous position and liberal Judaism has voiced forceful approval.

The legal status of a child conceived by donor insemination has not been clearly defined by the courts. Some legal minds think it is legitimate; while others have doubts. However, two state legislatures, Georgia in 1964 and Oklahoma in 1967, have passed statutes legitimizing children conceived through donor insemination, "if both husband and wife consent in writing to the use and administration of artificial insemination." It is high time other legislatures took similar action. Donor insemination should not be undertaken without serious, mature consideration by the couple in consultation with the doctor. It may be a splendid technique for couple "A" and ill advised for couple "B."

Should donor insemination be decided upon, the choice of the donor is of prime importance. Many doctors use semen from married house officers and medical students of known good heredity who, in addition to having normal semen, have proved their fertility by fathering their own children. Usually a donor is chosen for his similar body build and coloring to those of the husband. His blood Rh must also be in agreement with the recipient's.

To forestall any possible emotional complications the donor and recipient never know each other's identity. This is known only by the physician.

The physician selects the most fertile day or days of the cycle for the insemination on the basis of the woman's menstrual history, BBT chart, etc. If fresh semen is to be used the donor ejaculates the semen specimen directly into a bottle and the physician either calls for it, or it is delivered to his office. Within an hour, the recipient comes to the office, and by means of a glass syringe and metal cannula, the donated semen is deposited within and around the cervix. It is becoming increasingly common for the physician to buy donor semen from a sperm bank where it is stored at —195° C. The chief argument in favor of using frozen semen is the greater convenience—no prearrangements for collection have to be made. The frozen ampoule is thawed in a beaker of water at room temperature which requires less than half an hour. The rate of success appears to be the same for frozen and fresh semen, if the donor's ejaculate tolerates freezing well. I feel that fresh semen has the advantage that the physician has an opportunity to choose a donor with physical characteristics close to those of the legal father.

From one to three inseminations are carried out in one month, depending on the doctor's and the patient's preference. The greater the number of inseminations per month, the higher the likelihood for pregnancy. The rate of success in 690 cases of donor insemination, published by seven different clinicians, varied from 55 to 78 per cent, the average being 69 per cent. In my experience 80 per cent of my successful cases occurred during the first two months, using three inseminations per month, and 90 per cent during the first four months. Fetal results from donor-conceived pregnancies do not differ from normal pregnancies. A few studies report a disproportionately high number of males. Not infrequently couples return after successful A.I.D. for a second or third child. In my practice the record is four.

The semen is bought from the donor on a wholly impersonal basis, in the same way blood is purchased for transfusion.

There is a division in the medical profession concerning signed consents. Most physicians require the signature of the patient and her husband to a consent form. Some even require such papers from the donor and his wife. I belong to the minority requiring no signatures, because I feel such formal procedures tend to fix the procedure in the minds of the participants. I want it quickly forgotten, so that the couple have difficulty in remembering that the legal father is not the biological father. I pick my cases carefully and by no means consent to artificial donor insemination for all who request it. I try to make sure that there is equal enthusiasm for the treatment by husband and wife and that they have seriously considered all potential pitfalls. I also attempt to ascertain if the marriage is stable.

Finally let me point out that artificial insemination is no magical cure for all types of infertility. If the male has normal semen and the couple is capable of normal coitus, artificial insemination from the husband or a donor is rarely indicated.

A Message to the Infertile

If you are one of those luckless couples unsuccessfully trying to have a baby for a year or longer, what are your chances? A decade or two ago,

I would have said that if you seek expert medical counsel and help, your chance of having your baby is 25 per cent. Today I can say at least 33 per cent and more likely 40 per cent. Perhaps a decade hence the chances will rise to 50 per cent.

Above all, do not feel guilty or blame your mate if the news is bad and one of you is irremediably sterile. This is the way the dice fall. It's luck, just bad luck, not faulty management. Face up to your fate, and either adopt a child or remake your life and your point of view so that the two of you can live happily and fully without one. You have things in life—perhaps the love and respect you and your mate feel for each other—that other couples, though blessed with children, may lack.

20

The Newborn Baby

Stand back in the shadows of a hospital corridor and spy upon the first meeting between a baby and his family. The blanket is carefully peeled back, and for the first time the child and family meet. The grandmothers loyally out-coo each other, with "My, what a darling; it has the cute Smith nose. See the little Jones ears." The father, who may have seen his heir for one blurred moment in the recovery room or in one of the corridors, is speechless—not with pride but with anxiety. He has seen advertisements with new babies in them. They were beautiful—but this! In silent apprehension he waits for the doctor and takes him aside. "Frankly, Doctor, what's wrong with my baby? That's the funniest-looking thing I ever saw. Why, his head comes up to a point like an egg. When he cries, his face is all cockeyed, and his nose looks as though Muhammad Ali had taken a poke at it."

The doctor brusquely reassures him. "Perfectly normal! He'll be all right. Don't worry, just a case of primiparous molding with a slight paralysis of the facial nerve. Pressure by the forceps, you know. Oh, the nose! Many of them have that queer appearance at birth. Fortunately all babies improve." Off he goes. The dazed father retreats to an armchair to think and worry, worry and think.

In the next several pages I have attempted to answer some of the questions about the new baby which people would like to ask their doctor but do not for fear that they would sound silly to the busy man. This chapter is in no way intended to act as a guide in baby care after you leave the hospital. There are several excellent books written by highly competent pediatricians which cover this field with distinction, some very moderately priced.

The Molding Head

Molding of the fetal head was discussed in the chapter on "Difficult Labor." Let me restate the fact that it is a perfectly normal, harmless, process, most pronounced in first births. The heads of infants presenting by the breech, or delivered by Cesarean section before labor begins, do not have the opportunity to undergo molding, and are therefore rounded and normal in appearance. The egg-shaped, molded head rounds spontaneously within three or four days.

Swelling beneath the Scalp

In addition to distortion in shape of the head, the child is frequently born with a thick, softish swelling of that portion of the scalp which fitted into the aperture of the cervix when the latter was partially dilated. This swelling, termed caput (Latin: "head"), disappears spontaneously within a few days. Occasionally after spontaneous births, but more frequently after difficult operative deliveries, there may be a different type of swelling beneath the scalp; in this case a blood clot (cephalhematoma) accumulates between the bone and the attached membrane covering it. Usually a cephalhematoma does not appear for from twelve to twenty-four hours after delivery. It may continue to enlarge for a few days, then remains constant for several weeks, and eventually begins to disappear. A thin layer of new bone grows out from the edges of the fluidlike bump, compressing the clot between it and the old bone beneath. In the end it is merely an inconspicuous irregularity of the head, and when I sit in the balcony at a theater I fancy I can sort out the baldheaded men beneath who had cephalhematomas several decades ago. (May I point out that I have not attempted to prove or disprove this theory.) The clot, being external, outside the bone, of course cannot damage the brain.

The Nose

Since the baby usually faces back toward the mother's curved sacrum, it sort of skids out on its nose. At this period the nose is formed of malleable cartilage, the result being that any close resemblance between the nose at birth and the nose a week or two later is largely accidental.

Facial Palsy

The facial nerve, the nerve which innervates the muscles of expression, makes its exit from the brain on each side at the base of the skull, just below the ear. Not uncommonly one of the forceps blades makes pressure over it, causing temporary paralysis of the muscles it supplies. The infant is unable to close the eye on the affected side, and the paralyzed muscles of the mouth are pulled over toward the normal side, making the face look alarmingly askew. I have never seen a case which did not clear up completely; many within the first twenty-four hours.

Hemorrhage in the White of the Eye

Children are sometimes born with hemorrhages in the white of the eye; these clear up in about ten days. It is not unusual for a child to develop a pussy secretion in one or both eyes within the first twenty-four hours if silver nitrate was instilled in the eye as prophylaxis against gonococcus infection. It does not portend a cold or infection, but is the result of the chemical irritation which silver nitrate often sets up. Within a day or two the condition disappears without treatment. If penicillin ointment is instilled in the eyes for prophylaxis against the gonococcus this type of irritation is unlikely to occur.

Eye Color, Cross-Eyedness, Tears

The eye structure of the newborn is not completely matured. In the first place, the color is not fixed. Most children are born with a gray-blue or transparent liquid blue iris (the colored portion of the eye). The former type of iris usually begins to fleck with brown around the third month and gradually develops into a hazel or dark eye, while in babies destined to be blue-eyed the original blue shade is retained. Secondly, new babies are unable to focus the eyes properly; this causes them all to appear cross-eyed, but the vast majority are not. The ability to focus the eyes is gradually acquired, and the infant can progressively maintain a steady gaze for periods of increasing length. If by the end of the first year there is no marked improvement in eye coordination, an eye specialist should be consulted. A third difference between the eyes at birth and the same eyes a few months later is the presence of tears. No matter how lustily the newborn squalls, his cheeks remain dry. The first tears arrive when the child is about three months old, and from then on for several years there is rarely a dry day.

Ability to See and Hear at Birth

The question is frequently asked whether the infant sees at birth. The answer is, yes—at least it discriminates between light and darkness. This can be determined by flashing a light into its eyes. The pupils promptly contract, and when the light is removed they dilate. Furthermore, some infants follow a bright light when they are a day or two old, while others do not acquire this ability for a few weeks. There is no question that an infant hears almost immediately. He may appear deaf for a day or two, but soon demonstrates a "startle reaction" at a sudden loud noise such as the slamming of a door.

Retrolental Fibroplasia

This formidable name denotes what was a formidable disease. Beginning about twenty years ago, it was observed that 10 to 15 per cent of very small premature infants developed at the age of about a month a tragic eye condition involving the retina, which led to either complete or partial blindness. The conundrum was: why did this new disease suddenly appear? Some thought it was a new kind of viral infection; others thought it was due to some therapeutic agent newly given to these prematures, such as iron; and still others postulated a lack of a vitamin because of alterations in formulae—namely, vitamin E. Despite all the theories, the baffling curse continued to exact its cruel toll, and institutes for the blind are peopled with its victims. Within the past two decades the cause has been found; the villain, man's unsuspected benefactor, oxygen. It has been demonstrated without question that protracted exposure to oxygen concentration above 40 per cent will produce the lesion in newborn experimental animals. In addition, if the smallest human premature is given oxygen in a concentration less than 40 per cent it does not develop retrolental fibroplasia. To make safety doubly safe, in most premature nurseries they usually wean even tiny babies completely from supplemental oxygen within the first forty-eight to seventy-two hours by gradually diminishing the concentration from under 40 per cent to 0.

With the institution of these precautions, retrolental disease has become a completed and dramatic chapter in the history of medicine.

Sneezing, Hiccuping, and Snorting

Newborn babies sneeze at the least provocation or without any provocation, so that even a series of sneezes does not mean that the child has caught cold. As a matter of fact, it is almost unheard-of for a baby less than two weeks old to catch cold.

The hiccuping mechanism seems just as sensitive as the sneezing apparatus, and the hiccup is quite as benign. The infant may snort, grunt, and wheeze in a most disturbing fashion while it sleeps. This is due to a dropping back of the lower jaw, which places the tongue against the roof of the mouth, thus narrowing the airway. It is of no moment.

Skin

The skin of the newborn is marvelously sensitive, so that minor lesions are common.

Prickly heat due to overactivity of the sweat glands causes clusters of minute pink pimples surrounded by areas of pink skin. The application of calamine lotion or a weak solution of bicarbonate of soda, a bland powder, and—this should be especially emphasized—lighter clothes and covers, promptly cures the condition. There still seems to be a belief that a new infant must be kept very warm with layers of woolen clothing and several blankets. This is true only for premature infants, and the required temperature is provided them by heated incubator-cribs in which most small "premies" lie as naked as a jay bird, except for a diaper, while enjoying Florida warmth even in the winter.

A rash limited to the area covered by the diaper, called diaper rash, is quite common, and it usually means poor diaper hygiene. One of two things commonly causes it: either the soap in which the diapers have been rinsed is too strong, or the diapers have not been boiled long enough to kill the bacteria. If bacteria are present, they free ammonia from the urine, which irritates the skin. Stricter attention to the washing of the diapers and temporarily greasing the skin of the affected area with cold cream produce a prompt cure. The diaper should be changed only at each feeding, unless it is obviously soiled by a stool or dripping wet. Changing it more often disturbs the child.

The susceptibility of the baby's skin to infection at this time makes it obligatory that all nursery linen and clothes be sterilized. For the same reason, the attendants have to wash their hands carefully before touching each child. The most common of these skin infections is impetigo, which takes the form of little isolated, pea-sized blisters, each surrounded by a narrow red ring, occurring as early as the second or third day. When the blister is broken, a moist or dry red scab forms. The lesions appear in crops. Today the condition is most successfully treated with an antibiotic by mouth or injection. Since the condition spreads, if your child develops impetigo he may be banished to the isolation nursery.

Small strawberry marks are quite common on the forehead, above the bridge of the nose, on the upper lids, and on the nape of the neck. These pale in the course of months, and many disappear entirely; if they do not, the expert application of radium makes them fade away with the magic of Aladdin's lamp.

Fingernails

The nails of a small infant should be kept pared to prevent it from scratching its face with the purposeless, uncontrolled movements of its hands.

Thrush

Thrush, a fungous infection, coats the inside of the mouth with a white film resembling curdled milk, which can be peeled off, leaving a few bleeding points and an inflamed area. The infection causes no particular difficulty except in infants already in poor health. A ready cure is effected by swabbing the inside of the mouth three or four times with Mycostatin, an antibiotic specific for the causative fungus, *Candida albicans*.

Temporary Breast Enlargement

It is not unusual for the breasts of both boys and girls to enlarge on the third or fourth day of life. This is due to hormones received from the mother during intrauterine existence; these hormones had no effect at that time because they were neutralized by chemicals secreted by the placenta. Usually the enlargement begins to wane in a few days and is gone by the eighth or ninth day. No massage, ointments, ice, or any other treatment is necessary; in fact treatments do more harm than good. Sometimes the growth of breast tissue is so marked that a little secretion can be expressed from the nipple. This is called witch's milk, and during the medieval period it was accredited with miraculous healing properties. Infrequently one or both breasts become very red and tender. On two occasions I have seen abscesses form which cleared up a few days after incision.

Changes in Sex Organs

Female infants occasionally have a little bloody vaginal discharge toward the end of the first week. It is a form of menstruation, also hormonal in origin, which is of no significance and disappears, not to return until pubescence is reached.

In infants which present as frank breeches, buttocks first, marked swelling and discoloration of the scrotum and penis in the male and of the labia in the female may occur during labor and persist for a few days thereafter. Everything clears up without permanent damage.

Circumcision

Circumcision (Latin: "Around" + "cut"), the cutting off of the prepuce or foreskin, is probably the oldest surgical operation extant, except for omphalotomy, the severance of the navel cord. Some of the earliest Egyptian sculpture depict circumcisions. The operation was and still is practiced as a religious rite or tribal custom by peoples scattered all over the world. In some peoples it is practiced as a birth rite, in others as an adolescent ceremony, while in others it is reserved as a premarital ritual to be performed when the individual reaches sexual maturity. In such instances usually both sexes are circumcised; in the female the prepuce or fold of skin surrounding the clitoris is removed. Finally it is practiced by some upon old men as a rite of senescence.

Our chief concern is not its history but its present place in medicine. There are two distinct medical points of view: that which favors its routine use on all male infants, and that which would reserve it for babies in whom the foreskin cannot be drawn back readily. The believers in the first theory say that circumcision makes the care of the male infant a far simpler matter, for, if he is not circumcised the foreskin must be retracted during the bath and the penis beneath it washed carefully. In later years hygiene of the male organ is simplified. Infection and cancer of the penis in later life are decidedly less frequent in the circumcised. Those who oppose routine circumcision assert that it is an unnecessary surgical procedure and, even though its danger is slight, it carries with it a minimal risk.

The proponents of routine circumcision seem to be making wholesale converts, and among the private-patient group more than 75 per cent of newborn boys are circumcised today. In many hospitals it is a routine procedure unless the parents object, while in others it is done only on request or if difficulty in retracting the foreskin necessitates it.

Circumcision is performed at any time within the first week of life, provided the baby is in normal health and of term weight. If he weighs less than six pounds, circumcision is usually postponed until his weight attains this figure. Many obstetricians and surgeons give an intramuscular dose of vitamin K before the operation, just to make sure that the baby's blood clots well. The child is placed upon a padded Y-shaped board, to which it is secured by towels and safetypins, each leg being strapped to an arm of the Y. Under sterile precautions—the operative region is prepared with antiseptic solutions, and the operator scrubs as for any other operation—the foreskin is cut off with a knife or scissors, and sutures (stitches) are placed to control bleeding. If the Yellen (Gomco) clamp is used, no stitches are necessary, for postoperative bleeding is controlled by compressing the small blood vessels between two smooth steel surfaces for three to five minutes.

No anesthetic is used. Some pacify the child during the operation with a sponge dipped in wine, whisky, or sugar water. Convalescence is almost always prompt and uninterrupted. If the operation is done by a surgeon or an obstetrician, complications following it are extremely rare; they occur with slightly greater frequency after Jewish ritualistic circumcision, which is usually performed by a man without medical training.

It is noteworthy that the early Jews, who made many interesting observations in both medicine and hygiene, fixed the operation for the eighth day. This was probably arrived at by trial and error. Not an inconsiderable number of those done before the eighth day probably bled dangerously, while those done on the eighth day rarely bled excessively. Modern medicine has found a possible explanation in vitamin K. This vitamin, produced by bacterial action in the intestinal tract, contributes to the process of blood-clotting. The fetus does not manufacture its own vitamin K *in utero*, but some of the mother's passes across the placenta into the baby's circulation. At birth the level in the baby's blood is relatively low, and it drops even lower during the first few days of life, since the child cannot manufacture its own vitamin K until it swallows a healthy supply of germs. The baby's intestinal tract then begins to produce its own vitamin K, and the supply gradually rises until it reaches an adequate level when the baby is a week old.

Until the past decade or two, circumcision of the female was thought occasionally necessary in an adolescent or young woman, but it is never done any more. The pathological behavior for which it was deemed curative, excessive masturbation and nymphomania, are now more wisely handled through psychotherapy.

Physiologic Jaundice

About one-third of babies develop a transitory yellow tint of the skin and eyes (jaundice) between the second and fifth days of life. In premature infants physiologic jaundice is more common and usually more severe and prolonged than in term infants. The depth of color increases for two or three days and then begins to pale, and the normal skin color is soon restored. Ordinarily this "icterus neonatorum"— jaundice of the newborn—is of no significance. It can be distinguished from jaundice associated with hemolytic disease (erythroblastosis) because the latter appears on the first day of life, whereas icterus neonatorum does not occur before the second day.

Erythroblastosis—Rh Disease

Eighty-seven per cent of white Americans, 93 per cent of blacks, 99 per cent of Asian peoples, and 67 per cent of Basques are born with an inherited substance in the blood known as the Rh factor, so termed because an identical factor had been noted earlier in the blood of the Rhesus monkey. (An exception to United States white incidence is found among American Jews, 93 per cent of whom have the Rh factor in their blood.) Persons possessing the factor are called Rh-positive, and those lacking it, Rh-negative. The Rh factor is transmitted as a Mendelian dominant. If both parents of the husband and of the wife are Rh-positive (homozygous—pure Rh-positive), all the children will be Rh-positive. On the other hand, if the husband and the wife each had one Rh-positive and one Rh-negative parent, then both could be partial positives (heterozygous). If both are heterozygous for Rh, in every four children they produce one could be homozygous (pure) Rh-positive, two could be heterozygous (partial) Rh-positive, and one, Rh-negative. Possession or lack of the Rh factor does not make the slightest difference in health, vigor, or longevity.

Marriage between two Rh-positive people—whether pure or partial (homozygous or heterozygous)—and marriage between two Rh-negative people, as well as marriage between an Rh-positive woman and an Rh-negative man, never creates any difficulty in regard to the Rh factor. The only mating which can potentially cause trouble is the marriage of an Rh-negative woman to an Rh-positive man. Statistically this occurs in 13 per cent of United States white marriages, that is, once in slightly less than eight marital unions. Even then, in over 90 per cent of such unions, no Rh difficulty arises. In less than 10 per cent, the woman becomes sensitized by pregnancy to the Rh-positive factor in her husband's cells, a substance foreign to her body—just as foreign to her as typhoid bacilli or polio virus would be. Sensitization expresses itself by the creation of antibodies, chemical substances which attack the specific foreign protein to which the individual has become sensitized. For example, in the case of typhoid bacilli or polio virus, when an individual has been previously sensitized (immunized) either by having contracted typhoid fever or infantile paralysis or by a properly prepared vaccine, then whenever the live organisms of that particular disease enter his body an alarm bell rings which marshals the specific antibodies against the specific invader. In the case of an Rh-negative individual previously sensitized to the Rh factor, antibodies are ready and on the alert to be marshaled against Rh-positive cells. Some Rh-negative women who carry an Rh-positive baby develop antibodies after a first or a later pregnancy. The anti-Rh antibodies persist indefinitely and in subsequent pregnancies with a baby who possesses Rh-positive blood cells, the antibodies pass from the mother's blood stream via the placenta to the baby's blood stream and attack and destroy the baby's Rh-positive red cells. Ordinarily, fetal red cells, which are constantly being manufactured, survive fifty or sixty days in the fetus, but in severe Rh disease they are destroyed in five or six days. In such a situation the fetus cannot manufacture the red cells quickly enough to make up for the rapid rate of destruction, so that profound anemia develops. Sensitization to Rh affects one baby in every 120 births. If the mother is lightly sensitized, there may be little or no effect on the baby, but if the mother is highly sensitized, it may have a devastating result, even causing stillbirth.

How do Rh-negative women become sensitized? Rarely it follows transfusion or injection of blood from an Rh-positive donor; the common mechanism is bearing an Rh-positive fetus. For example, transfusion of Rh-positive blood into an Rh-negative seven-year-old girl at the time of tonsillectomy left her severely sensitized. An Rh-negative five-year-old was given an injection into the buttock of a small amount of blood from her Rh-positive father to transfer his immunity against measles. Seventeen years later she came to me in her first pregnancy, significantly sensitized.

However, most women are first sensitized by pregnancy and it makes no significant difference if pregnancy resulted in birth or abortion. When the husband is homozygous (pure) Rh-positive, all his fetuses will be Rh-positive; if he is heterozygous (partial) and his wife Rh-negative, half of the fetuses will be Rh-positive and half Rh-negative. For sensitization by pregnancy, Rh-positive red blood cells from the fetus must enter the maternal circulation. Such a transfer of red blood cells occurs frequently during the course of a nine-month pregnancy but far more frequently with the separation and delivery of the placenta. In a recent study fetal blood cells were found in the blood stream of 38 per cent of women during pregnancy and 60 per cent shortly after birth. It is difficult to ascertain the number of fetal red cells transferred to the mother's blood in any individual case, for the life of a baby's cells in the maternal circulation is no doubt brief. Unquestionably the main shower of fetal cells occurs with the separation and delivery of the placenta. Sensitization is more likely after a Cesarean section or a breech extraction, or when the placenta does not separate spontaneously and has to be peeled away from its attachment to the uterus by the doctor's fingers. It is also more likely after induced, rather than spontaneous, abortion. The conundrum remains as to why only one Rh-negative woman in ten, who conceive and bear Rh-positive infants, becomes sensitized.

What practical points come from all this theory?

The most exciting thing, which is relatively new, is that if you are Rh-negative and your husband is Rh-positive and if you have not been previously sensitized to Rh, you never will be because sensitization can now be prevented in 100 per cent of cases. If your baby is Rh-positive, you are given an intramuscular injection of Rhogam, human anti-Rh gamma globulin, within two to three days after delivery, so that you will not become sensitized. You can have baby after baby without any Rh problem, provided the Rhogam injection is repeated each time the baby is Rh-positive. Since the Rh of an abortion cannot be determined, you will require a Rhogam injection after spontaneous or induced abortion and after a tubal pregnancy.

Rhogam, which became commercially available in July 1968, was developed by Doctors V. J. Freda and J. G. Gorman of the Columbia Medical School and Dr. W. Pollack at the Ortho Research Foundation in Raritan, New Jersey. The preliminary scientific paper on its use was published in 1964. The reader cannot have the same sense of excitement at this discovery as the obstetrician. For him the possibility of the rapid elimination of one of nature's true tragedies came as a tremendous thrill, especially when through personal experience he could recall the heartache and anxiety that erythroblastosis so often caused in the past.

It is important to determine the presence or absence of the Rh factor early in pregnancy. If you are Rh-negative, the Rh of your husband is tested and if he is also Rh-negative, no Rh immunization as the result of such pregnancy can occur. If he is Rh-positive, by checking the Rh of his parents or—if this is impossible—the Rh of your other children, it may be possible to find out whether he is homozygous or heterozygous for the Rh factor. If either parent is Rh-negative or if one of the children is Rh-negative, your husband is heterozygous and your baby will have a fifty-fifty chance of being Rh-negative. If your husband is Rh-positive, whether homozygous or heterozygous, your blood will be checked for antibodies; if this is your first pregnancy most likely there will be none unless through some misadventure you received Rh-positive blood years back. Your blood will be rechecked for antibodies during mid-pregnancy and perhaps every four to six weeks during the last trimester. If no antibodies are found and almost certainly none will be, two or three days after delivery an injection of Rhogam will be given and everything will be kept under delightful control.

Suppose you have already been sensitized, probably by one or several pregnancies before the days of Rhogam, then what? Rhogam will be of no value to you for it cannot neutralize or eliminate the antibodies you already possess. If you are sensitized, your degree of sensitization must be determined; this is expressed in terms of the amount of titer. The lowest titer is 1:2, which means that your undiluted blood gives a positive Rh-antibody response, but when it is diluted by an equal volume of salt solution the antibody response disappears. Titers up to 1:16 are considered low, and 1:32 or 1:64 is moderate, but titers above 64 dilutions are high. Titers as high as 500 and more are occasionally recorded.

If within two weeks of the term date the titer is no higher than 1:16

and the baby appears to be thirty-six to thirty-eight weeks in size, labor is likely to be induced or a Cesarean section may be done at this time.

If the titer rises two dilutions during pregnancy or is more than 1:16 when you become pregnant, an amniocentesis will be performed at any time after the twenty-second week and repeated approximately every two weeks. As discussed in Chapter 5, amniocentesis consists of inserting a long spinal puncture needle using local anesthesia below the navel through the abdominal wall into the cavity of the uterus and aspirating about a teaspoon of the amniotic fluid which surrounds the baby. The procedure does not disturb the pregnancy. The aspirated amniotic fluid is centrifuged, and filtered, and a spectrographic tracing is made. The spectrogram, which analyzes the amount of bilirubin pigment present in the fluid, graphically records the amount of destruction which has already occurred of the baby's red blood cells. Tracings are graded from 2 to 4. A Number 1 tracing shows that the fetus is not in trouble; Number 2 means that the fetus is Rh-positive but not in immediate jeopardy, and Number 3 demonstrates that the fetus is in trouble. If the pregnancy has advanced to thirty-two weeks, an intrauterine transfusion (IUT) of the fetus is necessary to save its life. A Number-4 tracing is very ominous for the baby, and even if the pregnancy is as premature as thirty-two weeks, prompt delivery offers the best chance; earlier than thirty-two weeks, intrauterine transfusion is resorted to without likelihood of success.

Intrauterine transfusion was introduced by Dr. Liley of New Zealand in 1963. The mother is taken to the X-ray department and given heavy sedation, which not only makes her more comfortable and less apprehensive but also quiets the baby so that it is less likely to move during the procedure. The amniocentesis needle is guided by means of the fluoroscope through the uterus to the lower abdominal region of the fetus, which is punctured, and a transfusion of fresh packed red blood cells from an Rh-negative nonimmunized donor of the group O blood type, is given through it into the baby's abdominal cavity.

For easier determination of the position of the fetal abdomen, frequently amniocentesis is done twelve hours or so before the contemplated intrauterine transfusion and 15 cc of Renografin is instilled through the needle into the amniotic fluid surrounding the baby. This radio-opaque substance, which is swallowed by the fetus when it swallows amniotic fluid, as it always does, appears in the fetal intestines. Thus it shows the location of the fetal abdomen.

Donor blood is well absorbed from a baby's abdominal cavity into its own blood and in this way anemia created by the destruction of its own Rh-positive red cells can be corrected. Once an intrauterine transfusion is given, it is often necessary to repeat it every fourteen days until about the thirty-third week, when the fetus is likely to be large enough to survive delivery. An intrauterine transfusion is a complicated procedure which should be done only in a large teaching hospital and then only when a baby is in dire straits and too immature to survive delivery. One series of 238 cases requiring 399 transfusions showed an infant survival rate of 30.7 per cent, and in another study of 240 babies who had 400 transfusions, 40 per cent survived.

There are three forms of erythroblastosis of the newborn. In the least frequent and most serious, the fetus dies *in utero* at some time during the last third of pregnancy, or if born alive its tissues are so waterlogged (fetal hydrops) from heart failure, caused by its anemia, that it succumbs a few hours later. In the milder and more common forms the infants may be born already seriously anemic, or with a normal amount of hemoglobin that is rapidly destroyed postnatally. These two forms are almost always completely curable by one or several postnatal exchange transfusions.

The factor in erythroblastosis which damages babies after birth is the build-up of the yellowish pigment in their bodies, bilirubin, caused by the rapid destruction of red blood cells. This same pigment causes them to be jaundiced, or icteric. Important lesions may be produced in the brain, collectively known as kernicterus, some of the brain tissue being stained yellow and irreparably injured. Such infants frequently survive, but are likely to be spastics and mentally severely retarded. If the baby of a sensitized mother becomes jaundiced, blood samples are drawn frequently and the level of bilirubin in each serum sample determined. The critical level is 20 mg per 100 cc, and whenever this level is approached an exchange transfusion is given to reduce the amount of bilirubin. If and when the serum bilirubin approaches 20, again another exchange transfusion is carried out. Usually by the end of two to three days the level of bilirubin begins to recede spontaneously.

In an exchange transfusion a catheter (plastic tube) is threaded deep in the umbilical vein through the umbilical cord. In babies born to sensitized mothers, the cord is left longer than usual when it is cut. Twenty cubic centimeters (⅔ ounce) of the infant's Rh-positive blood are withdrawn, and 20 cc of Rh-negative donor blood injected, and repeatedly 20 cc is withdrawn and 20 cc injected until the infant has received at least 500 cc (1⅛ pints) of Rh-negative blood. By this time 85 per cent of the infant's Rh-positive red cells have been replaced by the donor's Rh-negative cells. At frequent intervals for the next thirty-six hours following transfusion, blood samples are checked to determine whether the hemoglobin is falling rapidly or whether the bilirubin is rising precipitately. At the end of forty-eight hours the infant's antibodies (with which it was born) begin declining spontaneously, the last trace being at four to eight weeks of age. Since new antibodies are not formed, the Rh-positive cells which its own bone marrow is forming go unmolested. The salvage of such children to completely normal health is another dramatic event in the history of recent medicine.

There are other blood factors besides Rh to which a mother may become sensitized and pass the sensitivity via the placenta to the baby. If she is blood group O and because of its father the fetus is A or B, she may develop antibodies against the blood type the fetus possesses; also in other cases antibodies may be developed against the so-called Kell factor or one of a large number of other blood subgroupings. Ordinarily this type of sensitization is mild, not requiring exchange transfusion. If the baby becomes deeply jaundiced and no Rh factor is at fault, other sources of isoimmunization are promptly investigated. In some of these cases exchange transfusion must be done. The donor blood is carefully selected so that it lacks the particular blood factor against which the baby has been sensitized.

Whether or not a woman should attempt another pregnancy after a fatal outcome to the fetus from erythroblastosis is difficult to answer. There are too many individual factors in each case to attempt to generalize. The patient's physician is in a much better position to advise. One factor which would be given weight in such a decision is whether the husband is homozygous or heterozygous Rh-positive. If he is heterozygous and by good fortune the sperm which fertilizes the egg transmits his Rh-negative factor, no difficulty will arise no matter how severely the wife is sensitized.

Successful pregnancies have been accomplished in highly sensitized women who have had a series of erythroblastotic stillbirths, by donor artificial insemination. The semen of an Rh-negative donor is substituted for the semen of the Rh-positive husband, with his knowledge and approval. Only some couples are emotionally attuned to this solution, but when they are it offers a foolproof answer.

Fractures

Bone fractures are uncommon at delivery; when they do occur they heal rapidly and perfectly. The clavicle, or collarbone, is the most frequent site; clavicular fracture is particularly common when difficulty is encountered in delivering the shoulders of excessively large infants. These fractures are often so benign that they go unrecognized until several weeks after birth, when the mother unexpectedly feels a bony ridge or stripe across the collarbone. Even when they are diagnosed at birth, usually no treatment is required other than temporarily immobilizing the arm by binding it to the child's chest.

Of the long bones, the thigh and upper arm bone are the most frequently fractured. These fractures must be set and splinted. Such accidents were more common when version was a popular obstetrical operation.

Occasional skull fractures are met, usually after difficult forceps or breech deliveries. If promptly diagnosed and treated by lifting up any bony fragments compressing the brain beneath, complete recovery may be anticipated.

Paralysis of the Arm

This is known as Erb's palsy, which is caused by excessive traction, sometimes necessary in breech extractions or delivery of a shoulder in vertex presentations. The baby's arm is flaccid and usually motionless, although there is finger movement. The likelihood of full recovery is good but not guaranteed, even with the care of competent specialists, neurologists, or orthopedists.

Newborn Mortality

Deaths of newborns are divided in two categories: fetal deaths (still-births—fetuses weighing more than fourteen ounces and born dead), and neonatal deaths (infants born alive weighing more than fourteen ounces but dying within the first four weeks of life). The summation of the two is termed the perinatal death rate, which is expressed as per 1000 live births.

Decline in the Perinatal Rate

The perinatal death rate in the United States in 1935 was 68.2; in 1940, 51.4; in 1950, 35.2; and in 1967, 31.1. The rate has been cut by more than half in thirty-two years. In 1967 there were 54,934 fetal deaths, and 58,127 live-born children died between birth and the end of the first four weeks. More than half of these deaths occurred during the first twenty-four hours of life.

Causes of Fetal Death

Until two decades ago syphilis was one of the primary causes of fetal death: now it has almost been eliminated. The prominent causes still remaining are antepartum hemorrhage late in pregnancy; accidents to the navel cord, such as prolapse, cord about the neck, and knots; maternal conditions, such as toxemia and diabetes; and fetal conditions, such as congenital malformations, birth injuries, and erythroblastosis.

Causes of Neonatal Death

The chief cause of death within the first week of life is prematurity. As stated in Chapter 10, only an occasional baby survives whose birth weight is less than 2 pounds, 3 ounces, and about 60 per cent of those between 2 pounds, 3 ounces, and 3 pounds, 5 ounces. Prematurity either causes, or is an associated cause, in 60 per cent of neonatal deaths. Other causes for neonatal death are imperfect expansion of the lungs, which interferes with breathing, and infections resulting in pneumonia, sepsis, or diarrhea. Causes of fetal death may also be causes of neonatal death, the main ones being birth injuries, congenital malformations, erythroblastosis, maternal diabetes, and hemorrhage complications of the mother before delivery.

Fetal Wastage

The 113,061 babies who died perinatally in 1967 would have populated a city, and with the addition of unrecorded abortions, a metropolis. Totaling the perinatal death rate of 31 and a spontaneous abortion rate of approximately 100, one derives a combined fetal wastage rate of about 130 per 1000 live births. In other words, the average woman when she becomes pregnant has an 87-per-cent chance of bringing a baby home from the hospital, a 10- to 11-per-cent possibility of aborting, a 1- to 2-per-cent chance of having her baby born dead, and a 1- to 2-per-cent likelihood of its being born alive but not surviving the first four weeks.

Congenital Abnormalities and Defects

This is a difficult subject to discuss with lay readers, for each prospective parent has a secret dread that his or her child may not be normal. Such fears cannot be helped; they distinguish the rational human from all other animals—it is unlikely that the pregnant bitch worries over the possibility that the pups she will whelp may be imperfect. Yet the worrying prospective human parent can gain reassurance from the fact that 97.5 per cent of human progeny are perfect at birth. Of the 2.5 per cent which are imperfect, half have only minor defects, such as hammer toes, extra digits, small appendages to the ear, birthmark, and pilonidal sinus at the base of the spine, so that they really need not be included in this category. Congenital abnormalities sufficiently serious to cause the child to be stillborn occur once in about 200 deliveries, and one in 200 babies born alive succumbs during the first year of life from birth defects. Of the 199 surviving babies less than 1 per cent have significant abnormalities, such as congenital heart disease, harelip, cleft palate, and clubfoot. A second source of solace is that many abnormalities which were very serious a few decades ago can be wholly eradicated by the miracles of modern medicine. A plaster cast applied within the first few days of life will straighten the clubfoot; the skillful use of the surgeon's scalpel will eliminate even so grave a lesion as an abnormal opening between trachea and esophagus, to say nothing of all the fantastic procedures being successfully done to correct congenital abnormalities of the heart. A third source of comfort must be the realization that in this enlightened era few obstetricians are cruel enough to fan the spark of life in a hapless monster unless sincere religious conviction dictates such a conservative policy.

Occasionally the diagnosis of a fetal abnormality can be made prenatally. Hydrocephalus, "water on the brain," demonstrates itself by excessive size of the fetal head. This is suspected by the doctor on palpation. Anencephaly, the absence of much of the skull and brain, is suggested to the doctor by his failure to feel the firm, rounded head at either fetal pole. Both suspicions can be confirmed or refuted by X-ray. When a fetal defect is diagnosed that is incompatible with life, labor is induced as soon as is technically possible, to spare the woman the weeks or months of unrewarding pregnancy which remain.

In truth little is known about the causes of congenital abnormalities. Some are unquestionably due to heredity, to genetic influences, such as hemophilia, the condition in which half the males bleed extravagantly from minor injuries and the females of the family transmit the defect. Others are due to environmental factors—such factors as German measles at an early stage of pregnancy or the application of ionizing radiation at critical periods of pregnancy by the use of therapeutic X-ray directly to the uterus, or a fallout from an atomic bomb when the pregnant woman is within three-quarters of a mile from its epicenter. There is probably an intermediate group among whom the effect of genetic influences is aided and abetted by environmental factors, perhaps the site of implantation within the uterus or the maternal age.

Many facts about congenital malformations defy exact explanation, though unproved, interesting hypotheses have been advanced. Let us consider the influence of maternal age. It is well documented that virtually all fetal abnormalities which are not transmitted in a clearly defined hereditary pattern increase in incidence with maternal age. Among these conditions are spina bifida (incomplete closure of the lower spinal canal), microcephaly (pin head), cleft lip and cleft palate, congenital heart defects, and hydrocephalus. Add to these the most clear-cut example, Down's disease, known as Mongolism because among other abnormalities such infants always have slanting eyes. In mothers younger than thirty years old, the risk of a Mongoloid birth is less than 1 in 1000. The risk increases to 1 in 100 at age forty, and 1 in 45 when the maternal age is forty-five or over. It has been shown in experiments on several different rodents, through a series of artificial inseminations at increasing intervals after proved ovulation, that when ova are overripe the litter size declines and the proportion of abnormal fetuses increases. Using this as a basis, Dr. James German of Cornell Medical School theorizes that the incidence of Mongolism may be correlated with coital frequency. Infrequent coitus makes it less likely that spermatozoa will be lurking in the tube to fertilize the ovum as soon as it is ovulated, so that with occasional intercourse the egg may be many hours old before fertilizing sperm cells arrive. As evidence for his thesis, Dr. German cites the fact that there is a lower incidence of Mongoloid births among newly married older women than among women of the same age group married several years.

A few years ago a study of two great Dublin hospitals, one Catholic and one Protestant, showed that the Catholic hospital reported twice as many abnormalities in its newborn. The researcher theorized that the difference may be due to the fact that a high proportion of the women in the Catholic hospital practiced the rhythm method of contraception and that a rhythm-failure pregnancy was more likely to be associated with coitus late in the cycle, and thus with the fertilization of an "old" egg—one ovulated hours before.

Another explanation for the increase in fetal abnormalities with maternal age is that the ova are all present at birth. Egg cells, unlike all other body cells, are not constantly being formed. Therefore, an egg fertilized at age forty is a much older cell than one fertilized at age twenty, and is more likely to have undergone chromosomal mutations or other deleterious changes than the egg cell from a younger woman. Spermatozoa, differing from ova, are constantly being formed and probably none is more than four weeks old when ejaculated.

Dr. Brian MacMahon of Harvard presents evidence that there may be ethnic and social factors in the incidence of two serious defects of the central nervous system, anencephaly (absence of brain cortex) and spina bifida. The prevalence rate for the two conditions in four Boston hospitals was 2.24 per 1000 live births. The rate for Boston parents born in Ireland was 4.9 and 3.1 for second and third generation Irish parents. The offspring of Jewish mothers had a rate of only 0.77. The Protestant rate was 2.01. However, when individuals came from the same socio-economic class these differences were less marked.

Dwelling on congenital abnormalities and defects may seem to some readers scary overemphasis. However, I feel that a scientist addressing the lay public should state the scientific facts as they exist, without alteration to gloss them over. To put the topic in better perspective, let me remind you that reliable data underscore the overwhelming likelihood of a normal infant at birth. Even mothers of forty-five have better than 10 to 1 odds that their newborn will be perfect.

PKU

Phenylketonuria, called PKU, is an inherited disease, transmitted as a Mendelian recessive, and affects about 1 in 20,000 newborn. It is characterized by mental deficiency and abnormal protein metabolism resulting in the excretion of phenylpyruvic acid. It accounts for 0.5 per cent of the serious mental defectives. PKU occurs mainly among Caucasians; black and Semitic groups show a lower incidence. In afflicted children an abnormally high level of phenylalanine (an amino acid present in protein foods) is found in the urine and blood, which permits a simple test for diagnosing the condition. Although the test may not be positive at birth, it becomes positive during the first few weeks. The test consists of adding a few drops of 5 per cent ferric chloride to a small amount of urine. A green color develops in positive cases which can be checked by determining blood levels. The importance of establishing an early diagnosis is that by instituting at once a special diet low in phenylalanine, brain damage can be prevented or largely eliminated. It is not yet possible to specify the optimum duration of dietary treatment. Perhaps after a few years a child may be able to tolerate a normal diet without impairment of mental function. Because of the gravity of the condition, its easy diagnosis, and the excellent therapeutic results achieved through prompt dietary restriction, it has become routine in many medical centers to test the urine of all young infants with ferric chloride.

Genetic Counseling

Genetic or inheritance counseling was at first limited to informing couples that they or their child had a disease or disorder that "ran in the family." With the acceptance and application of Mendelian genetics, which led to the linkage of selected diseases with specific modes of inheritance, genetic counseling became more exact. Doctors could then tell parents who had an infant with an identifiable genetic disorder the probable risk of its occurrence in their next child. For example, if a couple had a child born with cystic fibrosis (a fatal disorder of mucus-secreting and sweat glands) or Tay-Sachs disease (a fatal neurologic condition) there is one chance in four that subsequent children will have the affliction. There are three chances in four the children will be free of the disease, but two of the normal children will be recessive carriers or potential transmitters of the defect, while the third normal child will not be a carrier. If a male child suffered from crippling hemophilia one can prognosticate that half of subsequent sons will have the disease and all daughters will be carriers of the disease. With such information couples are able to make their decision about future childbearing. For some, a risk of one in four is a complete deterrant, while for others, it presents a justifiable gamble.

Several recent advances are changing the nature of genetic counseling from a drawing-board to a practical discipline.

In rare instances preconceptional genetic advice is available. For example, there is a serious form of anemia called sickle-cell disease, which is largely confined to the black race. One in twelve healthy Negroes has the trait and if two individuals with the trait mate, one quarter of their children will develop the disease, which is crippling and often fatal. Whether or not one is a carrier of the trait can be determined by one of several blood tests in which a drop of blood is exposed to low oxygen tension. Then under the microscope, the red blood cells of a carrier appear sickle-shaped, instead of remaining normally spheroidal.

The greatest advance has been the ability to detect prenatally the presence or absence of several genetic conditions early in pregnancy for parents bearing the risk of having a child with certain genetic disorders. If the test is negative the parents are given reassuring knowledge that the child will be normal, and if it is positive, in many political jurisdictions the parents can elect to have the pregnancy terminated by abortion. They are then in a position to try another pregnancy and again to test the normality of that fetus. Undoubtedly, in the future some genetic conditions will be susceptible to therapeutic correction while a fetus is still *in utero*, but now it is not possible. Therefore the only avenue of treatment is induced abortion and, therefore, unless a couple is willing to consider abortion if the test proves positive it makes no sense to assume the slight danger and inconvenience of taking the test.

What are high-risk pregnancies that justify these cytogenetic studies? The most common and important criteria are:

1. When a previous pregnancy produced an abnormal infant with a genetic defect that can be detected *in utero*.

2. When a previous pregnancy produced a genetic defect that is limited to males (X-linked recessive). It is possible to establish the sex of the fetus *in utero*, and then to abort a male fetus or to allow a female fetus to go to term.

3. If one parent is a known carrier of a translocated chromosome, to determine if the fetus's chromosomal pattern is normal or abnormal.

4. If the mother is over forty years of age when she conceives. Such a study is mainly to eliminate a Down's, or Mongoloid, fetus.

Using these criteria of high risk, in a study of 331 pregnancies forty-one affected fetuses (13 per cent) were found. Of these women, 119 were in the over-forty age group, and four Down's disease fetuses were discovered (3.4 per cent) and aborted.

To carry out such studies, an amniocentesis must be done, a technique discusssed previously in this book. After the fourteenth week of pregnancy, an abdomino-uterine puncture is made under local anesthesia and 10 cc or 2½ teaspoons of amniotic fluid aspirated with a syringe. The needle is then withdrawn. This simple procedure is usually performed by an obstetrician in his office.

There are different diagnostic tests employed depending upon the particular abnormality suspected. The chemistry and enzyme content of the amniotic fluid itself may be investigated, or the cells of the fetus studied. Amniotic fluid always contains cells from the fetus. The origin of the cells is presumably from the mouth cavity, vagina, skin umbilical cord, and fetal urine. One genetic condition, Pompe's disease, can be determined by electron microscopic examination of an individual cell, the immense magnification revealing the abnormalities of lysosome units within the cell that cause the disease. In sex-linked disorders the presence or absence of Barr bodies in individual cells permits diagnosis of the sex. To obtain a sufficient number of fetal cells for adequate cytological evaluation in order to diagnose other genetic conditions necessitates multiplication of the cells through tissue culture. This requires from three to forty days, with an approximate mean of three weeks. The cultured cells are then studied for their specific chromosomal pattern, as in Down's disease, for example, in which there are three chromosomes where normally there should be only a pair. Other conditions necessitate delicate chemical tests on a mass of cultured fetal cells to determine the absence or presence of an essential enzyme, a complicated organic substance which through catalytic action causes a specific cellular chemical reaction. One example is Tay-Sachs disease, which I mentioned earlier in this chapter. Now, instead of waiting until birth to find out whether this fatal disease will afflict the next child of a couple who have already produced a Tay-Sachs infant, cytological tests can reveal whether or not the fetal cells grown in tissue culture are producing a normal amount of the enzyme hexosaminidase A. If not, this second child will also be a Tay-Sachs victim, and abortion is indicated.

The field of cytogenetics is developing so rapidly and is so complex that it must be left in the knowledgeable hands of the professional genetic counselors. If you have a problem in this area, seek the most expert opinion you can get.

General Conclusions

The lay press has been flooded with sensational scare literature about congenital abnormalities. Much of it is largely conjecture and lacks proof. I know no proof that the minor amount of radiation to which a fetus is exposed while the mother undergoes diagnostic (not therapeutic) X-ray has ever done harm. Despite the fact that abnormal mice can be created by exposing the pregnant mother to an atmosphere as rarefied as Mount Everest for five hours, there is no evidence that an airplane trip in a pressurized cabin during early pregnancy has ever damaged a human fetus.

If a doctor desired to employ every conceivable precaution to reduce the incidence of malformations, he might issue the following suggestions. First I must stress that today the wisdom of some remains uncertain.

1. Encourage small children to get German measles and probably mumps and chicken pox while in nursery or grammar school (to develop natural immunity).

2. Never allow Rh-negative girls or women to receive Rh-positive blood by either transfusion or injection.

3. Control diabetes carefully during pregnancy and avoid excessive quantities of insulin.

4. Be sure you and your husband are in physical, nutritional, and reproductive prime before initiating a conception.

5. Avoid unnecessary diagnostic X-ray during pregnancy, especially to the pelvic region. Do not avoid essential X-ray.

6. When possible, substitute local anesthesia for general anesthesia in dental and surgical procedures during early pregnancy. Do not take gas alone as a general anesthetic.

7. Avoid air travel until after the twelfth week, unless the plane is pressurized. All commercial planes are pressurized.

8. Whenever possible, have children while you are both young.

9. Do not take drugs unless prescribed by your doctor, and don't ask for them unnecessarily.

10. If your situation can be catalogued as a genetic high-risk situation, consult a professional genetic counselor.

The Likelihood of Repetition of a Congenital Defect

If the defect is not due to an environmental influence such as German measles or ionizing radiation or a clear-cut inherited condition, for parents with one malformed offspring there is an average risk of 5 per cent of having a second malformed child. In half the cases such malformations duplicate the original one. With two malformed children, the risk of a third is increased to 15 to 25 per cent. However, since certain defects have a particular pattern of repetition, it is wise to consult an expert. Most large university medical centers have a division of medical genetics. Contact the one near you and make an appointment with the head of this special unit.

The Pediatrician

At this point it is wise to introduce the pediatrician, a physician whose services are fully as essential to you as the obstetrician's. In large maternities such as that at the Mount Sinai Hospital in New York, the newborn is the responsibility of the obstetrical staff until it leaves the delivery room, and from then on its medical needs and problems are taken over completely by pediatric colleagues. In private practice the patient's family or her obstetrician notifies a pediatrician within the first twenty-four hours and invites him to come to the hospital and examine the baby, to meet and advise the new mother about nursing, the layette, and similar problems. When possible, choose a pediatric specialist if one is available. Obviously he knows more about babies and children than most men in general practice, since he was specifically trained in this area. In case he does not arrive on time, I here give my views about the hospital care of the newborn, but if his views or advice differ from mine, by all means follow the guidance of the doctor who is going to take care of your baby at home.

Infant Feeding

"Shall I nurse my baby?" This is a very frequent question. I have earlier listed the advantages of breast feeding (page 96), and I myself am in favor of it. I think it is better for both mother and child. However, all the advantages when added together are not sufficient to justify the persuasion of a reluctant mother to nurse against her will.

Breast Feeding

Babies are offered nothing by mouth the first twelve hours. During the remaining twelve hours of the first day they nurse each breast for two or three minutes every four hours. Starting with a limited sucking time allows the nipples to become gradually adjusted to the process. If the mother takes a daily shower or bath and washes the nipple area with soap and water, no preliminary cleansing of the nipple before nursing need be done. It is important to be comfortable and relaxed while nursing. You may wish to lie on your side or you may find sitting up in bed or on a chair preferable. An infant instinctively turns its head toward anything touching his cheek, so by touching his cheek you can direct his mouth toward the breast. Both the nipple and the areola, the circular dark area, should be in his mouth while sucking. To aid him, pinch the nipple so that it erects, which allows him to grasp it more easily. If he imbeds his nose in your breast, try to shift your position or use your finger to hold the breast away. In most instances the child requires no preliminary training or encouragement to take the nipple but begins to suck promptly. Since it gets nothing but a scanty amount of colostrum, it may soon stop and go to sleep. Treat the baby roughly; wake it up, fleck the feet by snapping your fingers at its soles. On the second and third days the child suckles for three to five minutes on each breast, and ten minutes on each breast thereafter. A woman's milk generally comes in between the third and fifth days. Breast milk is bluish and looks watery compared to cow's milk. A baby can empty the breast in a short time. In the first several days infants get all they can from one breast in three to five minutes. Later they obtain 75 per cent of the milk in a breast in the first four minutes. Every four hours the baby is put to both breasts, alternating the starting breast. As long as the baby gets little milk it may be offered two ounces of 5 per cent glucose water after each nursing, especially in hot weather. Demand feeding has been discussed in an earlier chapter.

Stools of Breast-Fed Babies

Meconium, the initial tarry green, sticky intestinal contents of the baby, disappears around the third or fourth day with the establishment of lactation, its place being taken by feces which are bright yellow with a homogeneous consistency. For the first few days the stools, which have a characteristic sour-dough odor, are unformed, but soon take on a cylindrical shape. The bowels of the breast-fed infant move several times daily, not uncommonly toward the end of or after each nursing.

Mixed Feedings

If after several days the child does not get enough breast milk to satisfy its needs, discovered by weighing it before and after several nursings, the mother's breast milk is supplemented by offering the baby three ounces of formula. If after forty-eight hours of mixed feedings the mother's milk does not increase sufficiently to meet two-thirds of the baby's needs, it is wise to discontinue breast feeding and put the baby on full bottle feedings. Failure to gain weight and excessive wakefulness and crying may cause suspicion that the baby is not getting enough to eat.

Bottle Feeding

It is quite likely you will be told how to prepare a formula at the hospital before discharge by the nursery personnel or your own pediatrician, but in case you are not, I am including the following.

Utensils for Making Formula

1 one-quart measuring pitcher
1 measuring tablespoon
1 table knife
1 long handled spoon for stirring
1 funnel
1 sterilizer—with rack
1 bottle brush

1 can opener or ice pick
7 nursing bottles (8-oz. size),
    narrow or wide mouth, prefer-
    ably heat-resistant glass
7 nipples for nursing bottles
7 nipple caps—glass, bakelite,
    aluminum, or paper

Steps in Preparation

1. Wash all utensils to be used. Use the bottle brush to scrub the bottles, nipples, and nipple covers in hot, soapy water. Soap or a good detergent may be used. Rinse well in hot, clear water, and let drain—do not wipe. Squeeze water through nipple holes during washing and rinsing.

2. Measure the required* amount of warm water from the tap (water does not need to be boiled).

3. Pour into a pitcher or quart jar.

4. Measure the required amount of syrup or sugar in the measuring tablespoon. If syrup is used, pour it from the bottle or can into the spoon. If dry sugar is used, level off measuring tablespoons with back of table knife. Add syrup or sugar to water in pitcher. Stir until dissolved.

5. Scrub the top of the can of milk powder or milk with soapsuds and rinse in hot water from the tap. Open can by punching two holes in top if you are using evaporated milk.

6. Measure the required amount of milk in measuring cup, if evaporated, or by spoon if powdered.

7. Pour milk into water-sugar mixture and stir with long-handled spoon.

8. Use the funnel and pour the formula into the bottles. (Drinking water for the baby may be sterilized in a bottle at the same time you are sterilizing the formula.)

---

* Either the hospital or your pediatrician will instruct you on hospital discharge what kind of milk to use, the proportion and quantities of milk and water, and whether sugar or syrup should be added. The more popular milk brand names are Pet and Carnation.

9. Put the nipples on the bottles.

10. Place the nipple covers over the nipples. Three types are available: a glass bell-jar type for narrow-necked bottles; a hard bakelite screw-on cover for wide-necked bottles; and a brown-paper cap fastened with string or rubber band. Be sure covers are not pressed or screwed on so firmly as to form a tight seal. They should be loose enough to allow steam to circulate.

11. There are two different kinds of sterilizers. Either of them or a deep cooking utensil with lid may be used. The kinds are: a tall sterilizer (9 inches high, including lid) with rack for bottles; a standard-height sterilizer (7 or 8 inches high) for screw-cap-type bottles with nipples inverted. Can be used only with this type of bottle.

12. Place rack in bottom of sterilizer. Stand the bottles of formula on it, and then pour in 2 inches of water.

13. Cover the sterilizer with lid and place on stove. Turn on heat.

14. When water starts to boil, write down the time, or set your Minute Minder. Boil 25 minutes by the clock. After water has boiled 25 minutes, take sterilizer off the burner.

15. *Caution—do not remove lid from sterilizer.* Do not even lift the lid until sterilizer has cooled enough to allow you to hold your hands against the sides. Then remove bottles and press or screw the nipple covers down firmly over the nipples.

16. Place covered bottles in refrigerator until needed.

17. When it is time to feed the baby, warm the bottle in a pan of hot water (not boiling).

18. If screw-cap bottles are used, lift nipple and disk from bottle. Use disk to push shoulder of nipple through cap.

19. Remove disk and screw the cap on bottle.

20. Before giving the formula to the baby, test the temperature by shaking a few drops on the inside of your wrist. It should feel warm but not hot.

Ask your pediatrician about using a prepared formula such as Similac or Enfamil. They come all ready for use in sterilized bottles ready to feed. The one drawback is their expense. They are considerably less expensive if bought as milk concentrates in a can to which you add boiling water and then pour the mixture into sterilized bottles. Exact directions are on the cans.

I am very much in favor of having the mother give her baby each bottle herself while in the hospital, except the 2 a.m. bottle. She has more time than the average hospital nurse, and it is psychologically wise for both mother and child that she cuddle the infant against the warmth of her body while feeding it.

Stools of Bottle-Fed Babies

The stools of infants fed on most formulas are whitish-yellow, firm, well formed, and less frequent than those of breast-fed babies; two a day is the usual number. However, if Lactum is used, the stools are orange-yellow in color, and up to seven a day are normal.

Urine

The child usually voids a few minutes after birth and voids irregularly thereafter. The daily amount excreted depends upon the size of the baby, whether it is bottle fed or breast fed, its state of health, the temperature of the room, etc. The average breast-fed child excretes one ounce of urine on the second day of life, three on the fourth, five on the sixth, and seven on the eighth. The bottle-fed infant voids almost twice as much.

Weight Loss

Because of the excretion of meconium and urine and the evaporation of body water from the lungs and skin, the newborn loses about a half-pound, 7 to 8 per cent of its birthweight, in the first three or four days of life. Premature infants lose proportionately more than babies of normal size (10 to 12 per cent). In mature infants the weight loss is ordinarily regained by the tenth day, and from then on for several months the child gains an average of six to seven ounces per week. Birthweight is doubled by the time the child is five months old and trebled by the end of the first year.

Rooming In

Many hospitals have reintroduced rooming in for babies—reintroduced because nurseries are a twentieth-century refinement largely confined to the United States. I was surprised to find on a recent European trip that in most institutions the baby's crib was attached to the foot of the mother's hospital bed, where it had been for decades.

The ideal rooming-in setup is to have eight-bed central nurseries with rooms or wards opening into them. Then in the morning the baby's bassinet is wheeled next to the mother's bed, where it remains until ten at night, when the baby is taken back to the nursery so that the mother's night may be undisturbed except for the two-o'clock nursing. Various modifications are necessary and feasible in the absence of ideal facilities. If the mother has a private room, when the baby is twenty-four hours old the bassinet is kept constantly in her room until baby and mother are discharged together. In the case of a four-bed unit, only mothers desiring rooming in are placed in it and the babies kept constantly next to them.

I feel that rooming in should be wholly optional. It is ideal for some patients and unsuited to others. In the main, the woman with a first child desires it, while the woman with a fourth child objects on the basis that she has looked forward to the hospital stay for eight months as a period free of domesticity for solid, essential rest.

Arguments in Favor

The first thing to be said in favor of rooming in is that it allows mother and baby to become fully acquainted and makes the transition from hospital to home a natural and gradual one rather than a rude and sometimes dangerous shock. The mother has become accustomed to looking after the baby completely, she has learned to diaper and bathe it, and she is even able to interpret its noises and grunts. Let us not leave the father out, because under this plan he too becomes intimately acquainted with the baby before it leaves the hospital and probably becomes a "diaperer" of no mean skill. Usually the rooming-in program is combined with demand feeding, which means that the baby is either nursed or offered the bottle on its own terms, at the frequency it desires. When the baby cries and no obvious cause is apparent, it is fed. It soon learns to space its feedings quite regularly at three-, four-, or six-hour intervals, depending on the baby. Some child psychiatrists feel that rooming in, breast nursing, and demand feeding (that is, feeding the baby when it cries from hunger) give the new citizen a sense of security, a neurosis-free start in life which pays dividends all through the later years. Their thesis is that much of the insecurity of later life has its genesis in the nursery. A baby cries because it is hungry, yet no one pays attention to it. The infant lies alone in its chaste and impersonal surroundings, getting the idea that no one loves it. This earliest idea so deeply grooves the subconscious of some babies that the affection usually showered upon them later cannot erase it, and they are left insecure for the rest of their lives.

Arguments Against

In the rooming-in scheme visiting is restricted to the husband or to the husband and the mother, who must wear gown and mask and wash their hands before handling the baby.

Rooming in requires more nursing personnel and nurses who are capable and anxious to teach. The mothers must be carefully supervised at all times.

It is more difficult for hospitals to assign accommodations under the dual scheme—rooming in and rooming out.

Finally—the argument previously referred to—some women, particularly multiparas, do not want the inconvenience and the disturbance of rest and sleep.

Clothing

What Clothing to Bring to the Hospital for Baby When Going Home

3 diapers with diaper pins
1 nightgown
1 quilted pad or plastic pants
1 shirt

1 cotton receiving blanket, except in winter months when the blanket should be wool
1 wool blanket
1 sweater and cap

Layette

Now to answer the final question: What shall we get for the baby? The answer is: Only the absolute essentials. The normal tendency is always to get too much; the following includes only indispensable items:

Basic Layette

Diapers	3 or 4 doz.	Bird's-eye or gauze (keep a dozen on hand even if you have diaper service or use disposables)
Shirts	4 to 6	Cotton, open at side or front, six-months' size
Crib blankets*	1 or 2	Heavy wool, light wool
Sweaters*	1 or 2	Six-months' size
Receiving blankets	6	Cotton
Mattress protector	1	Water-resistant
Washcloths	2	Terry, soft
Towels	2	Terry, soft
Crib sheets	2	Make your own crib sheets from old bed sheets. Since crib sheets and bed sheets cost approximately the same, buy bed sheets for your own bed
Nightgowns	3 or 4	Cotton or flannel, open in front, six-months' size
Pads	3 or 4	Waterproof or quilted

Bunting	1	Not essential—receiving blankets and wool blankets may be used
Crib and mattress	1	Firm mattress
Bath equipment		Soap dish, milk soap, mineral oil, absorbent cotton, safety pins, talcum powder. Baby can be bathed in washstand or kitchen sink

* Since these are popular gifts, do not purchase until you have opened your baby presents.

As far as diapers are concerned you have three choices. It is cheapest to launder your own, but least convenient. According to Consumer Union reports, cloth diapers come to about 40 cents a week on the basis of fifty diapers used for eighteen months. Next in the expense ladder is a diaper service, which at the time of the survey cost $4.75 for a hundred per week, $4.30 for seventy, and $4.00 for fifty. The most expensive and most convenient way to handle the diaper problem was the disposable diapers: Pampers and Kimbies, a hundred of the small size per week costing $5.30, and of the medium size per week, $5.97; and Chux, for small size, $5.30, and for medium, $7.17. Pampers currently have 90 per cent of the disposable market, and disposables account for 15 to 20 per cent of the nation's diaper business. A statistician has figured that 540 million diaper changes are made each week in this country.

This concludes our story of the newborn. He is now ready to be taken home, whither we shall not follow him. Descriptions of his further care and progress can be found in popular books and free government pamphlets dealing with the first few years of life. Even if you are the best informed of the new mothers in your community, it does not relieve you of the privilege and necessity of visiting and consulting your pediatrician. In obstetrics and pediatrics, books should never be substituted for a doctor, they should be used only to supplement his care and wisdom.

Epilogue

This is a wonderful time to have a baby, wonderful for both mother and baby, for in the long history of man birth has never been so safe. The progress made in this area during the past several decades in much of the world—regrettably not in all the world—defies imagination. Yet the goal has not been reached, even among developed nations, though it is clear: no deaths for those who bring life, and no fetal wastage. What can be done to achieve this ideal?

Laymen must realize the importance of prenatal care; this means not merely registry with a doctor or a hospital for confinement, but also regular visits to the doctor from the early weeks of pregnancy until the time of delivery, and the carrying out of his advice to the letter. In some areas an acceptable substitute for the doctor is the expertly equipped nurse-midwife. To have had one or several babies without complications does not eliminate the possibility of complications in a later pregnancy, and therefore prenatal care is as necessary for the fifth as for the first pregnancy.

The choice of a doctor is important, and the well-trained obstetrical specialist is the best guarantee of safety. The danger of ill-equipped and badly supervised private obstetrical sanatoria is great, and a separate obstetrical pavilion attached to a general hospital, or a special obstetric hospital, is greatly to be preferred. There is sore and pressing need for additional obstetric beds, especially in the more remote regions of this country. These beds should be made available equally to rich and poor, black and white. Furthermore, the proper nutrition of the malnourished in this, the breadbasket of the world, must be improved—certainly the nutrition of many of its pregnant women. During the siege of Leningrad in 1942, with its attendant starvation, prematurity rose from 6.5

per cent to 41.2 per cent, stillbirths more than doubled, and the death rate for newborn infants soared to more than 100 per 1000.

The public must develop a standard of obstetric values. A simple delivery is the best recommendation for an obstetrician, much better than a long list of impressive operations. A completely painless labor may be bad obstetrics; the relief of pain is humane and necessary, but in some cases its obliteration may exact an excessive price.

The readers must realize that the vast majority of pregnancies have always ended successfully and they will continue to do so. This book, in trying to tell the whole story, may have given undue space and emphasis to abnormalities. It has not omitted the detailed story of the normal uncomplicated case, but as far as the number of pages is concerned the normal case is but a single story—abnormalities are so varied that they perforce occupy more printed lines. In actual obstetric practice the relative frequency of the normal to the abnormal is more than 9 to 1. The task of the future is to raise these odds still higher.

If you are going to have a baby, the previous paragraphs should have dissolved your doubts and fears. Believe me when I say that birth has become almost 100 per cent safe. Many modern obstetricians have practiced two decades or longer without a single maternal death.

In more than thirty years of obstetric practice, during which I have delivered something like 6000 private patients, I have seen three of my own patients die, one from a fatal blood disease (leukemia) at the fourth month, one from a clotting of a blood vessel in the brain several days after delivery, and one two weeks following birth from the effects of a recurrent breast cancer. Pregnancy and labor had little to do with any of the three. I do not recite these personal statistics boastfully, for they can be duplicated or improved by hundreds of doctors—probably by your own obstetrician—but their recitation must perforce be reassuring.

How shall we interpret this? It does not mean that all obstetrical problems and complications have disappeared. It simply means that the modern doctor, together with his modern hospital, is fully capable of handling problems and complications when they arise. Potential parents of the fourth quarter of the twentieth century are truly fortunate people.

Even granting these facts, obstetrical knowledge is far from complete. Many unsolved problems remain. Some day the laboratory will reveal the precise cause of the onset of labor; then we shall be able to initiate and retard it at will. No longer will patients carry a pregnancy long beyond term or babies be born prematurely; no longer will labors be lengthened by inertia. The malformed newborn of today will vanish tomorrow. A recital of the fields yet to conquer would cover page after page. Research worker and clinician are striving shoulder to shoulder: progress—in some decades slow, in others rapid—is inevitable. Among other goals of the future, I cannot omit the prevention of all unwanted conceptions. They are not only emotionally traumatic to the couples involved, but often rob a baby of its birthright to be eagerly anticipated by parents fully prepared to be responsible for its welfare.

This brief narration of obstetrics, past, present, and future, is now at an end. If these pages have instructed, advised, or encouraged, the author is well rewarded. To your baby not yet born, he wishes a triumphant entrance into this universe.

Index

Abdomen, care of, during pregnancy, 99–100; during puerperium, 242–43

Abdominal changes, during pregnancy, 27, 29–30, 31–32

Abdominal decompression, 190

Abdominal operations, and abortion, 132–33

Abdominal pain, as symptom, 130

Able, Luke, 256

Abnormalities, congenital, 37, 202–203, 272, 336–42, 352; anencephaly, 337; club foot, 337; and German measles, 158; hydrocephalus, 337; reducing incidence of, 342; repetition of, 342–43; in twins, 266; and vaccines, 102–103

Abortion (miscarriage), 24, 59, 69, 92, 94, 103, 268, 280

—induced: 140–50, 340; convalescence from, 148; danger from, 146; and diagnosis of sex, 66; and German measles, 161–62; and heart disease, 154; illegal, 88, 140, 142–43, 146; legal, 142, 143–46, 161–62; liberalized laws on, 141–46; psychic reactions to, 146; and religious groups, 140–41; and Tay-Sachs disease, 341

—spontaneous: 131–39; causes of, 132–136; complete, 138–39; danger from, 139; genetic basis for, 134–35; incomplete, 139; interval between, and another pregnancy, 137; late, 135; preventing, 136–37; repetition of, 138; surgery to prevent, 316

Abscess, breast, 246–47

Abstinence, 292

Accidents, 123–24, 133; and premature labor, 56

Addiction, maternal, 59–60

Adolescents, and sex, 6

Afterbirth, 50

Afterpains, during puerperium, 241

Age, maternal: 172–73; and absence of menstruation, 25; and congenital abnormalities, 337–38; and death rate, 88; and family planning, 272–73; and fertility, 308; and length of first labor, 171–72; and twinning incidence, 253

Agency for International Development, 296

Alcohol, and fetus, 62; and milk production, 237

Ambulation, early, after Cesarean section, 233; after delivery, 240; after multiple birth, 265

Amenorrhea, 25–26, 238, 276

American Birth Control League, 270

American College of Obstetrics and Gynecology, 89

American College of Surgeons, 178

American Fertility Society, 309

American Indians, 274

American Law Institute (A.L.I.), 143–144

American Society for Psychoprophylaxis in Obstetrics, 186

Amnesics, for labor pain, 181, 183

Amniocentesis, 68, 332, 341

Amniotic fluid, 56–57, 72, 170, 341

Amphojel, 119

Analgesia, 177, 194; for labor pain, 181, 183, 184, 191; in twin pregnancy, 264

Anemia, 88, 248, 262, 263; iron in diet to prevent, 106, 107; and Rh factor, 330, 333

Anencephaly, 337, 338

Psychic shock, and abortion, 133
Psychologic methods, of pain relief, 181, 184–89
Psychological factors, and absence of menstruation, 26; and infertility, 316–317
Psychoprophylaxis, 186–88; choosing doctor and hospital for, 189–90
Psychotherapy, 138, 328
Ptyalism, 28, 115
Pudendal block, 191–92
Puerperal fever, 244–45
Puerperium, 234–50; complications during, 244–49
Pyelonephritis, 247–48

Quadruplets, 253, 255
Queen Mary I (England), 43
Quickening, see Fetus, movements of
Quinine, 150
Quintuplets, 252, 255, 261

Rabbit test, for pregnancy, 41
Race, and twinning incidence, 253
Radiation, 37; and congenital abnormalities, 337; see also X-rays
Rat test, for pregnancy, 41
Rats, cannibalism among, 29; fertilization among, 20, 21–22; on protein-deficient diets, 106–107
Reagan, Ronald, 144
Referring Planned Parenthood affiliates, 146
Renografin, 332
Reproduction, sexual, advantages of, 4–5
Respiration, fetal, 57, 74
Rest, during pregnancy, 95; during puerperium, 239–40
Resuscitation, of baby (birth), 199–200
Retrolental fibroplasia, in newborn, 324
Rh factor, 84, 328–34; and artificial insemination, 317–18, 334; control of, 342; and Rhogam, 149, 224, 330–31
Rhesus monkeys, 329
Rhinitis, allergic, 118–19
Rhogam, 149, 224, 330–31
Rhythm method, with basal body temperature (BBT), 274, 292, 293–94; with calendar, 274, 292–93
Rickets, 210–11
Rockefeller, John D., III, 91
Romer, Thiele, 252
Rooming in, 347–49
Rubella, see German measles
Rubin, I. C., 313
Rubin test, 313

Sabine vaccine, 162
"Safe period," 16; see also Rhythm method
Salivation, exessive, see Pytalism
Salk vaccine, 162
Salt, in diet, 109, 111, 128, 263
"Salting out," 129–30, 148, 224
Sanger, Margaret, 269
Sanger, Margaret, Research Bureau, 309
Sänger, Max, 228
Scopolamine, 182, 183, 184, 194
Seconal, 121, 183
Sedatives, for insomnia, 121–22
Semen, 7–8, 11–12, 17; and male sterilization, 304
Sensitization, of mother to Rh factor, 329–34
Septuplets, 252
Sex, chromosomes, 65–68; and heredity, 66
Sex-linked disorders, 341
Sex organs, female, function and structure of, 13–14; male, function and structure of, 12–13
Sex ratio, 69, 267; for twins, 266
Sexual activity, and sterilization, 297, 304–305
Sexual difficulties, origin of, 6
Sexual Inadequacy (Masters-Johnson), 316
Sexual intercourse, and fertilization, 15; frequency of, and fertility, 12, 308; and insemination, 267; and ovulation, 67; during pregnancy, 102
Sexual pleasure, see Libido
Sexual reproduction, advantages of, 4–5
Shettles, Landrum, 66–67
Siamese twins, 256–58
Sickle cells, 58–59; disease, 340
Simpson, James Young, 182
Sims-Hühner test, see P.C. test
Single-celled organisms, 3
Six Practical Lessons for an Easier Childbirth (Bing), 186
Size of baby, and maternal diabetes, 156
Sleep, during pregnancy, 29, 95; "twilight," 182–83, 184
Sleeping pills, 121–22
Smallpox, immunization against, 103
Smoking, cigarette, 61–62
Sneezing, of newborn, 324
Socioeconomic factors, and birth weight, 63; and toxemia, 105, 128
Soranus, 140, 149, 271
Sparine, 183
Sparteine, 49, 205, 225
Spermatozoa, 3, 4, 5, 7–8, 260; fertile